TRAUMA
and MOBILE
RADIOGRAPHY

TRAUMA and MOBILE RADIOGRAPHY

SECOND EDITION

Michael W. Drafke, EdD
Professor and Radiographer
College of DuPage
Glen Ellyn, Illinois

Harry Nakayama, BS, RT(R)
Clinical Instructor
Kapiolani Community College
Honolulu, Hawaii

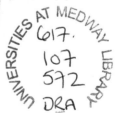
F. A. DAVIS COMPANY
Philadelphia

F. A. Davis Company
1915 Arch Street
Philadelphia, PA 19103

Printed in Canada

Last digit indicates print number: 10 9 8 7 6

Acquisitions Editor: Lynn Borders Caldwell
Developmental Editor: Sharon Lee
Production Editor: Jessica Howie Martin
Cover Designer: Louis J. Forgione

As new scientific information becomes available through basic and clinical research, recommended treatments and drug therapies undergo changes. The authors and publisher have done everything possible to make this book accurate,
up to date, and in accord with accepted standards at the time of publication. The
authors, editors, and publisher are not responsible for errors or omissions or for
consequences from application of the book, and make no warranty, expressed or
implied, in regard to the contents of the book. Any practice described in this
book should be applied by the reader in accordance with professional standards
of care used in regard to the unique circumstances that may apply in each situation. The reader is advised always to check product information (package in-
serts) for changes and new information regarding dose and contraindications
before administering any drug. Caution is especially urged when using new or
infrequently ordered drugs.

Library of Congress Cataloging in Publication Data

Drafke, Michael W.
   Trauma and mobile radiography / Michael W. Drafke, Harry
Nakayama.—2nd ed.
      p. : cm.
   Includes bibliographical references and index.
   ISBN 0–8036–0694–X (soft cover : alk. paper)
   1. Wounds and injuries—Radiography—Handbooks, manuals, etc. 2.
Diagnosis, Radioscopic—Handbooks, manuals, etc. 3. Surgical
emergencies—Handbooks, manuals, etc.
   [DNLM: 1. Wounds and injuries—radiography—Handbooks. 2. Emergency
Treatment—methods—Handbooks. WO 39 D758t 2000] I. Nakayama,
Harry, 1947– II. Title.
   RD93.7 .D73 2000
   617.1'07572—dc21

                              00-034605

Dedicated to
our families,
students, and
patients everywhere

PREFACE

Trauma and Mobile Radiography, second edition, is a concise introduction to radiographing trauma patients. Mobile radiography fundamentals are also included because much trauma work is performed using portable units. The book is dedicated to trauma *radiography*—not trauma radiology—and is designed to be equally useful in classroom settings and during trauma examinations.

The first five chapters develop supporting concepts that radiographers must draw upon in order to work successfully with trauma patients. Chapter 1 surveys vital signs and patient assessment as they apply to trauma situations. Because a trauma patient is typically in a precarious physical condition, Chapter 2 reviews supportive measures for medical emergencies and Chapter 3 describes drugs that often affect a patient's ability to cooperate during the radiographic examination. Trauma terminology and fractures are covered in Chapter 4, and Chapter 5 describes the injuries that result from fractures.

The heart of *Trauma and Mobile Radiography* is Chapter 6, which presents 131 trauma radiographic procedures. The method of presentation is unique. Whereas standard texts carefully specify the position of the patient or part for each exam, the format here gives no such specifications. Rather, the exams are described by how the film and central ray are positioned in relation to the part. The positioning directives will work whether the patient is supine, prone, lateral recumbent, upright, or immobile. Chapter 7 discusses portable radiography and rounds out the coverage provided by the book.

Trauma radiographers need certain types of information at their fingertips. A quick reference card is included that provides the following information:

- Physical signs indicating fractures
- Basic information for a patient history
- Evaluation areas for patient assessment
- Evaluating the patient's mental status
- Checklist for portable radiography
- Description categories for non-routine positions
- Special considerations during portable radiography of the chest
- SID conversion chart

This book was written to benefit students and practicing radiographers. However, equally importantly, *Trauma and Mobile Radiography* was written to benefit patients. No book covering such a variable topic can be complete. The hope is that, by studying the procedures presented here, radiographers will be able to produce better images in difficult situations and thus avoid much of the "learning by accident" at the one time when it is least advisable to do so. One further note: This book was designed to be easy to read and not to sound as "dry" as many textbooks. So, if it seems as though someone is talking directly to you, that was what was intended!

ACKNOWLEDGMENTS

A good book is always made better by careful peer review. I would like to thank the following individuals whose professional experience and insights guided me in writing the first edition:

Patricia A. Bynum, MEd, RT(R)(N)
Howard University
Mary Jane Clarke, MS, RT(R)
Quinnipiac College
Emily Hernandez, MS, RT(R)
Indiana University
Albert Michael Snopek, BS, RT(R), CXT, CRT
Middlesex County Community College
Judy Carol Southern, MA Ed, RT(R)
The University of Alabama at Birmingham

I also wish to thank Caryn Wiseman, Mary Baratta-Raimundi, and my wife Kathleen for their help with the original drawings.

I must also thank my parents for somehow teaching me to think, especially my father, who forced me to learn to always look a few steps ahead—a skill that is invaluable in trauma radiography.

Finally, I thank the only person to endure more than I had to during the original writing of this book, my wife Kathleen.

Michael W. Drafke

CONTENTS

2 Aid for Medical Emergencies **39**

3 Drugs that May Affect Patient Cooperation **61**

4 Trauma Terminology and Fractures **83**

5 Injuries from Types of Trauma **111**

6 Radiographing Trauma **145**

7 Portable Radiography **277**

INTRODUCTION TO THE RADIOGRAPHY OF TRAUMA

A patient lies strapped to a backboard. Blood is caked on his face and in his hair. He is semiconscious and breathing heavily. The front of his chest is caved in, and his right leg is injured in several places. The emergency room physician has sent the patient to radiography with an order for more than half a dozen examinations. The radiographer is alone with the patient, and every second counts. This is trauma radiography, and this is no time for "learning by accident."

Some people may say that it is not possible to teach trauma radiography; that it cannot be learned from a book, nor can a book or class on trauma radiography cover all of the possibilities. The belief is that the radiographer can learn only by performing the examinations. It is true that all possible situations caused by trauma cannot be presented along with the exact methods needed in each. It is also true that experience is extremely important. However, it is not true that trauma radiography cannot be taught. It is, in fact, critical that it be taught because there are too many things radiographers should know before they even begin to acquire experience.

1

▪ ▫ PREPARING FOR TRAUMA RADIOGRAPHY

In order for radiographers to radiograph trauma victims effectively, they must prepare. The following topics must be covered before starting trauma and mobile radiography:

- Anatomy
- Routine positioning
- Basic patient care
- Basic image production

A thorough knowledge of anatomy is essential to all radiographic positioning, especially trauma. The radiographer must know anatomy in order to perform normal radiography, to alter routine positions, and to create new positions when the other positions fail. Knowledge of routine positioning is necessary because many routine positions can be used in trauma with little or no alteration. Sometimes larger changes are required, but the radiographer still needs to know routine positions as a basis for new or varied positions. Although patient care and medical emergencies are covered, they are covered as they relate to trauma patients. The radiographer should have covered the basics before progressing to more specific applications. Basic image production should include standard radiographic equipment (e.g., the x-ray unit, cassettes, intensifying screens, grid) and an introduction to exposure factors. With this background, the radiographer should be technically prepared for trauma radiography.

The radiographer should also prepare mentally. In addition to the technical abilities required, there are nontechnical skills that the radiographer should possess or should work toward acquiring as preparation for trauma radiography. These include:

- Organizational skills
- Planning skills
- Nonverbal communication skills

Many trauma patients need a number of radiographic examinations performed in a small amount of time. The radiographer must be organized in accumulating the supplies and equipment needed to perform all of the examinations and in executing those examinations. For example, a patient may need femur, knee, and lower leg examinations. The radiographer will need sufficient films and positioning aids for these. All the anteroposterior (AP) projections should be performed first, and then the lateral projections (rather than having the patient supine for an AP lower leg, then lateral recumbent for the lateral lower leg, then back to supine for the AP knee, and so forth). The radiographer will also need organizational skills to record the technical factors used (in case repeats are needed) and to guarantee that all required radiographs are taken. Finally, an organized review of the patient's condition should be performed throughout the time he or she is in the radiographer's care.

The radiographer will need planning skills to save time. In many trauma cases, time is of the essence. The radiographer must be able to think ahead, to plan the next step while performing the current one. When a requisition is received, the radiographer should immediately place the required positions in a logical order. If a cervical spine fracture is suspected, the lateral cervical spine radiograph is made first. If the patient is having difficulty breathing, a chest examination may need to be performed first. The radiographer should begin to form the plan of action while moving the patient to the x-ray room. If the radiographer is called to a portable examination before he or she is needed, the time should be used to establish a plan, to select methods to be used, and to decide on technical factors.

The ability to plan ahead requires conscious effort and practice. When a radiographer is observing or assisting with trauma cases, he or she should envision a plan and compare it with what is actually done. The comparison should include checking for areas where the two methods were similar and where they were different. Another method for developing planning skills also involves observing or assisting a more experienced trauma radiographer. Here the less experienced radiographer should try to predict what the more experienced radiographer will need or will do next. The less experienced radiographer should try to look ahead to the next step and, if possible, obtain the film, sponge, sandbag, or other equipment that is needed. Using this method ensures that the less experienced radiographer receives the maximum benefit from the observational/assisting phase of learning. If the less experienced radiographer is trying to predict needs or actions, he or she will have to be concentrating on the business at hand, actively processing the information, and evaluating the results.

Radiographers should attend to their skills in receiving and sending nonverbal communication. Receiving the patient's nonverbal messages correctly is important in understanding when the patient is confused, anxious, or aggravated. It is also important in gauging the patient's condition (as will be seen in Chapter 1).

The nonverbal messages that the radiographer sends to the patient should also be of concern—especially with trauma patients. The radiographer must be careful not to show alarm, shock, or surprise at the patient's condition. This is particularly true when the trauma has caused facial disfigurement. The radiographer must convey compassion and concern, not shock.

■ ■ REQUIREMENTS OF TRAUMA RADIOGRAPHY

Before studying and practicing trauma radiography, the radiographer should be familiar with the preparatory material just mentioned. To perform trauma work, the radiographer also needs a knowledge of:

- Trauma patient care, patient analysis, and observation
- Procedures for responding to medical emergency
- Drugs that may affect a patient's ability to participate in radiographic examinations
- Trauma terminology
- Common injuries from different types of trauma
- Methods for radiographing trauma patients
- Portable radiographic methods

Separate chapters are devoted to each of these topics.

Chapter 1 covers patient care that applies to trauma victims, vital signs and other evaluations of the patient's condition, and patient observation methods. The chapter discusses how vital signs, evaluations, and observations are performed, as well as why the radiographer should be performing them. The medical and legal aspects of documentation are also covered.

Chapter 2 covers radiographer responses to medical emergencies that can arise with trauma patients. Methods of identifying the specific type of medical emergency the patient is having are included.

Chapter 3 contains a list of drugs that may interfere with the patient's mobility, the patient's ability to cooperate with radiographic examinations, or the patient's ability to provide a medical history. Some of these drugs may be given to trauma victims. Others may have been taken by the patient before the trauma occurred. Some are not recommended for trauma patients but may be encountered by the radiographer in mobile or in routine radiography.

Chapter 4 discusses trauma terms, fracture terms, fracture identification, and fractures that have acquired names. These terms will enable the radiographer to communicate better with fellow health-care workers.

Chapter 5 covers the types of injuries that typically result from common trauma situations. With this knowledge, the radiographer will have some idea of what to expect and will be able to select methods with the best chance of demonstrating the area with the least chance of causing further injury.

Chapter 6 explains and diagrams various positions for trauma radiography. The basics of positioning and trauma radiography are discussed. The position descriptions are free from any reference to patient position, so they are applicable to anyone regardless of any restrictions in movement caused by trauma or patient condition. Over 100 methods are included, some of which have never been published before. Methods for creating new positions are also included.

Chapter 7 covers portable, or mobile, radiography. This is included because many trauma cases must be performed with a mobile x-ray unit, and the positions discussed in Chapter 6 are applicable to trauma and routine portable x-ray examinations. Methods for routine portable radiography are fully discussed.

■ ■ EXPERIENCE

The intention of this book is to give each radiographer the benefit of the years of experience of other radiographers so that he or she does not have to rediscover this information during serious or life-threatening situations. It is not intended to replace all experience. It *is* intended to give radiographers a head start that will improve their trauma experience and provide better patient care sooner.

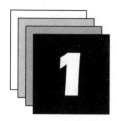

VITAL SIGNS AND PATIENT ASSESSMENT

■ ■ INTRODUCTION

The trauma patient's condition must be evaluated before any x-ray examination. The patient's condition affects the methods the radiographer uses to obtain the required radiographs. Furthermore, changes in the patient's medical status cannot be known if his or her initial status was not noted. Finally, the trauma patient's condition on entering and exiting the department should be documented for legal purposes. Such documentation can provide evidence that the patient did not receive additional injuries while in the radiography department or, if the patient did, that the injury was detected and managed properly.

This chapter first reviews the procedure for taking the patient's vital signs and the clinical significance of these signs in trauma patients. It then outlines procedures and principles for establishing the observational baseline that influences the radiographic methods used and that determines how closely the radiographer must monitor the trauma patient.

▪ ▪ STANDARD PRECAUTIONS

Universal Precautions (UPs), guidelines designed to protect health workers from bloodborne pathogens, were introduced by the Centers for Disease Control and Prevention (CDC) in 1985 in response to the need to guard against human immunovirus (HIV) infections. In this system, barriers, such as masks or gloves, were to be used whenever there was a possibility of contact with certain body fluids. The type of interaction with the patient determined the type of barrier to be used, regardless of the patient's condition.

Because UPs did not address the transmission of disease through feces, saliva, and other bodily sources such as tears or sputum, a system called Body Substance Isolation (BSI) was introduced in 1987. This system was designed to protect health workers from all pathogens and their sources of transmission, but did not specifically address contact, droplet, and airborne disease transmission.

Because the implementation of UPs and BSI caused some confusion, especially in the area of which body fluids were covered under which system, the CDC introduced a new system called Standard Precautions in 1996. A combination of UP and BSI, Standard Precautions is applicable to all patients and includes barriers to blood, body fluids, excretions, secretions, mucous membranes, broken skin areas, and contaminated items regardless of the presence of visible blood. Standard Precautions are summarized in Box 1–1.

When a highly transmissible disease is confirmed or suspected in a patient, Transmission Based Precautions are implemented along with Standard Precautions. Transmission Based Precautions are designed to reduce infections caused by the airborne, droplet, or contact route.

Airborne pathogens are suspended in the air for a relatively long period of time. Dust particles and small droplets, 5 μm or less, provide the means of transport. Airborne isolation consists of taking special ventilation precautions and using special masks capable of stopping airborne particles.

Droplets, which are larger than 5 μm in size, are formed by sneezing, coughing, or talking and do not usually travel

BOX 1–1
STANDARD PRECAUTIONS

PROCEDURE

For the following, the term "body fluids" shall also include blood, secretions, and excretions.

1. Wash hands after touching body fluids or contaminated items even if gloves are worn. Hands should be washed right after gloves are removed.
2. Wear gloves when contact with body fluids or contaminated items is likely. Also, wear gloves when touching mucous membranes or broken skin areas.
3. Wear mask, gown, eye, and face protection when performing procedures that may cause splashing or spraying of body fluids.
4. Handle sharp items such as needles and scalpels carefully. Never recap or remove used needles from syringes by hand. Always use a designated puncture-resistant container when disposing sharp items.

more than 3 feet. Droplets can also be formed during suctioning or other procedures involving the respiratory system. Infection occurs when these droplets come in contact with the conjunctivae or mucous membranes of the nose or mouth. Masks capable of stopping droplet particles should be used when working within a 3-foot radius of the patient.

Contact transmission occurs through direct or indirect means. Direct contact implies skin-to-skin or physical contact, whereas contaminated inanimate objects, such as instruments or facial tissues, serve as the vehicles of transmission in the indirect route. Gloves should always be worn in this isolation environment and removed before leaving. Hands should be washed immediately after gloves are removed. Be sure not to touch contaminated objects with bare hands. Remember to use paper towels or disposable sponges to turn the water on and off, and rub hard when soaping; friction is the key to removing germs.

When performing mobile radiography in isolation, two radiographers should be available. One radiographer performs only duties concerning the positioning of the patient and the bagged cassette. The other operates the x-ray machine and handles the clean cassettes (puts them in protective bags and removes them once they have been used). This system reduces the chances of contamination because one radiographer never makes contact with the x-ray machine or unprotected cassette.

Remember that isolation patients feel exactly that way—isolated. Carry out your duties in a friendly manner without hurrying or showing fear (acting as if you cannot wait to leave the environment). In this way, your patient will not incur added feelings of rejection and reduced self-worth.

PULSE

OVERVIEW

The pulse indicates how fast the heart is beating and reflects the patient's general physical condition. Of equal significance to the trauma radiographer is that the patient's pulse can also reveal hidden injuries, such as blood vessel damage. When first taking charge of a trauma patient, the pulse reading should be noted from the history or taken immediately by the radiographer. Whenever a pulse rate is taken, it should be documented, along with the time it was taken. The strength, weakness, or absence of pulse should also be noted.

LOCATING PULSE POINTS

Figure 1–1 shows locations for taking pulse rates. The radial artery is the most common location for taking a pulse. The index and middle fingers are placed on the anterior surface of the patient's wrist on the lateral side (at the distal end of the radius, near the navicular). Alternate locations for determining pulse rates are the carotid, femoral, temporal, dorsalis pedis, and popliteal arteries. Of

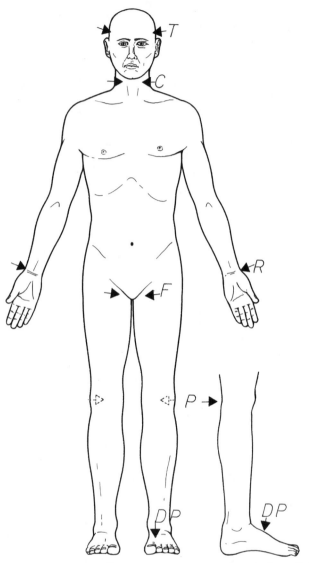

FIG. 1–1. Pulse points. T, temporal; C, carotid; R, radial; F, femoral; P, popliteal; DP, dorsalis pedis.

these, the carotid artery is most often used. It is found on either side of the thyroid cartilage. The femoral pulse is located about 2 inches medial and 3 inches inferior to the anterior superior lilac spine (ASIS). The temporal pulse is about ½ inch anterior and ½ inch superior to the external auditory meatus (EAM). The dorsalis pedis pulse is on the dorsal surface of the foot, at the top of the arch, on the medial side of the first metatarsal. The popliteal pulse is in the middle of the posterior surface of the knee.

In suspected fracture patients, the pulse should be taken distal to the fracture site. It is important to document the presence or absence of pulses distal to fractures. Lack of a pulse may mean that fracture fragments have severed blood vessels. If a pulse is present, it should be checked whenever the patient is moved and during the exit evaluation to ensure that an artery has not been severed.

OBTAINING PULSE READINGS

Box 1–2 describes a standard procedure for obtaining the patient's pulse reading. The radiographer should refrain from using excess pressure on the artery to avoid collapsing it and obliterating the pulse. The radiographer should practice taking pulse rates to maintain competency.

THE SIGNIFICANCE OF PULSE RATES

The typical pulse rate for men is 70 to 72 beats per minute (bpm), and it is 78 to 82 beats per minute for women. These rates vary, however, according to the patient's age, height, physical condition, and body position.

Higher pulse rates are seen in pediatric patients (often 110 to 120 bpm), in patients who are standing, in those who have fevers, and in those who have just exerted themselves. Simply entering a hospital may raise some patients' heart rates. Being nervous, having just been in an accident, or the onset of shock also may raise the pulse rate. A pulse rate faster than 100 bpm in an adult is considered unusually rapid and is called tachycardia. A

BOX 1–2
OBTAINING PULSE READINGS

PROCEDURE

1. Patient must be at rest, either sitting or lying down. Pulse is usually taken over the radial or brachial artery, but the carotid, dorsalis pedis, or femoral arteries can also be used when necessary.
2. Apply gentle pressure over the artery with the tips of the first two fingers. When the palm is turned upward, the radial pulse can be detected by following the thumb to its base on the wrist.
3. Count the beats for 30 seconds and multiply by two when the pulse is regular. If irregular, count the pulse for a full minute.
4. Record the readings immediately. *Example:* TPR 98.6-72-16.

Source: Modified from Frew, MA, and Frew, DR: Comprehensive Medical Assisting: Administrative and Clinical Procedures, ed 2. FA Davis, Philadelphia, 1988, p 362, with permission.

rate of 170 bpm or higher is extremely serious and must be reported immediately.

Pulse rates lower than normal are sometimes found in tall patients, geriatric patients, resting or recumbent patients, and those in excellent physical condition. Bradycardia, a heart rate of less than 60 bpm, sometimes follows tachycardia as the heart weakens from maintaining an accelerated pace.

The strength or weakness of the pulse should be noted, in addition to its speed. A strong, rapid pulse may be caused by nervousness, whereas a weak and rapid pulse may be a symptom of shock. Experience with normal pulses is needed to differentiate between a strong and a weak pulse.

Absence of a pulse can be caused by several conditions. As noted previously, too much pressure on an artery may cause it to collapse, giving the appearance of no pulse. More significantly, the pulse may be obliterated by trauma-induced pressure on an artery between the pulse point and the heart or by the severing or rupture of an artery. Of course, cardiac arrest is also a cause of an absent pulse.

RESPIRATION

OVERVIEW

The trauma patient's breathing should be constantly monitored. The initial observation is best done after taking the pulse. If the patient's breathing changes noticeably during the radiologic examination, the respiration rate should be counted again and the results recorded.

OBTAINING RESPIRATION RATES

Box 1–3 summarizes the procedure for determining the patient's respiration rate.

Remember that you must not let the patient know that his or her respiration rate is being watched to prevent the patient from consciously altering the respiration rate. Also, one respiration consists of one inspiration *and* one expiration.

THE SIGNIFICANCE OF RESPIRATION RATES

Normal breathing varies from 12 to 20 respirations per minute, with the average being 15 or 16. Children younger than 5 years old normally breathe more rapidly than adults do. In normal breathing, inspiration lasts about twice as long as expiration.

Tachypnea (rapid breathing) is 25 or more respirations per minute. Exertion, disease, or nervousness may cause this condition. The patient may become dizzy or lightheaded if tachypnea continues, possibly resulting in syncope (fainting). Patients exhibiting tachypnea caused by stress or anxiety (also called hyperventilation) should be told to control their breathing consciously in order to slow it down. If this method fails, having them either

BOX 1–3
OBTAINING RESPIRATION RATES

PROCEDURE

1. Patient should be at rest in a sitting or lying position. The respirations are counted after the pulse has been counted for 30 seconds and while the fingertips remain on the pulse as though the rate of pulsation were still being measured.
2. Observe the rise and fall of the chest, and count each complete cycle as a single respiration. Count for 30 seconds and multiply by two.
3. Count irregular respirations for 1 full minute while keeping fingertips on the radial pulse so as not to call the patient's attention to the procedure.
4. Record the respirations accurately. *Example:* 98.6-72-18.

[NOTE: Respirations in infants are easier to count by using a stethoscope and continuing to observe the rise and fall of the chest or clothing over the chest.]

Source: Modified from Frew, MA, and Frew, DR: Comprehensive Medical Assisting: Administrative and Clinical Procedures, ed 2. FA Davis, Philadelphia, 1988, p 364, with permission.

breathe into a paper bag or close the mouth and shut off one nostril can restore normal breathing by returning carbon dioxide and oxygen levels to normal. Rapid breathing that is also shallow may indicate the onset of shock or may indicate severe blood loss. Fewer than 12 respirations per minute is called bradypnea. If this condition continues, it may produce cyanosis (blue skin color) or syncope.

Dyspnea is difficult, or labored, breathing and has many causes. Having the patient sit upright may ease dyspnea. Brief periods of dyspnea should be recorded, noting the time, duration, and rate of respiration. Persistent dyspnea requires a physician's attention. Apnea (absence of breathing), when seen in trauma situations requires immediate action by the radiographer or the calling of a cardiac arrest code (often called a "code blue").

TEMPERATURE

OVERVIEW

General or local, formal or informal, the taking of patient temperatures may be needed to monitor the trauma patient's condition. General temperature refers to the internal temperature of the body. Local temperature refers to the temperature of a segment of the body. An extremity, for example, may have a depressed local temperature due to a loss of circulation produced by a fracture fragment severing an artery, or an elevated local temperature may be due to a local infection. A formal temperature is one recorded in degrees Fahrenheit (F) or Celsius (C) using a glass, electronic, or strip thermometer. An informal temperature is a subjective assessment made by the radiographer noting that the patient felt hot or cold to the touch, or that the patient reported feeling chilled or warm. Shivering (the body trying to generate heat) and sweating (the body trying to cool itself) also are informal indicators of temperature.

OBTAINING TEMPERATURE READINGS

If a formal temperature is needed, the patient will generally prefer the oral method (Box 1–4). Oral temperatures should not be taken if the patient has had a hot or cold drink within the last 10 minutes because this will alter an oral reading. Typical adult oral temperature is 98.6°F (37°C), with the normal range being plus or minus 1 degree. A more accurate temperature reading can be obtained from a rectal measurement (Box 1–5). A rectal temperature reading is also the preferred method for infants (Box 1–6). Normal rectal temperature is ½° to 1°F (¼°–½°C) higher than oral temperature. The least accurate

BOX 1–4
TAKING AURAL AND ORAL TEMPERATURES

PROCEDURE

1. Wash hands.
2. Select an electronic thermometer and attach a new disposable cover (lens), or select an oral thermometer. If the oral thermometer has been stored in a chemical solution, rinse it with cool water and wipe it dry with a cotton ball, moving from the end of the stem to the bulb.
3. If the electronic thermometer is off, turn it on and wait until it indicates that it is ready. If using an oral thermometer, check the level of mercury by holding the thermometer with the calibration toward you and at eye level. Shake the thermometer down to 95°F (35°C) if the mercury level is above these calibrations. The thermometer is shaken down by holding the thermometer firmly between the thumb and forefinger and shaking downward with a snapping wrist action.
4. Identify the patient and explain the procedure. Pull the earlobe down gently and carefully insert the electronic thermometer into the patient's ear canal. If using an oral thermometer, have the patient in a sitting or lying position. Ask the patient if he or she has recently consumed a hot or cold drink, or has been smoking. If so, wait 15 minutes for a more accurate reading. Instruct the patient not to bite down on the thermometer and to avoid talking.
5. Aim the electronic thermometer slightly anterior and slightly cephalic. Click the button and hold for 1 second. With an oral thermometer, position the thermometer under the patient's tongue and leave in place 3 to 5 minutes. Instruct the patient to keep the mouth closed.
6. Remove the thermometer. If using an oral thermometer, wipe it with a cotton ball once from the end of the stem down to the bulb, using a firm, twisting motion. Discard the cotton ball.

BOX 1–4
TAKING AURAL AND ORAL TEMPERATURES
(continued)

7. Read the thermometer. For an oral thermometer, hold the thermometer between the thumb and index finger at the tip end, away from the bulb. Rotate the thermometer until the silver mercury line can be identified and follow the line until it becomes opaque. Once the temperature reading is obtained, shake the mercury to 95°F (35°C).
8. Record the reading on the designated form or chart. Patient's name, date, time, and reading are included. Abbreviation for temperature is T. *Example:* T-99.
9. Wash hands.

Source: Modified from Frew, MA, and Frew, DR: Comprehensive Medical Assisting: Administrative and Clinical Procedures, ed 2. FA Davis, Philadelphia, 1988, p 356, with permission.

is the axillary (armpit) measurement (Box 1–7). Axillary temperature is usually ½° to 1°F lower than an oral temperature. All temperatures should be taken for a minimum of 3 to 5 minutes, if possible.

THE SIGNIFICANCE OF TEMPERATURE READINGS

Areas of higher local temperature often indicate infection and may be evidenced by erythema (reddening of the skin). Areas of low local temperature are caused by decrease in, or absence of, blood flow and can be accompanied by cyanosis. In trauma situations, especially with fractures, the chance of decreased blood flow from a severed artery is quite possible. If this situation arises suddenly—especially after the patient has just been moved—it must be brought to the physician's attention.

BOX 1–5
TAKING RECTAL TEMPERATURES

PROCEDURE

1. Wash hands.
2. Assemble a rectal thermometer, petroleum jelly–based lubricant, and cotton ball or gauze 4 × 4.
3. Close door to examining room.
4. Identify the patient and explain the procedure.
5. Assist the adult patient to assume a Sims' (side-lying) position and drape properly.
6. Select a rectal thermometer and check the mercury at eye level. If necessary, shake down the mercury. If the thermometer has been stored in a chemical solution, rinse with cool water and wipe dry with a cotton ball from bulb to the tip end.
7. Lubricate the thermometer with a petroleum jelly–based substance by pressing the tube of lubricant and allowing a small amount to fall on the mercury tip while rotating to obtain even lubrication. Lubricate to 1 inch above the bulb. Separate the buttocks so that the anal sphincter is seen clearly, and insert the thermometer gently for approximately 1½ inches. Allow the buttocks to fall back into place.
8. Hold the thermometer in place for 2 to 3 minutes. *Do not* leave the patient for any reason before removing the thermometer.
9. Remove the thermometer and wipe it once with the cotton ball, from the fingers to the mercury bulb, using a firm, twisting motion.
10. Read thermometer and record on designated form or chart as you would for oral. When recording rectal temperature, add an R next to the numerals. *Example:* 99R. After shaking the thermometer below 96°F (35.5°C), wash the thermometer in cool, sudsy water and place in receptacle containing disinfectant solution with gauze at the bottom.
11. Wash hands.

Source: Frew, MA, and Frew, DR: Comprehensive Medical Assisting: Administrative and Clinical Procedures, ed 2. FA Davis, Philadelphia, 1988, p 357, with permission.

BOX 1–6
TAKING AN INFANT'S TEMPERATURE

PROCEDURE

1. Wash hands.
2. Identify the patient and explain the procedure to the adult who is present. Select the rectal thermometer. Check the level of the mercury. If the reading is above 96°F (35.5°C), shake down the mercury.
3. Place the infant on his or her stomach on a firm surface. Have an adult hold onto the infant during the procedure.
4. Lubricate the thermometer with a petroleum jelly–based substance by pressing the tube of lubricant and allowing a small amount to fall on the mercury tip while rotating to obtain even lubrication.
5. Using the left hand, separate the buttocks. Using the right hand, insert the thermometer (lubricated end) into the rectum approximately 1 inch.
6. Using the right hand, hold the buttocks together firmly, the thermometer lodged between the fingers of the same hand.
7. Place the left hand in the small of the infant's back. Keeping the elbow of this arm straight, lean slightly on the infant.
8. Keep the thermometer in place for 3 to 4 minutes.
9. Continuing to hold the child, remove the thermometer, place it in the cotton or gauze, and set it aside out of the infant's reach. Position the infant safely in an adult's arms after assisting with diapering and dressing.
10. Wipe the bulb end of the thermometer. Read and record. *Example:* 99R.
11. Wash hands.

Source: Frew, MA, and Frew, DR: Comprehensive Medical Assisting: Administrative and Clinical Procedures, ed 2. FA Davis, Philadelphia, 1988, p 358, with permission.

BOX 1–7
TAKING AXILLARY TEMPERATURES

PROCEDURE

1. Wash hands.
2. Select an oral thermometer. Rinse off disinfectant solution with a cotton ball or gauze 4 ×4. Check the level of mercury. If above 96°F (35.5°C), shake down.
3. Identify the patient and explain the procedure.
4. Dry the area with tissue or gauze. Insert the thermometer in the axilla. Instruct the patient to hold the thermometer by tightly pressing the arm against the chest.
5. Leave the thermometer in place for 10 minutes.
6. Remove the thermometer. Wipe dry with a cotton ball in a twisting, downward manner from stem to bulb.
7. Read the thermometer, shake it down below 96°F (35.5°C), and place it in the proper container. Record, using an A after the numerical value. *Example:* 99-A.
8. Record on designated form or chart. Include patient's name, time, date, and reading. Indicate that the temperature reading is axillary by placing an A after the numerals.
9. Wash hands.

Source: Frew, MA, and Frew, DR: Comprehensive Medical Assisting: Administrative and Clinical Procedures, ed 2. FA Davis, Philadelphia, 1988, p 357, with permission.

■ ■ BLOOD PRESSURE

■ OVERVIEW

Blood pressure (BP) measures the high and low points of a patient's pulse. It is recorded with the high number (systole) first, then a slash, and then the low number (diastole). An example is 120/80, and this is read as "one-twenty over eighty." The difference between the two numbers is the pulse pressure. For a blood pressure of 120/80, the pulse pressure is 40.

Shock, cardiac arrest, and respiratory arrest are the common situations when radiographers take blood pressure readings on trauma patients.

▦ OBTAINING BLOOD PRESSURE READINGS

A sphygmomanometer, or blood pressure cuff, and a stethoscope are needed to measure the patient's blood pressure. The cuff measures pressure in millimeters of mercury. The abbreviation of millimeter is mm, and the chemical abbreviation of mercury is Hg, so the reading may be written 120/80 mm Hg. Box 1–8 lists a standard procedure for obtaining a blood pressure reading.

▦ THE SIGNIFICANCE OF BLOOD PRESSURE READINGS

Typical adult male blood pressure is 120/80. The range for normal systolic pressure is 100 to 140. The normal diastolic range is 60 to 90. Female, pediatric, and geriatric patients generally have lower normal blood pressures. Blood pressure increases with exertion, excitement, or nervousness. Therefore, it should be taken with the patient at rest.

Blood pressure is considered abnormal when the systolic pressure is consistently above 140, the diastolic pressure is consistently above 100, or the pulse pressure is consistently above 50. Pulse pressure is obtained by subtracting the diastolic pressure from the systolic pressure. High blood pressure is termed hypertension; low blood pressure is hypotension. Falling or low blood pressure is one indication of shock.

BOX 1–8
OBTAINING BLOOD PRESSURE READINGS

PROCEDURE

1. Identify the patient and explain the procedure.
2. Assemble necessary equipment: sphygmomanometer and stethoscope.
3. Assist the patient to assume a comfortable position sitting or lying with the forearm and palm at heart level.
4. Wrap the cuff around the upper arm about 1 inch above the elbow, placing the tubing toward the outer aspect of the arm. Cuff must fit snugly around the arm.
5. Place stethoscope in ears.
6. Palpate the brachial pulse and place the diaphragm of the stethoscope over it.
7. After tightening the valve to prevent leakage, squeeze the (pump) inflator bulb with quick, even strokes until the mercury level rises to approximately 180 mmHg. An alternative method is to place the fingertips on the radial pulse while inflating the cuff. When the radial pulse is obliterated, the cuff is inflated to a level 30 mmHg higher than the point at which the radial pulse was obliterated. After the cuff is deflated and the stethoscope placed over the brachial artery, the procedure, then continues as described.
8. With thumb and forefinger regulating the valve, slowly release the pressure in the cuff.
9. Note the first distinctly audible pulse sound heard—the systolic pressure. Read the gauge at eye level and remember the corresponding number on the pressure gauge.
10. Note the last distinctly audible sound heard—the diastolic pressure. Remember the corresponding number on the gauge.
11. Allow the remaining air to escape by completely opening the control valve.

BOX 1–8
OBTAINING BLOOD PRESSURE READINGS
(continued)

12. Remove equipment, put in order, and record immediately as systolic over diastolic. *Example:* 120/80 left arm.

Source: Frew, MA, and Frew, DR: Comprehensive Medical Assisting: Administrative and Clinical Procedures, ed 2. FA Davis, Philadelphia, 1988, p 369, with permission.

■ ▨ VITAL SIGNS AND TRAUMA RADIOGRAPHY

The trauma patient's vital signs should be monitored throughout the radiographic procedure. Some trauma patients may require only a quick visual check between positions. Severely injured patients require more active care. It is with these patients that experience is invaluable. Knowing how to check vital signs and knowing what to look for can be easily taught. Knowing when to apply this knowledge is mostly a function of experience. The radiographer should begin by practicing one vital sign or making limited observations on routine or slightly injured patients. While observing examinations on the more severely injured patients, the radiographer should take the opportunity to practice these skills. Practice and experience prepare the trauma radiographer for the times when he or she will have to work alone.

■ ▨ BASELINE OBSERVATIONS

Any trauma patient can develop complications while in the radiography department. Patients with seemingly minor injuries, such as dislocated fingers, have suddenly turned white and fainted during postreduction filming. A patient receiving a routine chest x-ray examination may suddenly develop a pneumothorax. In view of such possibilities, every trauma patient should receive an initial evaluation and be monitored while he or she is under the radiographer's care. It is time well spent, and with practice, it can be done quickly.

THE PURPOSE OF PATIENT HISTORIES

Although the radiographer's discussion with the trauma patient is typically brief, it has five important goals:

1. Obtaining the patient's medical history. Does the patient have old fractures? Has he or she undergone any surgical procedures? How was he or she injured? The answers to patient history questions help the radiographer select the most effective methods and help the radiologist interpret the radiographs.
2. Verifying that the correct examinations were ordered. Was a left knee examination accidentally ordered when the right knee was injured? Does the patient need a shoulder, humerus, clavicle, or scapula examination?
3. Assessing the trauma patient's mental status and physical condition. Will the patient be able to stand? To cooperate? To be left alone?
4. Taking the trauma patient's vital signs. This goes hand in hand with baseline observations; both are part of patient care and assessment.
5. Conveying a caring and empathetic attitude.

THE PATIENT HISTORY

The more information radiographers gather about their cases, the better they will be able to help their patients. The requisition and patient's chart should be reviewed. Emergency room personnel and the patient's family can be consulted, especially if the patient is unable to give a history. Information gathered from these sources should be verified with the patient by questioning and observation, or observation alone if the patient cannot answer questions.

The following questions represent the minimum amount of information that the radiographer should try to elicit:

- What happened? What type of accident happened?
- Where is the patient injured? Where is his or her pain?
- When was the patient injured?
- Has the patient had previous injuries, fractures, or surgery in the same location as the current injuries?

Determining what type of accident occurred indicates to the radiographer and radiologist the typical kinds of injuries that result (this will be discussed in Chapter 5). Knowing what types of injuries are common from different accidents guides the radiographer in selecting the methods to be used. Knowing where the patient is injured aids the radiologist by giving him or her a starting point in interpreting the radiographs. Therefore, the radiographer should try to be as specific as possible as to the location of the injuries, impact point, or pain. It also helps the radiographer select methods and verify the correctness of the examinations that were ordered. Knowing when the patient was injured and if there have been previous injuries mainly assists the radiologist.

If the patient reports that there are no symptoms, the radiographer should write "asymptomatic" on the history. The history sheet should not be left blank in these cases. Writing "asymptomatic" tells the radiologist that a history was taken but that the patient reported no symptoms. Leaving the history blank could mean that there were no symptoms, but it could also mean that no history was taken, or that the patient was physically unable or unwilling to give a history, or that the patient could not speak English. In short, the radiographer should report exactly what happened during the history.

▨ VERIFYING THE CORRECTNESS OF THE EXAMINATION

It is the radiographer's responsibility to ensure that the examination he or she is about to perform is the one that is needed. The radiographer can accomplish this by obtaining a history from the patient and comparing the results to the requisition. The most common reason an incorrect examination is ordered is clerical error. For example, some requisitions contain a list of all the radiographic examinations available. This can be 50 or more. It is easy to circle the one just above or below the examination that is needed. It is also common to order an examination of the left side when one for the right side is needed. Sometimes there is unfamiliarity with the exact anatomy that will be demonstrated, and a knee examination may be ordered when a patella examination is needed. When there is doubt, the radiographer must confirm the order with the physician. Sometimes there is a perfectly good reason why the examinations were ordered in a certain way. Often it was a simple error. In either case, it takes only a few seconds to check and saves the patient from excess radiation and a needless examination.

▨ ▨ THE PROCEDURE FOR PATIENT ASSESSMENT

Seven major areas should be evaluated during patient assessment:

1. Mental status
2. Respiration
3. Skin color
4. Presence of open wounds or bleeding
5. The degree of sensation or the presence of pain
6. Musculoskeletal integrity
7. Patient mobility

▓ MENTAL STATUS

The patient's level of consciousness and mental status can be checked while his or her history is obtained. Determine whether the patient is alert, drowsy, or unresponsive. Will he or she be able to cooperate or not? Decide whether the patient can move without assistance and whether the patient can be left alone.

The Alert Patient

IF the trauma patient

- Is aware of himself or herself
- Answers questions without unusual delay
- Follows commands well
- Is cooperative
- Knows where he or she is
- Knows the time and date (or at least whether it is night or day)

THEN the patient can be considered alert, should be able to attain typical radiographic positions, and can be left alone during film development, if necessary.

The Drowsy Patient

IF the trauma patient

- Is sleepy or drowsy
- Is irritable or restless
- Has slurred speech
- Is uncertain of the time or date
- Answers questions in a rambling or halting manner

THEN the patient may be able to attain routine positions but will probably require additional support or immobilization. The patient should not be left alone. It may be necessary to ask a relative or friend to stay in the x-ray room with the patient if the radiographer must leave.

The Unresponsive Patient

IF the trauma patient

- Is lethargic
- Falls asleep but can be aroused verbally
- Provides a sketchy history, if any
- Follows commands only with some help or maintains positions only with added immobilization

THEN a medical person should always be present. The patient should be closely observed. If the patient loses consciousness and cannot be aroused verbally, a physician should be notified immediately and the radiographer should check the patient's vital signs.

If the patient is unconscious and unresponsive, he or she cannot be left without medical care. Such patients must always be observed closely. The unconscious patient, or the patient who slips in and out of consciousness, can *never* be left alone. If the patient is not alert and cooperative, this fact should be recorded on the history. Vital signs, especially breathing, must be monitored throughout the procedure. Preparations should be made for the possibility that the patient could go into cardiac or respiratory arrest.

▦ MONITORING RESPIRATION

If the trauma patient's breathing rate is noticeably fast or slow, then respirations per minute should be counted. Also note if the patient's breathing seems difficult or labored, shallow or deep, or if he or she is panting. Watch for hemoptysis (coughing up blood). Blood that is coughed up is usually bright red and frothy, whereas blood that is vomited (hematemesis) appears dark red and clotted.

▦ SKIN COLOR

Check the color of the face and injured extremities. In the face, look for pallor (lack of color, whiteness or grayness), cyanosis, or redness. For the extremities, check areas distal to the injury, especially for cyanosis or pallor. Cyanosis or pallor can be caused by loss of blood flow to the body part. It can be a precursor of syncope or shock, or it may indicate a severed or punctured artery. Circulatory damage may also occur while the patient is being moved or positioned. For this reason, monitor the patient's skin color and pulse should be monitored distal to the injury throughout the procedure. For legal reasons document both normal and abnormal findings.

BLEEDING

Even though bleeding is almost always under control by the time a radiographer takes charge of a patient, bleeding sites must still be noted. Mentally note bandaged areas. Check for bleeding from the nose, mouth, and ears. Bleeding from the ears can indicate deep, severe head injury. If bleeding from the ears has not been previously noticed, it should be brought to a physician's attention. Do not wipe up and discard the blood, because it is often needed for testing to determine whether it contains cerebrospinal fluid. Recheck any bleeding sites if the patient or an extremity is moved. In severe trauma cases, occasionally check the patient during the examination. Again, any changes in the patient's condition should be documented.

SENSORY EVALUATION AND PAIN

The trauma patient should be checked for pain and sensation. Note the location and, if possible, the intensity of any pain. The degree of sensation in the extremities and torso should be checked. Complaints of lack of sensation, or a tingling sensation, in a body part indicate possible spinal cord damage. In such cases, it is as important to record that the patient has feeling as to record that the patient does not. This sign should be checked when the patient enters and leaves the department. The other senses should also be evaluated. Any vision or hearing problems are important. The patient's complaint of double vision or blurred vision, as well as hearing difficulties or ringing in the ear (tinnitus), should be noted.

▦ MUSCULOSKELETAL INTEGRITY

In addition to asking about pain or lack of sensation, check the patient's skeletal system. This procedure is necessary to verify that the correct examination was ordered and to determine patient mobility. If any joints will have to be flexed or extended, determine whether this will be possible. *Never force a joint.* A good procedure to follow is to ask the patient to bend the joint. If the patient replies that he or she cannot, ask the patient to try again and to try moving it slowly. The radiographer might apply *gentle* pressure and encourage the patient to relax. If this method does not work, another way should be found to obtain the projection. To this day, there are still some radiographers who force joints to move with a strong, quick jerk. *They are wrong.* As is noted in later chapters, there is almost always an alternative.

▦ PATIENT MOBILITY

Determine whether the patient's injuries prevent the patient from physically attaining a position or from moving. Any trauma patient with a *suspected* cervical spine injury should not be moved until a horizontal beam lateral cervical spine radiograph has been interpreted by a physician. Lower extremity and head injuries generally prevent the patient from standing for an examination. Pelvic and abdominal injuries often stop the patient from sitting upright. A physician should be consulted before having a patient with thoracic trauma sit up. It may also be difficult for patients with upper extremity injuries to lie down on an x-ray table. Many times, patients can sit or lie down but find it difficult to perform the movement of lying down. As is noted in later chapters, these patients can be examined in a seated upright position at a vertical cassette holder, or they can stand on an upright fluoroscopy table and be slowly lowered to a recumbent position. Assistance with lifting the patient is needed if the patient cannot move himself or herself or cannot be moved by a single radiographer. A minimum of four people is needed for light, minimally injured patients. A minimum of six people—preferably eight—is required for heavier or more severely injured patients.

THE EXIT EVALUATION

One last check of the patient's condition should be made before the patient leaves the department, and the findings should be recorded. This is especially advisable when the patient is greatly injured. Although it is to the patient's benefit to be periodically checked, medicolegal reasons necessitate this practice as well. Having documentation that a patient left the x-ray department at a certain time, that the patient's general condition was reevaluated, and that, for example, the patient could still move his or her toes and fingers would provide significant support in a malpractice case against a radiographer or the department. For the few moments it takes, an exit evaluation is well worth the time.

LEGAL ASPECTS

References to legal considerations have been made throughout this chapter. The radiographer should give careful consideration to following them. The suggested approach is to:

- Evaluate and document the patient's condition on entering the radiography department

- Constantly monitor the patient (the more severe the injuries or the more unstable the patient's condition the closer the observations)
- Evaluate and document the patients condition upon leaving the department

Ideally, the patient will leave the department in the same condition as when he or she entered it. However, if the patient's condition does change, the documentation should show that the patient received prompt and proper treatment.

The two major aspects of these methods are active patient evaluation and monitoring, and documentation. Many radiographers engage in a more passive method of patient care. The patient's condition and any changes in that condition are noted subconsciously. In contrast, the method suggested here advocates a more conscious effort not only to notice changes but also to notice and measure them immediately. Accurate evaluation of changes in a patient's condition can be noted only if the patient's initial condition is known.

Active, accurate patient evaluation and observation are essential to good, professional patient care. Documentation is good patient care and good legal practice. Trauma cases have an increased chance of becoming legal cases. Documentation that the radiographer did everything possible to care for the patient will support his or her case. For example, a patient is involved in an automobile accident. A cervical spine fracture is suspected, and, in fact, the patient is found to have a fracture and the spinal cord is severed. The patient is now quadriplegic. The question in a subsequent court case is: When did it happen? During the automobile accident? When the paramedics extricated him from the car and placed him on a backboard? When he was moved from the ambulance cart to the emergency room (ER) cart? When he was moved from the ER cart to the radiographic table and back again? Or when he was placed in a hospital bed that night? If the radiographer can show that the patient's condition did not change while he was in the radiography department, there will be little to worry about.

Showing that the patient's condition did not change requires documentation. That documentation should include three items:

1. Specific details about the patient's condition. A history that does not mention that the patient could move his toes and fingers does not necessarily mean that he could; maybe the radiographer never checked.
2. The time and date. Writing a history on a piece of paper the day before the trial will not count. The history should be on the history sheet or requisition in the patient's file. If this is not a practice of a department, the radiographer should have a special notebook for this purpose with entries in chronological order.
3. The radiographer's signature or initials.

For many radiographers, it may be a personal decision to follow these procedures. Some believe that it takes too much time. It should be remembered that the patients deserve the highest level of care possible, that with practice these procedures can be accomplished in a few moments, and that following them is another mark of a professional radiographer.

SUMMARY

Although many radiographers are not routinely called on to perform the tasks outlined in this chapter, they must be prepared to do so. Also mentioned in this chapter is one of the most difficult jobs in health care: conveying a caring attitude in the hurried, high-stress atmosphere and the short amount of time in which radiographers have to perform their duties. To accomplish this goal, radiographers should perform their job not only efficiently but also with care and compassion. Radiographers need to have patience, to maintain eye contact, and to talk to the patient—not to the x-ray tube or Bucky tray. They should remember that the patient is probably scared—scared of the procedure and scared of what the procedure will find. The examination should be explained to reduce this fear and anxiety, even if it is explained in only brief, general terms. At least the patient will know what to expect of the next few minutes. Carrying out these procedures with efficiency and empathy advances the professional status of all radiographers.

■ ■ SELF-ASSESSMENT TEST

DIRECTIONS: Supply answers to each of the following questions.

1. List and describe the locations for taking a patient's pulse.
2. What procedure for taking a patient's pulse should be followed when a fracture of an extremity is suspected?
3. What is the typical pulse rate for male and female patients?
4. What terms describe higher than normal and lower than normal pulse rates?
5. What types of patients tend to have higher than normal pulse rates?
6. What types of patients tend to have lower than normal pulse rates?
7. What characteristics of pulses should be noted and recorded?
8. What is the normal respiration rate?
9. What terms describe a higher than normal breathing rate, a lower than normal breathing rate, difficult breathing, and an absence of respiration?
10. What is a normal oral temperature reading for an adult in degrees Fahrenheit and Celsius?
11. What is the typical adult male and adult female, blood pressure reading?
12. List and explain the five goals of taking a patient's history.
13. What is the minimum amount of information a radiographer should try to obtain during a patient history?
14. List the seven major patient areas a radiographer should assess, and describe the assessment for each.
15. Describe the legal considerations for radiographers when making patient assessments and observations.

▨ ▨ BIBLIOGRAPHY

Ehrlich, RA, et al: Patient Care in Radiography, ed 5. Mosby, St. Louis, 1999.

Garner, JS: Guidelines for Isolation Precautions in Hospitals, 1996. Hospital Infection Control Practices Advisory Committee, Centers for Disease Control, Atlanta, 1996.

Thomas, CL (ed): Taber's Cyclopedic Medical Dictionary, ed 18. FA Davis, Philadelphia, 1997.

Torres, L, Linn-Watson, T, and Dutton, AG: Basic Medical Techniques and Patient Care for Radiologic Technologists, ed 5. JB Lippincott, Philadelphia, 1997.

2

AID FOR MEDICAL EMERGENCIES

PREREQUISITE

Before starting this chapter, the radiographer should be familiar with taking vital signs, observing patients, and methods of patient care. The radiographer should have had training in cardiopulmonary resuscitation (CPR) and the abdominal-thrust maneuver (formerly called the Heimlich maneuver) and should know cardiac arrest code procedures. He or she should know how oxygen administration equipment and suctioning devices function and should be acquainted with the contents of crash carts.

OUTLINE

▨ ▨ INTRODUCTION

A trauma patient's condition can change at any moment. Radiographers must be prepared to recognize and react to these changes. This chapter lists the indicators of common medical emergencies, methods of verifying the type of emergency, immediate aid and actions for the radiographer, and supporting actions after additional assistance has arrived.

Warning signs give the first clue that the patient may be in distress. For example, the patient's skin color may change to grayish white. This suggests a number of possible medical emergencies. Verification helps prove and identify the type of emergency. Immediate actions can be used once an emergency has been confirmed. These are actions the radiographer should take whether additional medical help will be needed or not. Finally, supporting actions are those a radiographer may use to assist other medical professionals after they have arrived.

▨ ▨ IMPAIRED BREATHING

One of the primary concerns of first aid and patient care is breathing and maintaining a patent (open) airway. Baseline patient respiration should be established and should be constantly observed for changes. Patients with significant chest trauma require closer observation because of the importance of the underlying organs and the high mortality associated with thoracic injuries. Nauseated or vomiting patients should not be left alone in a recumbent position, because they could aspirate foreign matter. Unconscious patients must never be left alone, especially on an x-ray table.

Symptoms that indicate dyspnea (difficulty breathing) and respiratory failure are obvious in conscious patients but may not be so in the unconscious. The unconscious patient must be watched closely, most notably for respiratory arrest. Because indications of dyspnea are usually quite noticeable, there are few confirming actions to be taken. Other breathing problems include choking and asthma attacks, both of which can restrict breathing. Boxes 2–1

BOX 2–1
DYSPNEA

WARNING SIGNS
    Labored breathing
    Gasping
    Anxiety
    Dilated nostrils
    Expansion of the chest
    Protrusion of the abdomen

VERIFICATION
    Same as **Warning Signs**, and possibly:
        Cyanosis (check fingernails and lips)
        Hemoptysis (usually frothy pink or red)

IMMEDIATE ACTIONS
    Ensure airway is clear. (Sit patient up. If he or she cannot sit up, tilt the head back. If there is a possible cervical spine injury, check mouth for obstruction. Use a gloved finger or tongue depressor to remove obstruction or to press the tongue down.) If the dyspnea continues, call for assistance.
    If the onset of dyspnea is very severe, call for assistance immediately.

SUPPORTING ACTIONS
    Remove any interfering radiographic equipment.
    Prepare for possible suctioning, oxygen administration, and epinephrine injection.
    Document symptoms, actions, and time.

BOX 2–2
CHOKING

WARNING SIGNS
Grasping at throat
Agitation

VERIFICATION
Patient unable to speak

IMMEDIATE ACTIONS
Perform the abdominal-thrust (Heimlich) maneuver.

SUPPORTING ACTIONS
Remove any interfering radiographic equipment.
Prepare for possible suctioning, tracheotomy, or oxygen administration.
Document symptoms, actions, and time.

BOX 2–3
ASTHMA ATTACK

WARNING SIGNS
Labored breathing
Wheezing

VERIFICATION
Tightness in throat

IMMEDIATE ACTIONS
If patient carries a nebulizer, assist in its use.
If attack is severe or if symptoms persist, call for assistance.

SUPPORTING ACTIONS
Remove any interfering radiographic equipment.
Prepare for possible epinephrine or other injectable drug administration.
Document symptoms, actions, and time.

WARNING SIGNS

Lack of chest/abdomen movement
Unconsciousness

VERIFICATION

Lack of air exchange (check by holding back of hand by the patient's mouth and nostrils to detect air movement).

Pulse continues for a few moments, gradually weakens, then ceases. [NOTE: In CARDIAC arrest, the pulse does NOT continue; it ceases immediately.]

IMMEDIATE ACTIONS

Get assistance—quickly (call a code).

Ensure airway is clear. (Sit patient up. If patient is unable to sit up, tilt head back. If there is a possible cervical spine injury, check the mouth for obstructions. Use a gloved finger or tongue depressor to remove obstructions or to press the tongue down.)

Begin artificial respiration. [NOTE: Consider using an S-tube airway or Ambu-bag with ventilating patients with communicable diseases.]

SUPPORTING ACTIONS

Remove any interfering radiographic equipment.

Prepare for possible suctioning, oxygen administration, and drug administration.

Document symptoms, actions, and time.

through 2–4 describe the symptoms and actions a radiographer may take for dyspnea, choking, asthma attacks, and respiratory arrest.

■ ■ CARDIAC ARREST

Fast action is required if the radiographer suspects that the patient's heart has stopped beating. The brain can survive undamaged for less than 5 minutes without its blood

43

supply. The patient must be constantly observed for warning signs. Although it is used infrequently, knowledge of the cardiac arrest code procedure and CPR competency are essential. Box 2–5 diagrams the procedure for possible cardiac arrest situations.

BOX 2–5
CARDIAC ARREST

WARNING SIGNS
> Loss of consciousness
> Respiration stops

VERIFICATION
> Absence of pulse—check carotid artery. [NOTE: In RESPIRATORY arrest, the pulse continues for a few minutes.]

IMMEDIATE ACTIONS
Call a cardiac arrest code.
Mentally note the time.
Begin CPR:

1. Clear airway.
2. Place palms 2 inches superior to xiphoid process.
3. Compress chest and heart once every second.
4. If alone, give two artificial respirations for every 15 compressions.
5. If assistance is available, 1 respiration is given for every 5 compressions.

SUPPORTING ACTIONS
> Remove any interfering radiographic equipment.
> Assist in obtaining supplies.
> Keep spectators away from the area.
> Document the time the cardiac arrest began, the time the code team arrived, and other information as requested by the team.

▪ ▪ SHOCK

Shock often accompanies trauma. It is caused by insufficient circulation. The types of shock that are related to trauma are hypovolemic, neurogenic, and traumatic. The patient may be conscious or unconscious, and the onset of shock may be immediate or delayed. Shock may also affect witnesses to accidents or the friends and family of the patient. Shock is a serious, possibly life-threatening, medical emergency and requires quick diagnosis and treatment.

▪ HYPOVOLEMIC SHOCK

Hypovolemic means low volume, and hypovolemic shock means shock caused by a decrease in the quantity of circulating blood. This can be caused by both external and internal bleeding, and sometimes by dehydration or diarrhea. Even the bleeding into the thigh from a femur fracture can cause hypovolemic shock. A decrease in the amount of blood causes the heart to beat faster, so the pulse rate rises, but it also makes the pulse weak or difficult to detect. The patient's breathing will be similar—rapid but shallow.

▪ NEUROGENIC SHOCK

Neurogenic shock may include mental and physiologic shock caused by overwhelming the nervous system. Excessive fear, grief, pain, or stress may cause it. What constitutes excessive, however, varies with each patient. Fear of the unknown (not knowing what an x-ray examination involves or fear of the unknown diagnosis) combined with the stress of an accident may be enough to send a patient with relatively minor injuries into shock. Therefore, every patient must be observed for the symptoms of shock. Neurogenic shock also may strike the patient's visitors or family, uninjured accident victims, or witnesses. Just the sight of blood or an injury causes

BOX 2–6
SHOCK

WARNING SIGNS

Skin and face—white, gray, pale, cyanotic
Patient feels faint or light-headed
Rapid but shallow respiration
Patient stares or is uninterested in surroundings
Possible restlessness or anxiety
Possible extreme thirst
Cool, clammy (moist) skin

VERIFICATION

Pulse is rapid but weak.
Pupils are dilated.
Blood pressure (BP) and pulse pressure decrease.
(However, there may not be enough time for the radiographer to check the patient's BP. Most of the
time, immediate action should be taken. The physician or a nurse will then check the BP.)

IMMEDIATE ACTIONS

Place the patient supine (if he or she is not already).
Place the patient in the Trendelenburg position by el-
evating the feet or tilting the x-ray table or cart so
that the head is down and the feet are up, unless
the injuries prevent this. Place a blanket over the
patient if it is readily available. Ensure that the patient has a clear airway.
Get a physician (in severe cases call a cardiac arrest
code). While waiting for assistance to arrive, control any external bleeding and do NOT give the
patient fluids.

SUPPORTING ACTIONS

Obtain a crash cart.
Obtain a blood pressure cuff.
Prepare for possible IV or IM drug administrations
(such as epinephrine).
Prepare for possible oxygen administration.
Prepare to write down physician orders for labora-
tory exams, blood transfusions, or other services.
Document the incident, the time, and the actions taken.

many to faint or go into shock. To avoid this, it is best to keep the radiographic room door closed and injuries covered. When the radiographer is working alone, visitors should probably be left in the emergency room waiting area.

TRAUMATIC SHOCK

Traumatic shock—shock caused by an injury—has many causes, and radiographers should closely watch trauma patients for the warning signs of shock. In general, the degree of traumatic shock is proportional to the severity of the injury. Crushing injuries and compound fractures are more likely to induce shock. Abdominal and cerebral injuries also produce shock. Abdominal injuries cause shock mainly from damage to internal organs. Shock from cerebral trauma is mainly from edema and hemorrhage. Traumatic shock also can be caused by damage to highly sensitive nerves such as those in the eye or celiac (solar) plexus. Box 2–6 outlines the symptoms of and actions for shock.

BLEEDING

Bleeding (hemorrhage) may be external or internal, arterial, venous, or capillary. External bleeding will be under control when the patient arrives in the x-ray department but may start again as a result of moving the patient. Internal bleeding is less noticeable and may send the patient into shock before it is detected. Arterial blood is bright red because of its high oxygen content. It pulses from arteries near the surface but may appear to flow steadily out of a wound when a deep artery is involved. Venous blood is dark red and has a constant flow. Capillary bleeding oozes from tissue. Severe bleeding must be controlled immediately, and all fresh bleeding should be reported. Box 2–7 is concerned with external bleeding, and Box 2–8 is devoted to internal bleeding.

BOX 2–7
EXTERNAL BLEEDING

WARNING SIGNS
Arterial—bright red, usually pulsing
Venous—dark red, steady flow
Capillary—reddish color, oozes from tissue

VERIFICATION
Same as **Warning Signs**

IMMEDIATE ACTIONS
Apply direct pressure, with fingers. For capillary or
mild venous bleeding in an extremity, raise the
limb above the heart.
If bleeding cannot be stopped in less than 5 minutes,
call for assistance.

SUPPORTING ACTIONS
Document symptoms, actions, and time.

BOX 2–8
INTERNAL BLEEDING

WARNING SIGNS
In general: shock with weak, rapid, irregular pulse
Extremities: possible swelling
Abdomen: rigidity
Chest: dyspnea
Intracranial change in level of consciousness

VERIFICATION
Same as for shock (see Box 2–6)

IMMEDIATE ACTIONS
If it is present, treat for shock (see Box 2–6).

SUPPORTING ACTIONS
Document symptoms, actions, and time.

▓ ▓ IMPAIRED CONSCIOUSNESS

▓ SYNCOPE

A temporary loss of consciousness due to insufficient blood supply to the brain may cause fainting (syncope). The causes are many, including stress from trauma. The radiographer should carefully observe trauma patients for the warning signs of syncope, especially those who are standing or sitting. Ampules of ammonia should be readily available. It is good practice to have ammonia ampules taped to the walls near upright cassette holders, near the ends of the x-ray table, and on the collimator. They should

---

BOX 2–9
SYNCOPE

WARNING SIGNS
> Pallor
> Cool, moist (clammy) skin

VERIFICATION
> Dizziness or light-headedness
> Possible nausea

IMMEDIATE ACTIONS
> If the patient is upright, place him or her supine on the floor, on a cart, or on the radiographic table.
> If the patient is conscious, place him or her in the Trendelenburg position.
> If the patient is unconscious, administer ammonia.
> If the patient fails to regain consciousness, call for assistance.

SUPPORTING ACTIONS
> Check for respiratory arrest (see Box 2–4), cardiac arrest (see Box 2–5), and shock (see Box 2–6).
> Prepare to respond to each of these.
> Document symptoms, actions, and time.

never be carried in a pocket, where they can be easily broken. Ammonia should be administered briefly by waving it under the patient's nose. The radiographer's head should not be over the patient's when doing this because the fumes rise and can be quite strong. Box 2–9 is concerned with syncope identification and actions.

VERTIGO

Dizziness is sometimes called vertigo, but dizziness and vertigo are actually two different problems. Vertigo is a balance, or orientation, problem linked to central nervous system problems, inner ear problems, and intoxication.

BOX 2–10
VERTIGO

WARNING SIGNS

Patient grasping at objects to maintain balance, or patient falling

VERIFICATION

Sensation of room spinning (as opposed to dizziness)
Possible severe nausea
Possible vomiting

IMMEDIATE ACTIONS

If the patient is upright, assist him or her to a recumbent position.
Provide an emesis basin.
If the vertigo is severe, report it to a physician before continuing the exam.

SUPPORTING ACTIONS

Ensure that the patient cannot fall.
If the patient is vomiting, ensure that vomitus is not aspirated.

Patients suffering from vertigo report a sensation of the room spinning around them. Because vertigo affects the patient's balance, he or she should not be placed in upright positions without assistance. Vertigo should be reported to a physician, especially if the patient has not experienced it before. Box 2–10 diagrams the radiographer's actions for suspected cases of vertigo.

■ ■   NAUSEA AND VOMITING

Nausea or vomiting may accompany head injuries, intoxication, or nervousness. There should always be several emesis basins close at hand in every x-ray room. The patient should be positioned to reduce the chance of as-

---

BOX 2–11
NAUSEA AND VOMITING

WARNING SIGNS
Patient reports upset stomach or nauseated feeling.
Facial color turns white, gray, or greenish.
Vertigo.

VERIFICATION
Same as **Warning Signs**

IMMEDIATE ACTIONS
Try to relieve the nausea by having the patient take short, shallow breaths through an open mouth.
Place the patient in a lateral recumbent, Trendelenburg, or seated position.
Obtain an emesis basin.
Maintain a patent airway.

SUPPORTING ACTIONS
If vomiting is so severe or uncontrollable that the exam cannot be continued, notify a physician.

pirating vomitus. The recommended positions are lateral recumbent, Trendelenburg, and seated. In the seated position, the patient should lean over the basin, and the forehead should be supported. If the patient must remain supine, the head should be turned to the side. If the patient's head cannot be turned because of a possible cervical spine or other injury, then fast action with a suctioning machine is required. Box 2–11 outlines the procedures for nausea and vomiting.

■ ■ MEDICAL EMERGENCY SYMPTOMS

Patient-care and first-aid books often cover medical emergencies just as they have been covered in Boxes 2–1 through 2–11. Each emergency is followed by a discussion of its potential symptoms and treatment. In real life, however, a radiographer first notices a symptom (or symptoms), determines which medical emergency the patient is experiencing, and selects the appropriate supportive measures. The following tables are arranged according to this experiential pattern.

Tables 2–1 through 2–8 are headed by symptoms that may appear in more than one type of medical emergency. The clusters of verifying signs listed after the initial heading should help you pinpoint the most likely medical emergency. The entries alongside each column then direct you to the immediate and supporting actions portions of Boxes 2–1 through 2–11.

Table 2–9 is a quick-reference, alphabetical index of symptoms that a radiographer is likely to notice first in a patient experiencing a medical emergency. If a symptom listed here is typically associated with only one type of medical emergency, you will be directed to consult the verifying signs and appropriate actions in Boxes 2–1 through 2–11. If a symptom is frequently associated with more than one type of medical emergency, then you will first be directed to one of the symptom lists in Tables 2–1 through 2–8 in order to pinpoint the exact emergency.

TABLE 2–1. PATIENT SHOWS CYANOSIS

And
- labored breathing   *See* Box 2–1. DYSPNEA
- gasping
- dilated nostrils
- chest expansion
- protruding abdomen
- anxiety

And
- rapid, shallow breathing   *See* Box 2–6. SHOCK
- cool, moist skin
- rapid, weak pulse
- dilated pupils
- anxiety

TABLE 2–2. PATIENT SHOWS WHITE, GRAY, OR PALE COLOR

And
- rapid, shallow breathing   *See* Box 2–6. SHOCK
- rapid, weak pulse
- cool, moist skin
- dizziness
- thirst
- anxiety

And
- nausea   *See* Box 2–9. SYNCOPE
- cool, moist skin

And
- nausea   *See* Box 2–11.
- vertigo   NAUSEA AND VOMITING

TABLE 2–3. PATIENT SHOWS UNCONSCIOUSNESS

And
- no respirations   *See* Box 2–4.
- steadily weakening pulse   RESPIRATORY ARREST

And
- no respirations   *See* Box 2–5.
- no pulse   CARDIAC ARREST

And
- evidence of head trauma   *See* Box 2–8.
- irregular pulse   INTERNAL BLEEDING

And
- cool, moist skin   *See* Box 2–9. SYNCOPE
- pallor

And
- rapid, shallow breathing   *See* Box 2–6. SHOCK
- rapid, weak pulse
- cool, moist skin
- dilated pupils
- thirst
- anxiety

TABLE 2–4. PATIENT SHOWS COOL, MOIST SKIN

And
- dizziness   *See* Box 2–9. SYNCOPE
- nausea
- pallor
- unconsciousness

And
- dizziness   *See* Box 2–6. SHOCK
- rapid, shallow breathing
- rapid, weak pulse
- dilated pupils
- thirst
- anxiety

TABLE 2–5. PATIENT SHOWS NAUSEA

And
- dizziness   *See* Box 2–9. SYNCOPE
- cool, moist skin
- pallor

And
- evidence of head trauma   *See* Box 2–8.
- irregular pulse   INTERNAL BLEEDING

And
- reports room spinning   *See* Box 2–10. VERTIGO
  or moving

TABLE 2–6. PATIENT SHOWS LABORED BREATHING

And
- gasping   *See* Box 2–1. DYSPNEA
- chest expansion
- protruding abdomen
- dilated nostrils
- cyanosis
- hemoptysis
- anxiety

And
- wheezing   *See* Box 2–3.
- throat tightness   ASTHMA ATTACK

And
- evidence of thoracic injury   *See* Box 2–8.
- irregular pulse   INTERNAL BLEEDING

TABLE 2–7. PATIENT SHOWS ANXIETY

And
- labored breathing   *See* Box 2–1. DYSPNEA
- gasping
- dilated nostrils
- chest expansion
- protruding abdomen
- cyanosis
- hemoptysis

And
- rapid, shallow respirations   *See* Box 2–6. SHOCK
- rapid, weak pulse
- cool, moist skin
- dilated pupils
- thirst

TABLE 2–8. PATIENT SHOWS NO CHEST OR ABDOMINAL MOVEMENT

And
- steadily weakening pulse   *See* Box 2–4. RESPIRATORY ARREST

And
- no pulse   *See* Box 2–5. CARDIAC ARREST

TABLE 2–9. QUICK-REFERENCE LIST

Symptom	Reference
abdomen, protrusion of	Box 2–1
abdomen, rigidity of	Box 2–8
agitation	Box 2–2
	(continued)

TABLE 2–9. QUICK-REFERENCE LIST *(continued)*

Symptom	Reference
anxiety	Table 2–7
bleeding, external	Box 2–7
bleeding, internal	Box 2–8
breathing, labored	Table 2–6
breathing, rapid and shallow	Box 2–6
breathing, stopped	Table 2–8
chest, expansion of	Box 2–1
chest, no movement of	Table 2–8
choking	Box 2–2
consciousness, loss of	Table 2–3
cyanosis	Table 2–1
dizziness	Box 2–9
fainting	Box 2–9
gasping	Box 2–1
grasping at throat	Box 2–2
hemoptysis	Box 2–1
light-headedness	Box 2–9
nausea	Box 2–11
nostrils, dilated	Box 2–1
pallor	Table 2–2
pulse, irregular	Box 2–8
pulse, none	Box 2–5
pulse, rapid and weak	Box 2–6
pupils, dilated	Box 2–6
skin color, blue	Table 2–1
skin, cool and moist	Table 2–4
skin color, white/gray/pale	Table 2–2
speaking, suddenly unable to	Box 2–2
staring, uninterested in surroundings	Box 2–6
swelling	Box 2–8
syncope	Box 2–9
thirst	Box 2–6
throat, grasping at	Box 2–2
throat, tightness in	Box 2–3
unconsciousness	Table 2–3
vertigo	Box 2–10
vomiting	Box 2–11
wheezing	Box 2–3

■ ■ SUMMARY

This chapter presented the medical emergencies that a radiographer might encounter during trauma radiography and appropriate responses. The emergencies, a means for identifying them, and a radiographer's actions were presented three different ways to enable a radiographer to access the information they need quickly in real situations.

■ ■ SELF-ASSESSMENT TEST

DIRECTIONS: Identify the patient's medical emergency, if any, and the radiographer's course of action in each situation.

1. Initial evaluation:
   a. The patient is unconscious.
   b. Pulse rate is 63.
   c. Respirations are shallow.
   d. The patient's chest is severely injured.
   After bringing the patient into the radiography room, you notice that the patient's chest is not moving. There does not seem to be any air coming out of the patient's mouth or nose. You quickly check the patient's pulse and it is present but seems to be deteriorating.

2. Your patient was brought to the emergency room with a shoulder injury. Your initial radiographs demonstrate an anterior dislocation of the shoulder. The shoulder has been relocated, and the patient has returned to radiography for postreduction films to rule out avulsion fractures. On his return, the patient's color, breathing, and pulse were normal. He was not particularly attentive throughout the follow-up examination. When you return to your room after developing the films you notice the following:
   a. His breathing is fast, but not deep.
   b. His face is pale.
   c. His skin is damp and cool.
   You check his pulse, and it is fast but not very strong.

3. Your patient was involved in a motorcycle accident in which she fractured her left femur. The femur

has broken through the skin, but the only other injuries appear to be abrasions from skidding across the pavement. When she was first brought to the radiography department, you checked for a popliteal pulse, which was present and had a rate of 87. After moving the patient's leg for a lateral projection of the femur, you notice fresh bleeding from the thigh. The blood is bright red.

DEFINE THE FOLLOWING TERMS:

4. Dyspnea
5. Patent
6. Trendelenburg position
7. Hemorrhage
8. Shock
9. Syncope
10. Pallor

11. Explain the differences between respiratory arrest and cardiac arrest.
12. Explain the differences between hypovolemic, neurogenic, and traumatic shock.
13. List the visible differences between arterial, venous, and capillary bleeding.
14. Explain the differences between vertigo and dizziness.
15. What are the differences between one-person and two-person CPR?

▪ ▪ BIBLIOGRAPHY

Ehrlich, RA, et al: Patient Care in Radiography, ed 5. Mosby, St Louis, 1999.

Thomas, CL (ed): Taber's Cyclopedic Medical Dictionary, ed 18. FA Davis, Philadelphia, 1997.

Torres, L, Linn-Watson, T, and Dutton, AG: Basic Medical Techniques and Patient Care for Radiologic Technologists, ed 5. JB Lippincott, Philadelphia, 1997.

3

DRUGS THAT MAY AFFECT PATIENT COOPERATION

PREREQUISITE

Before starting this chapter, the radiographer should be familiar with drug classifications and drug administration routes including the intravenous (IV), intramuscular (IM), subcutaneous (SC or subq), oral, and rectal methods.

OUTLINE

■ ■ INTRODUCTION

This chapter outlines the reasons radiographers should be informed of the drugs that patients have received. The speed with which drugs take effect and how the administration method affects the speed are reviewed. A table of drugs that can affect the patient's ability to cooperate with radiographic procedures is included at the end.

■ ■ RADIOGRAPHER CONCERNS

Medications are of concern to the radiographer because they may affect the patient's mobility and mental state. Whether the patient will be able to stand, walk, sit, or maintain radiographic positions affects routine, trauma, and portable radiography. Drugs that alter the patient's mental condition can make his or her history unreliable. A release or consent form may be worthless if the patient is under the influence of certain drugs like morphine or meperidine. Therefore, the radiographer should know what drugs the patient has been given and how they may affect the examination.

■ ■ LEGAL CONCERNS

Besides professional reasons to check the patient's chart to see what medications have been given, there are legal considerations. As mentioned earlier in this book, a release or consent form signed by the patient while he or she is under the influence of drugs—including analgesics, narcotics, barbiturates, preoperative medications, and others—may not be ruled as an informed consent. If there is any question as to a patient's ability to give consent, the radiographer should consult the patient's physician or a radiologist.

Another legal concern is liability. For example, a patient is given a drug that carries a warning for orthostatic hypotension. The radiographer neglects to check the patient's chart. While getting off the cart, the patient faints, falls to the floor, and is injured. The radiographer is guilty of malpractice. The hospital and the radiographer are liable for the patient's injuries and possibly for damages. The radiographer could not claim that he or she did not know the patient had been given a drug; the radiographer *should* have known. Similarly, if a trauma patient is given a drug but the emergency room personnel forget to tell the radiography personnel, the hospital would still be liable. It would be held that it is the hospital's fault—not the patient's—if its communication system fails. Radiographers should acquire the habit of checking drug administrations to their patients so that appropriate safety precautions can be used.

■ ■ RADIOGRAPHER ACTIONS

Knowing what drugs a patient has been given is just a beginning. Many drugs have the *potential* to alter a patient's mental state but do not do so in any noticeable way. Also, patients react differently, even when given the same drug by the same method. For example, some drugs that sedate most people produce the opposite effect in others. When a patient has been given a drug from the list provided in this chapter, the radiographer should read the warning and take it under advisement. Observe these patients more closely. Get them up more slowly. Give them extra assistance when moving, or extra immobilization. Do not leave them alone if the drug's effects are particularly strong. In short, be more aware—although nothing may happen, the chances that something will happen have been increased.

Besides knowing what drug the patient has been given and looking up any warnings, the radiographer should know the method and time of administration. The typical administration routes for the drugs listed in this chapter are injection, oral, and rectal. Knowing the method and time of administration is another guide to how impaired the patient may be. Injected drugs work the fastest. IV injections work in less than 1 minute, with maximum effectiveness. IM and SC injections work within a few minutes. Rectally administered drugs work in 15 to 30 minutes. Oral drugs, although common, are slowest to take effect. They begin to affect the patient in 30 to 60 minutes. However, some oral drugs are designed for immediate release (IR) and take effect in about 30 minutes. Other oral drugs are designed for slow release (SR) and give off controlled amounts of the drug over a longer time (usually 8 to 12 hours).

▓ ▓ DRUG TABLES

The drug tables in this chapter have been compiled as a guide to the radiographer. They were compiled mainly from the *Physicians' Desk Reference (PDR)*. They are not, however, all-inclusive. They include drugs from the major categories that can affect the patient's ability to cooperate with radiographic examinations. If a drug is on this list, the radiographer should make an extra effort to watch for conditions listed from the manufacturer's warnings. If a drug is not on this list, it still may affect the patient. Generic names have also been included to help guide the radiographer with drugs not listed. When in doubt, a physician, pharmacist, a pharmacist's *Drug Facts and Comparisons,* or *PDR* should be consulted.

Two tables are provided. Common analgesics, tranquilizers, and so forth have been listed alphabetically by brand name in the trade drug table (Table 3–1). The generic name in brackets refers to the component of the drug that may cause the effects in the warning. The warnings are those provided by the manufacturer that may affect the behavior of the patient during an examination. The second table lists drugs by their generic name, also alphabetically (Table 3–2).

The most common warning is that the drug may impair the mental or physical abilities, or both, of the patient to carry out potentially hazardous activities such as operating machinery or driving a car. This side effect has been abbreviated as "may impair" in this list. The ambulatory warning generally means the same as the orthostatic hypoten-

TABLE 3–1. TRADE DRUG TABLE

Brand Name [Generic Name]	Warnings	Typical Administration Method
Actifed with Codeine [codeine]	dizziness, may impair	oral
Alfenta [alfentanil]	hypotension	injection
Alurate [aprobarbital]	may impair	oral
Ambien [zolpidem]	mental alertness, drowsiness	oral
Anafranil [clomipramine]	mental alertness	oral
Anaprox [naproxen]	dizziness, vertigo, drowsiness	oral
Ascriptin with Codeine [codeine]	may impair	oral
Anexsia [hydrocodone]	may impair	oral
Aquachloral [chloral hydrate]	mental alertness, drowsiness	oral, rectal
Asendin [amoxapine]	mental alertness	oral
Astramorph [morphine]	orthostatic hypotension	injection
Atarax [hydroxyzine]	dizziness	oral
Ativan [lorazepam]	avoid ambulation for 8 hours, may impair for 24–48 hours	injection

(continued)

TABLE 3–1. TRADE DRUG TABLE *(continued)*

Brand Name [Generic Name]	Warnings	Typical Administration Method
Aventyl [nortriptyline]	mental alertness, dizziness	oral
Axotal [butalbital]	may impair	oral
B & O Supprettes [opium]	drowsiness, may impair	rectal
Bancap [hydrocodone]	drowsiness, mood changes, may impair	oral
Benadryl [diphenhydramine]	may impair	injection, oral
Buprenex [buprenorphine]	drowsiness, sedation, may impair	injection
Butisol Sodium [butabarbital]	may impair	oral
Ceta Plus [hydrocodone]	may impair	oral
Codiclear DH [hydrocodone]	drowsiness, may impair	oral
Codimal DH [hydrocodone]	drowsiness, may impair	oral
Co-Gesic [hydrocodone]	may impair	oral
DHC Plus [dihydrocodeine bitartrate]	ambulatory warning, may impair	oral
Dalgan [dezocine]	may impair	injection

TABLE 3–1. TRADE DRUG TABLE *(continued)*

Brand Name [Generic Name]	Warnings	Typical Administration Method
Dalmane [flurazepam]	may impair	oral
Damason-P [hydrocodone]	may impair	oral
Darvocet-N [propoxyphene]	ambulatory warning, may impair	oral
Darvon; Darvon-N [propoxyphene]	ambulatory warning, may impair	oral
Demerol [meperidine]	orthostatic hypotension, may impair	injection, oral
Desyrel [trazodone]	orthostatic hypotension, syncope	oral
Dilantin with Phenobarbital [phenobarbital]	may impair	injection, oral
Dilaudid [hydromorphone]	ambulatory warning, orthostatic hypotension, drowsiness, mood change	injection, oral, rectal
Dolacet [hydrocodone]	may impair	oral
Dolophine [methadone]	may impair	injection, oral
Duocet [hydrocodone]	may impair	oral

(continued)

TABLE 3–1. TRADE DRUG TABLE *(continued)*

Brand Name [Generic Name]	Warnings	Typical Administration Method
Duraclon [clonidine]	severe hypotension, drowsiness, may impair	injection
Duramorph [morphine]	orthostatic hypotension, may impair	injection
Elavil [amitriptyline]	mental alertness, dizziness	oral
Empirin with Codeine [codeine]	may impair	oral
Equanil [meprobamate]	drowsiness, dizziness, mental alertness	oral
Esgic with Codeine [codeine, butalbital]	may impair	oral
Eskalith [lithium]	may impair	oral
Etrafon [perphenazine]	may impair	oral
Fioricet [butalbital]	may impair	oral
Fiorinal [butalbital]	may impair	oral
Fiorinal with Codeine [codeine, butalbital]	may impair	oral
Haldol [haloperidol]	may impair	injection, oral
Hydrocet [hydrocodone]	may impair	oral

TABLE 3–1. TRADE DRUG TABLE *(continued)*

Brand Name [Generic Name]	Warnings	Typical Administration Method
Hydrogesic [hydrocodone]	may impair	oral
Hy-Phen [hydrocodone]	may impair	oral
Infumorph [morphine]	may impair	injection
Inapsine [droperidol]	orthostatic hypotension	injection
Innovar [fentanyl, droperidol]	hypotension	injection
Kadian [morphine]	may impair	oral
Levo-Dromoran [levorphanol]	hypotension, dizziness	injection, oral
Levoprome [methotrimeprazine]	orthostatic hypotension, sedation, fainting, dizziness, supervise ambulation for 6 hours post administration	injection
Libritabs [chlordiazepoxide]	mental alertness	oral
Librium [chlordiazepoxide]	mental alertness	injection, oral
Limbitrol DS [chlordiazepoxide]	mental alertness	oral

(continued)

TABLE 3–1. TRADE DRUG TABLE *(continued)*

Brand Name [Generic Name]	Warnings	Typical Administration Method
Lithane [lithium]	may impair	oral
Lithobid [lithium]	may impair	oral
Lorcet [hydrocodone]	may impair	oral
Lortab [hydrocodone]	may impair	oral
Margesic-H [hydrocodone]	may impair	oral
Marinol [drobinol (THC)]	mood changes, may impair	oral
Mebaral [mephobarbital]	may impair	oral
Mellaril [thioridazine]	orthostatic hypotension (especially in women), may impair	oral
Mepergan [meperidine]	orthostatic hypotension, may impair	injection
Miltown [meprobamate]	drowsiness, dizziness, mental alertness	oral
MS Contin [morphine— continuous action]	may impair	oral
MSIR [morphine— immediate release]	orthostatic hypotension, sedation, may impair	oral

TABLE 3–1. TRADE DRUG TABLE *(continued)*

Brand Name [Generic Name]	Warnings	Typical Administration Method
Nembutal [pentobarbital]	may impair	injection, oral
Neuramate [meprobamate]	drowsiness, dizziness, mental alertness	oral
Norflex [orphenadrine]	ambulatory warning, syncope, dizziness, may impair	injection, oral
Norpramin [desipramine]	mental alertness	oral
Nubain [nalbuphine]	may impair	injection
Numorphan [oxymorphone]	orthostatic hypotension, sedation, may impair	injection, rectal
OMS Concentrate [morphine]	may impair	oral
Oramorph SR [morphine]	may impair	oral
Oxycontin [oxycodone]	may impair	oral
OxyFAST [oxycodone]	may impair	oral
PMB 200 [meprobamate]	may impair	oral
Pamelor [nortriptyline]	mental alertness, dizziness	oral

(continued)

TABLE 3–1. TRADE DRUG TABLE *(continued)*

Brand Name [Generic Name]	Warnings	Typical Administration Method
Panacet [hydrocodone]	may impair	oral
Paral [chloral hydrate]	mental alertness, drowsiness	oral, rectal
Paxipam [halazepam]	may impair	oral
Percocet [oxycodone]	may impair	oral
Percolone [oxycodone]	may impair	oral
Percodan [oxycodone]	may impair	oral
Permitil [fluphenazine]	may impair	oral
Phenaphen with Codeine [codeine]	may impair	oral
Phenergan [promethazine]	may impair	injection, oral
Phenergan with Codeine [promethazine, codeine]	orthostatic hypotension, drowinsess, dizziness, may impair	injection, oral
Phrenilin Forte [butalbital]	may impair	oral
Placidyl [ethchlorvynol]	drowsiness, dizziness	oral
Prolixin [fluphenazine]	may impair	injection, oral

TABLE 3–1. TRADE DRUG TABLE *(continued)*

Brand Name [Generic Name]	Warnings	Typical Administration Method
Propacet [propoxyphene]	may impair	oral
RMS [morphine]	may impair	rectal
Roxanol SR [morphine]	hypotension, dizziness, sedation	oral
Roxicet [oxycodone]	may impair	oral
Roxicodone [oxycodone]	may impair	oral
Roxilox [oxycodone]	may impair	oral
Roxiprin [oxycodone]	may impair	oral
Ru-Tuss with Hydrocodone [hydrocodone]	drowsiness, may impair	oral
Salutensin [reserpine]	orthostatic hypotension, dizziness	oral
Sedapap [butalbital]	may impair	oral
Serax [oxazepam]	may impair	oral
Serentil [mesoridazine]	hypotension	injection, oral
Sinequan [doxepin]	drowsiness	oral
Stadol [butorphanol]	sedation	injection

(continued)

TABLE 3–1. TRADE DRUG TABLE *(continued)*

Brand Name [Generic Name]	Warnings	Typical Administration Method
Stagesic [hydrocodone]	may impair	oral
Stelazine [trifiuoperazine]	hypotension	injection
Sublimaze [fentanyl]	orthostatic hypotension, dizziness, euphoria	injection
Sufenta [sufentanil]	hypotension	injection
Synalgos-DC [dihydrocodeine]	ambulatory warning, may impair	oral
Talacen [pentazocine]	sedation, dizziness, euphoria, hallucinations, disorientation	oral
Talwin [pentazocine]	sedation, dizziness, euphoria, hallucinations, disorientation	oral
Tegretol [carbamazepine]	dizziness, drowsiness, may impair	oral
Tencet [butalbital]	may impair	oral
T-Gesic [hydrocodone]	may impair	oral

TABLE 3–1. TRADE DRUG TABLE *(continued)*

Brand Name [Generic Name]	Warnings	Typical Administration Method
Thorazine [chlorpromazine]	may impair	injection, oral, rectal
Tofranil [imipramine]	may impair	oral
Tranxene [clorazepate]	mental alertness	oral
Trilafon [perphenazine]	may impair	injection, oral
Tylenol with Codeine [codeine]	may impair	oral
Tylox [oxycodone]	may impair	oral
Ultram [tramadol]	dizziness, somnolence, orthostatic hypotension, may impair	oral
Valium [diazepam]	mental alertness	injection, oral
Versed [midazolam]	hypotension, may impair	injection
Vicodin [hydrocodone]	may impair	oral
Wellbutrin [bupropion]	mental alertness	oral
Wygesic [propoxyphene]	may impair	oral
Xanax [alprazolam]	may impair	oral
Zydone [hydrocodone]	may impair	oral

TABLE 3–2. GENERIC DRUG TABLE

Generic Drug Name	Warnings	Typical Administration Method
alfentanil	hypotension	injection
alprazolam	may impair	oral
amitriptyline	mental alertness, dizziness	oral
amoxapine	mental alertness	oral
aprobarbital	may impair	oral
buprenorphine	sedation, may impair	injection
bupropion	mental alertness	oral
butabarbital	may impair	oral
butalbital	may impair	oral
butorphanol	sedation	injection
carbamazepine	may impair	oral
chloral hydrate	mental alertness, drowsiness	oral, rectal
chlordiazepoxide	mental alertness	injection, oral
chlorpromazine	syncope, dizziness, may impair	injection, oral
clomipramine	mental alertness	oral
clonidine	severe hypotension, drowsiness, may impair	oral
clorazepate	mental alertness	oral
codeine	ambulatory warning, may impair	injection, oral

TABLE 3–2. GENERIC DRUG TABLE *(continued)*

Generic Drug Name	Warnings	Typical Administration Method
desipramine	mental alertness	oral
dezocine	may impair	injection
diazepam	mental alertness	injection, oral
diphenhydramine	mental alertness	injection, oral
doxepin	drowsiness	oral
droperidol	hypotension	injection
ethchlorvynol	drowsiness, dizziness	oral
fentanyl	hypotension	injection
fluphenazine	may impair	injection, oral
flurazepam	may impair	oral
halazepam	may impair	oral
haloperidol	may impair	injection, oral
hydrocodone	may impair	oral
hydromorphone	orthostatic hypotension, drowsiness, mood change	injection, oral, rectal
hydroxyzine	dizziness	oral
imipramine	may impair	oral
levorphanol	hypotension, dizziness	injection, oral
lithium	may impair	oral
lorazepam	avoid ambulation for 8 hours, may impair for 24–48 hours	injection
loxapine	may impair	injection, oral

(continued)

TABLE 3–2. GENERIC DRUG TABLE *(continued)*

Generic Drug Name	Warnings	Typical Administration Method
meperidine	orthostatic hypotension, may impair	injection, oral
mephobarbital	may impair	oral
meprobamate	may impair	oral
mesoridazine	hypotension	injection, oral
methadone	orthostatic hypotension, increased effects in ambulatory patients	injection, oral
methocarbamol	dizziness	injection, oral
methotrimeprazine	orthostatic hypotension, sedation, fainting, dizziness, supervise ambulation for 6 hours post administration	injection
midazolam	hypotension, may impair	injection
midodine	drowsiness, dizziness, mental alertness	oral
morphine	may impair	injection, oral
nalbuphine	may impair	injection

TABLE 3–2. GENERIC DRUG TABLE *(continued)*

Generic Drug Name	Warnings	Typical Administration Method
naproxen	dizziness, vertigo, drowsiness	oral
nortriptyline	mental alertness, dizziness	oral
orphenadrine	ambulatory warning, syncope, dizziness, may impair	injection, oral
oxazepam	may impair	oral
oxycodone	may impair	oral
paraldehyde	mental alertness, drowsiness	oral, rectal
pentazocine	sedation, dizziness, euphoria, hallucinations, disorientation	oral
pentobarbital	may impair	injection
perphenazine	may impair	oral
phenobarbital	may impair	injection, oral
propoxyphene	ambulatory warning, may impair	oral
secobarbital	may impair	oral
sufentanil	hypotension	injection
thioridazine	orthostatic hypotension	oral

(continued)

TABLE 3–2. GENERIC DRUG TABLE *(continued)*

Generic Drug Name	Warnings	Typical Administration Method
trazodone	orthostatic hypotension, syncope	oral
tramadol	dizziness, somnolence, orthostatic hypotension, may impair	oral
trifluoperazine	hypotension	injection
zolpidem	mental alertness, drowsiness	oral

sion warning. The patient may feel light-headed or dizzy on sitting or walking but may not feel this way while seated. Therefore, with these warnings, even if the patient states that he or she can sit, stand, or walk, the radiographer should maintain a firm grip on the patient. If the patient is recumbent in bed, on a cart, or on the x-ray table, he or she should sit up slowly, then pause for a minute or two before standing or walking. Warnings about sedation and drowsiness may caution the radiographer against leaving the patient unattended on the table or on a cart.

■ ■ SUMMARY

For patient safety and for legal reasons, radiographers should review the warnings for drugs given to their patients. Although any patient may be on prescription medication, particular attention should be given to trauma patients, surgical patients (before and after surgery), pa-

tients restricted to bed (portable x-ray patients), and patients who appear to be sleepy or confused. If the patient
has been given a medication, the radiographer needs the
following information:

- the name of the drug
- when it was given
- what administration method was used

The warnings on the drug tables in this chapter should
then be reviewed, and appropriate precautions or extra
observation used. Finally, if the patient is acting unusual
and has not been medicated, or if there is any doubt as
to the warning or the action of a drug, the radiographer
should consult a physician.

▓ ▓ SELF-ASSESSMENT TEST

DIRECTIONS: Locate the warning for each of the
drugs listed below. Then evaluate the patient's possible
level of impairment as ascertained by the drug and its
warning, the administration method, and the time of
administration.

Drugs:

1. Fluphenazine, oral administration, 25 minutes ago
2. MSIR, oral administration, 35 minutes ago
3. Sublimaze, IM injection, 15 minutes ago
4. Lorazepam, IM injection, 40 minutes ago
5. Thorazine, rectal administration, 20 minutes ago
6. Donnatal, oral administration, 95 minutes ago
7. Benadryl, oral administration, 10 minutes ago
8. Talacen, oral administration, 120 minutes ago
9. Methadone, IV injection, 50 minutes ago
10. Valium, IV injection, 5 minutes ago
11. Methotrimeprazine, IM injection, 5 hours ago
12. Margesic, oral administration, 9 hours ago
13. Tramadol, oral administration, 75 minutes ago
14. Cloridine, IV injection, 25 minutes ago
15. Aquachloral, oral administration, 13 hours ago

Evaluate the level of impairment as:

1. Possible HIGH level of impairment
2. Possible MODERATE level of impairment
3. Possible LOW level of impairment
4. No impairment, or very little impairment

■ ■ BIBLIOGRAPHY

Drug Facts and Comparisons. Facts and Comparisons, St. Louis, 1999.

Hitner, H, and Nagle, B: Basic Pharmacology for Health Occupations, ed 4. McGraw-Hill, Boston, 1998.

Huff, BB (ed): Physicians' Desk Reference, ed 53. Medical Economics Company, Oradell, NJ, 1999.

4

TRAUMA TERMINOLOGY AND FRACTURES

OUTLINE

▪ ▪ INTRODUCTION

This chapter defines trauma terms. The terms used to describe trauma, fractures, and other injuries are explained. The observable signs of fracture are presented so that the radiographer may better select the methods to be used in the radiographic examination of trauma patients. The basics of the fracture and healing processes are also included. This material will improve the radiographer's understanding of fractures and dislocations and better enable him or her to perform radiographic examinations. Communication with other health-care workers also will be improved.

▪ ▪ DEFINITION OF TRAUMA

Trauma injuries are those caused by external force or violence. They cover a wide range—from a minor bruise to amputation. Sometimes the damage is obvious (as with an amputation); other times the damage is not so apparent (as with some concussions). Some patients have a single injury, such as the softball player's dislocated finger. At the other extreme, automobile accident victims often have multiple injuries. To prepare for these possibilities, the radiographer should know the types of trauma injuries and types of fractures (discussed in this chapter), as well as which incidents tend to produce which injuries (see Chapter 5).

▪ ▪ TRAUMA TERMINOLOGY

Listed below are the basic, general trauma terms and abbreviations.

A/A: abbreviation for automobile accident.
abrasion: an area where a portion of skin (or mucous membrane) has been scraped away (as if with sandpaper). The slang term *road rash* is sometimes used to de-

scribe abrasion caused by the patient (often a motorcycle rider) skidding across pavement.

amputation: the complete removal of a body part.

concussion: injury from a blow or from striking an object. Usually means a blow to the head that causes unconsciousness and damage to the brain. Can also be used in reference to the spine or inner ear.

crepitus or **crepitation:** the sound made by the broken ends of a bone grating against one another.

dislocation: a bone no longer in its normal articulation; "out of joint."

Fx or **fracture:** a break in a bone. It may or may not break across the entire width of the bone (see later discussion of fracture and dislocation types).

hematoma: a mass of blood (often clotted) restricted to an area. Also called a bruise or contusion.

laceration: an opening or tear through the skin or through an organ.

luxation: displacement of organs or dislocation of a joint.

sprain: a stretching or tearing of a ligament. In a severe sprain, all the fibers of the ligament may tear. Usually, surrounding capillaries are torn also, causing swelling and pain.

subluxation: a partial dislocation, usually meaning one bone has moved inferiorly (caudally) from its normal position.

▪ ▪ THE FRACTURE PROCESS

When a bone fractures, there is damage to the surrounding area (except in the case of some stress and pathologic fractures). This may include damage to muscles, tearing of blood and lymph vessels, severing of nerves, damage to nearby organs, and laceration of the skin. Swelling is usually present because of the infiltration of blood, lymph, and tissue fluids. The swelling or fracture, or both, cause pain by pressing on nerves. Shock may be present either from the trauma or from blood loss.

■ ■ SIGNS OF FRACTURE

Having an indication of a fracture, and its location, can aid the radiographer in the choice of methods or positions to be used to demonstrate the area. The objective should be to demonstrate the anatomy without further injury to the patient and with minimum discomfort. As will be seen in Chapter 5, the radiographer may have an indication of the patient's injuries from the type of trauma. There are also physical signs to look for. The indications of a fracture or dislocation are:

- Limited movement, or no movement, of a limb
- Swelling at the site of the injury
- Pain at the injury or distal to the injury
- Bruising at the injury site
- Deformity of a limb
- No pulse distal to the injury
- Loss of feeling at, and distal to, the injury

When any one of these signs is present, the radiographer should take extra precautions in moving and positioning the patient. The more signs that are present, or the more severe a sign, the more conservative the methods should be. The radiographer must *never* force a joint or limb into position. Also, if crepitus is heard, the radiographer must stop immediately and find another way of radiographing that area.

■ ■ FRACTURE HEALING

The radiographer should have a general knowledge of the healing process of fractures because most patients have follow-up films taken to check on their progress. Healing is beginning when swelling occurs. The blood, lymph, and tissue fluids form a fibrin clot around the fracture. Soon fibroblasts appear and begin granulation. The granulation process helps stabilize the fracture. Calcium is then deposited around the fracture, forming a callus. The callus is the first phase of healing (other than swelling) that can be demonstrated radiographically. Initially, the calcified area is larger than the original bone. Once the patient resumes normal use, the body may reduce or reshape the initial deposit, and the bone will have a more normal appearance. Still, the final product is often larger than the original. Because the new bone is just as strong as the original bone but is wider, the fracture site may end up being stronger than before. Last, the healing process is dependent on four factors: patient age, general health, nutrition, and circulation at the fracture site. The younger the patient, and the better the patient's health, nutrition, and blood supply to the fracture site, the faster the fracture will heal.

FRACTURE AND DISLOCATION TYPES

It is possible to use 10 or more terms to describe a single fracture. Knowing each will improve communication between the physician or radiologist and the radiographer. It will also help the radiographer select the best methods for demonstrating specific injuries.

GENERAL FRACTURE DESCRIPTORS

Fractures may be complete (Fig. 4–1) or incomplete (see Fig. 4–10). A *complete fracture* involves the entire cross section of the bone. An *incomplete fracture* does not break the bone into separate pieces.

In a *closed fracture* (Fig. 4–2), the fragments have not broken through the skin. Simple fracture is a less accepted term for closed fracture. When a fracture fragment has broken through the skin (Fig. 4–3), it is called a *compound fracture*. When moving a patient or positioning a part, the radiographer must take care not to make a closed fracture compound.

TERMS DESCRIBING FRACTURE LOCATION

The terms direct fracture and indirect fracture are not used often in conversation but are quite important to

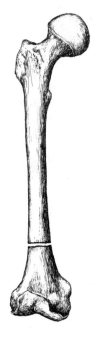

FIG. 4–1. Transverse, complete fracture.

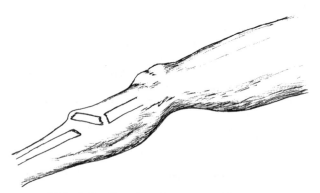

FIG. 4–2. Closed and segmented fracture.

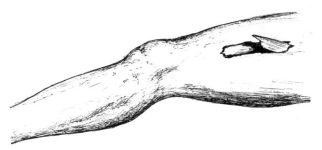

FIG. 4–3. Compound fracture.

radiographers. A *direct fracture* is one that occurs at the site of the trauma. An *indirect fracture* is one that occurs away from the impact point. For example, the patient may twist the ankle, resulting in a direct fracture of the distal lower leg and an indirect fracture of the proximal lower leg. The procedure used for moving the patient and positioning of the part, and the film size, all may need to be changed when there is a chance of an indirect fracture. Situations that may produce indirect fractures are covered in Chapter 5.

Fractures are also described by their location. Besides *proximal* or *distal*, they may be *midshaft*, which is also called *diaphyseal*. Children may have *epiphyseal* fractures, which the radiologist may classify in degrees from 1 to 4 using the Salter-Harris method. If a fracture extends into the joint cavity, it may be called *intra-articular*.

▧ TERMS DESCRIBING THE POSITION OF FRACTURE FRAGMENTS

The relationship of fracture fragments is another way to categorize them. *Displacement*, or *apposition*, is shown in Figure 4–4 and may also be called *alignment*. The job of a muscle is to contract, and when there is a fracture, shortening of the limb may result (Fig. 4–5). This is also referred to as a *bayonet fracture*, or an *overlapping fracture*.

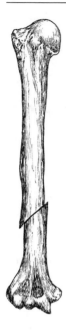

FIG. 4–4. Displaced fracture.

Figure 4–6 shows *angulation*—another way to describe a fracture. Here the proximal fragment remains aligned (to the femur) and the distal fragment is angled internally. *Varus* is another name for the distal fragment being angled toward the midline of the patient. *Valgus* is the opposite of varus, meaning external angulation. Last, one fragment may be rotated, as when the patient is supine but the toes point to the floor (the unfortunate condition of a patient radiographed after a pile of telephone poles rolled down on his legs).

■ FRACTURES DESCRIBED BY FRACTURE LINE TYPE

Often the fracture line is used to describe the various types. Figures 4–7 and 4–8 show *transverse fractures.* The name comes from its being parallel to the transverse

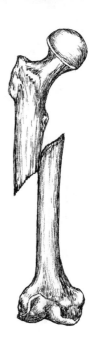

FIG. 4–5. Bayonet or overlapping fracture.

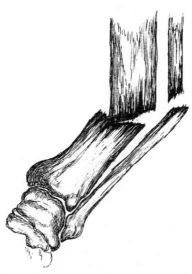

FIG. 4–6. Fracture showing varus angulation.

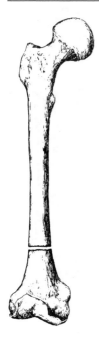

FIG. 4–7. Transverse, complete fracture.

plane of the body. It is found in the long bones (e.g., metacarpals, femurs).

The *linear fracture* is similar to the transverse in that both are straight lines. The linear fracture, however, is usually reserved for incomplete, straight line fractures. As seen in Figure 4–9, these fractures are often found in the skull. Figure 4–10 shows another type of linear fracture, sometimes called a *cleft fracture.* The cleft fracture is also called a *longitudinal fracture* because it runs parallel to the long axis of a bone.

If a fracture runs in a straight line but at an angle, it is an *oblique fracture* (Fig. 4–11). Like the transverse fracture, it is found in long bones. Actually, few fracture lines run straight across a bone, so the oblique fracture is much more common than the transverse. Care should be taken so that closed oblique fractures do not become compound.

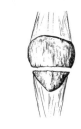

A

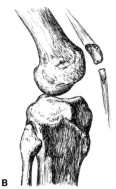

FIG. 4–8. Transverse fracture of the patella. (A) Anterior view. (B) Lateral view.

B

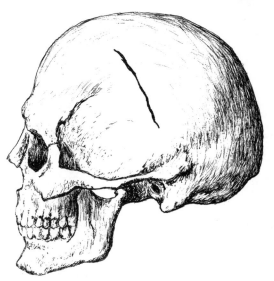

FIG. 4–9. Linear fracture.

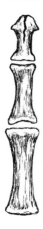

FIG. 4–10. Cleft fracture.

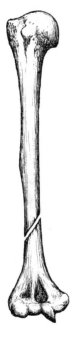

FIG. 4–11. Oblique fracture.

When a twisting force is applied to a bone, a *spiral fracture* may result. The fracture line rotates around the bone (Fig. 4–12). The oblique fracture appears similar, but it is different in that its line runs straight (the bone is truncated). The line of the spiral fracture runs up and around the bone. The sharp ends of the spiral fracture's fragments require careful patient movement and positioning to avoid further damage.

The transverse, oblique, and spiral fractures described thus far have divided bones into two fragments. A more complex type is the *comminuted fracture* (Fig. 4–13). A comminuted fracture is defined as any fracture with two or more fracture lines. This will result in three or more fracture fragments. If the two fracture lines form a V, re-

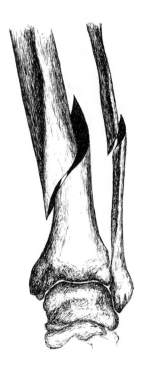

FIG. 4–12. Spiral fractures.

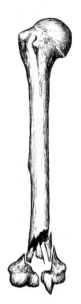

FIG. 4–13. Comminuted fracture.

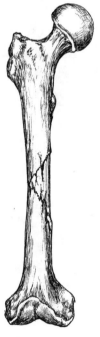

FIG. 4–14. Butterfly fracture.

sulting in a triangular fragment, it is sometimes called a *butterfly fracture* (Fig. 4–14). A comminuted fracture that occurs at two different levels (Fig. 4–15) (see also Fig. 4–2) is called a segmented fracture. Severe comminuted fractures are sometimes called *crush fractures.* It is typical to find comminuted fractures at the ends of long bones, but they can also appear on the patella or the calcaneus.

An *impacted fracture* (Fig. 4–16) can result when the trauma occurs down the long axis of a bone. The shaft of the bone is forced, and imbedded, into the end of the bone. The distal femur and distal humerus are typical locations for this type of fracture.

Figure 4–17 is a rare fracture, usually caused by a gunshot wound. The bone fragments are thin shards, or splinters, similar to wood, hence its name *splinter fracture.*

The term *stellate fracture* is usually reserved for a special fracture of the patella (Fig. 4–18). Here the lines

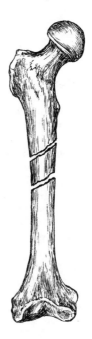

FIG. 4–15. Segmented fracture (a type of comminuted fracture).

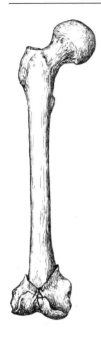

FIG. 4–16. Impacted fracture.

radiate outward from the center point in a starlike pattern. Stellate means starlike. These fractures usually result from a direct blow to the patella, as when a knee hits a dashboard.

When a vertebral body collapses (Fig. 4–19), it is called a *compression fracture*. Most often it is the anterior section of the body that is reduced in height. Such a fracture can be caused by trauma or it may result from demineralization of bone due to old age.

A *burst fracture* (Fig. 4–20) is a special fracture of a vertebra. The vertebral ring is broken, and the fragments move outward. The first cervical vertebra can burst from something hitting the top of the patient's head or from the patient diving into shallow water and hitting the head on the bottom.

A tennis ball, or other object, penetrating past the bony orbit and striking the eyeball can cause a *blowout fracture*

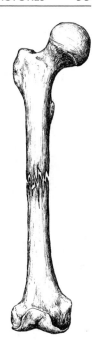

FIG. 4–17. Splinter fracture.

of the orbit (Fig. 4–21). If an object hits the eyeball, it may push it back hard enough to force the fatpad surrounding the eye to break through the bone at its weakest point. That weak point is the floor of the orbit. Blowout fractures are extremely difficult to demonstrate radiographically. Because the floor of the orbit is also the roof of the maxillary sinus, a blowout fracture can sometimes be diagnosed by the history and by an opacified maxillary sinus. Frequently, tomography or computed tomography is needed to show these fractures.

A *depressed fracture* is one in which a section of bone is pushed in toward the center of an area. The skull (Fig. 4–22) and the sternum are the usual locations. On the skull, the appearance is the same as that of pushing in the shell of a hard-boiled egg or of making a dent in a Ping-Pong ball.

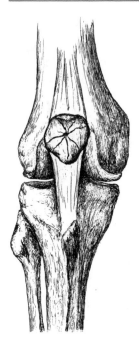

FIG. 4–18. Stellate fracture.

■ OTHER TYPES OF FRACTURES

Few classifications would be complete without a category called "Other." It is under this heading that the complicated, pathologic, stress, avulsion, and greenstick fractures may be placed.

A *complicated fracture* is one that involves not only a bone or bones but also damage to an internal organ.

Pathologic fractures are nontraumatic. They are defined as fractures caused by normal stress being placed on abnormal bone. Pathologic fractures happen when the bone is being used normally but has been weakened by a disease, such as cancer, osteomalacia, osteomyelitis, or Paget's disease (Fig. 4–23). Sometimes they are called *spontaneous fractures*.

Stress fractures are caused by abnormal stress applied to normal bone. These fractures can thus be defined as

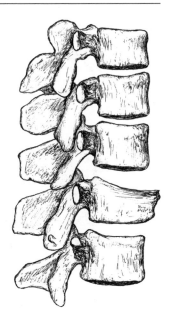

FIG. 4–19. Compression fracture.

opposite in origin. Like pathologic fractures, however, they are nontraumatic. Stress fractures can be caused by marching (as in the military), in which case they are usually found midshaft in the metatarsals. Running can also cause stress fractures. In runners they are commonly found on the distal third to midshaft of the tibia. There

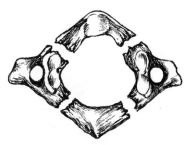

FIG. 4–20. Burst fracture of the atlas (C-1).

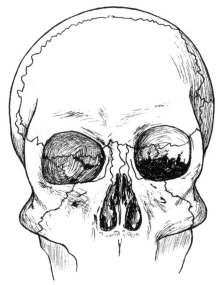

FIG. 4–21. Blowout fracture of the left orbit.

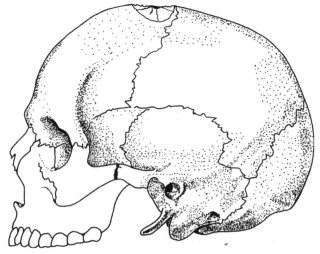

FIG. 4–22. Depressed fracture.

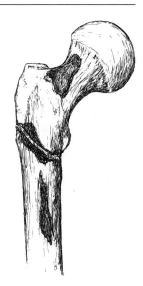

FIG. 4–23. Pathologic fracture.

was at least one incident of a man having a severe stress fracture of the femur while running a marathon. He was able to complete the run because the strength of his thigh muscles held the fragments in place. Once he stopped, however, he immediately collapsed.

Most stress fractures are extraordinarily difficult to radiograph. Often they can be diagnosed only by the history. They may not become radiographically visible until the callus forms. The best method for demonstrating them is to use detail screens, a small focal spot, and a long source-to-image receptor distance (SID) for maximum detail. Stress fractures are sometimes referred to as fatigue fractures.

There are two fractures that can occur only in pediatric patients. One is the previously mentioned *epiphyseal fracture*. The other is the *greenstick*, or *torus, fracture* (Fig. 4–24). A greenstick fracture is an incomplete fracture. Because a child's bones are more flexible, they may break on one side and not the other. When the bone is bent, the break will occur on the outer edge. When the bone straightens out, a faint fracture line may be seen on the outer edge,

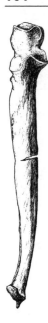

FIG. 4–24. Greenstick (torus) fracture.

and the inner edge may have a slight wrinkle-like defect. Like stress fractures, these fractures can be difficult to radiograph. The same methods should be applied as in stress fractures.

■ DISLOCATIONS AND FRACTURES WITH DISLOCATIONS

Avulsion, or *chip, fractures* (Fig. 4–25) are often seen with dislocations. Avulsion fractures are caused by stress to a joint or tendon. Instead of the tendon breaking, it pulls a piece of the bone away. In some dislocations, the bone moves out of joint but the tendon holds fast to its anchoring place, pulling it away from the main bone. It should be noted that the damage is caused when the bone dislocates. It does not matter whether the bone stays dislocated or if it relocates itself; the damage has been done.

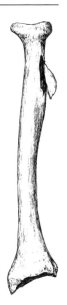

FIG. 4–25. Avulsion fracture.

Therefore, all dislocations should be radiographed. Also, dislocation postreduction films should be taken not only to document successful relocation but also to check for avulsion fractures that may have been superimposed with bone on the original films.

Figure 4–26 shows one of the most common dislocations. It is feasible that any joint may dislocate, but the typical ones are the interphalangeal joints of the fingers, the shoulder, hip (Fig. 4–27), elbow, and patella. Finger dislocations may be posterior, medial, or lateral. Shoulder dislocations can be interior, posterior, or luxatio erecta. About 90 percent of shoulder dislocations are anterior. The *luxatio erecta* is rare—the shoulder dislocates with the arm pointing straight up to the sky. Hip dislocations are usually superior or posterior. When elbows dislocate, the arm is shortened as the radius and ulna are shifted proximally. A patella usually dislocates medially or laterally. The joints of the spine can also dislocate, but subluxation

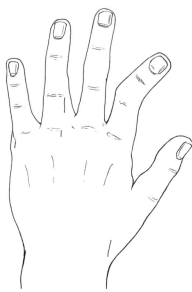

FIG. 4–26. Dislocation of the proximal interphalangeal joint of the index finger of the left hand.

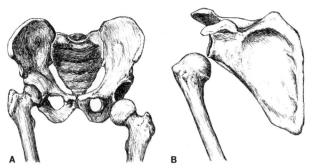

FIG. 4–27. Dislocations of the hip (A) and shoulder (B).

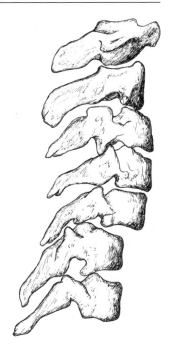

FIG. 4–28. Subluxation of the fifth cervical vertebra.

(especially in the cervical spine—Fig. 4–28) is seen more often.

■ ■ SUMMARY

Terminology for trauma, fracture, and dislocation has been presented to improve understanding and communication. The fracture and healing processes also have been described to improve the radiographer's understanding. External indicators of fracture have been included to minimize the chance of causing further injury to the patient during radiographic examinations. As professionals, radiographers should strive to apply this material and to use the correct terminology at all times.

■ ■ SELF-ASSESSMENT TEST

DIRECTIONS: Define each of the following terms:

1. Trauma
2. A/A
3. Fx
4. Dislocation
5. Concussion
6. Callus
7. Compound Fx
8. Closed Fx
9. Apposition
10. Comminuted Fx
11. Stellate Fx
12. Compression Fx
13. Depressed Fx
14. Stress Fx
15. Greenstick Fx
16. Torus Fx
17. Avulsion Fx
18. Subluxation

DIRECTIONS: Supply answers in your own words to each of the following questions:

19. Differentiate between transverse, oblique, and spiral fractures.
20. Differentiate between compound, comminuted, complicated, and compression fractures.
21. What are the names of the two nontraumatic fractures?
22. What are the names of the two fractures that only pediatric patients can have?
23. What are the seven physical signs that indicate a possible fracture?
24. Differentiate between direct and indirect fractures.
25. What is the significance of indirect fractures to radiographers?

26. Your patient arrives from the emergency room for a radiographic examination of the ankle. His history indicates that he had been running, had stepped into a depression, had twisted his ankle, and had fallen. While radiographing the ankle, you notice swelling on the lateral portion of the ankle joint. After the routine examination is done, the patient complains of pain in the corresponding knee area. What do you think may have happened? Write this patient's history using the terms in this (and previous) chapters.

27. During your lunch break, you hear of an attempted bank robbery in which shots are exchanged between the robbers and the police. The robbers escape. A few hours later you radiograph a patient whose history indicates that he was involved in an industrial accident, suffering blunt trauma to his leg. You put up his radiographs on the viewbox and see a splinter fracture. What do you think may have happened? What should you do?

■ ■ **BIBLIOGRAPHY**

Feison, B (ed): Roentgenology of Fractures and Dislocations. Grune & Stratton, New York, 1978.

Huckstep, RL: A Simple Guide to Trauma, ed 3. Churchill Livingstone, New York, 1995.

Kilcoyne, RF, et al.: Handbook of Orthopedic Terminology. Year Book Medical Publishers, Chicago, 1991.

Kilcoyne, RF, and Fartar, E: Handbook of Radiologic Orthopedic Terminology. Year Book Medical Publishers, Chicago, 1986.

Thomas, CL (ed): Taber's Cyclopedic Medical Dictionary, ed 18. FA Davis, Philadelphia, 1997.

5

INJURIES FROM
TYPES OF TRAUMA

OUTLINE

111

▨ ▨ INTRODUCTION

By knowing or deducing how a patient has been injured, the radiographer is better able to select which methods to use or to avoid. Knowing what types of injuries commonly result from each type of trauma affects taking the patient's history, moving the patient (or not moving the patient), observing the patient, and selecting or creating positions to show (or to rule out) the typical injuries. However, it must be emphasized that anything can happen. The injuries mentioned here are typical. Other injuries will occur, and the severity of the injuries will vary greatly. One must begin somewhere, however. Trauma radiography is too serious for the uninitiated, and the risks are too great to begin without this information.

A more thorough history can be taken if the radiographer knows beforehand what types of injuries to expect. By asking more specific questions, the radiographer should try to improve the information for the radiologist, obtain baseline information for patient observation, and determine whether routine radiographic methods can be used. Knowing the typical injuries will also guide the radiographer in monitoring the patient's condition, documenting the condition for medical and legal purposes, and deciding whether assistance will be needed. After obtaining the history, if there is any doubt, the most conservative methods of moving and positioning the patient should be chosen.

The radiographer should know of, and take into account, associated injuries when moving and positioning a trauma patient. An obvious example is not flexing the knee and hip to obtain a routine anteroposterior (AP) foot radiograph when there is a possibility of transverse fracture of the patella or a fractured femoral neck. Locating the impact point and direction of the force can often identify the area that might be injured. Many factors enter into injuries, so one can never be certain of their prediction, but again, it helps to have a logical place to start. This chapter includes descriptions of injuries that are important to radiographers. It does not include injuries such as burns and abrasions, which do not significantly affect the radiographic process or the care of the patient while he or she is in the radiography department. Chapter 6 outlines the methods to use when these injuries are suspected.

▨ ▨ AUTOMOBILE ACCIDENTS

Automobile accidents are one of the most frequent sources of trauma victims. By knowing the type of impact, the radiographer can vary the procedures to minimize the chance of additional injury and to limit pain for the patient. This knowledge can also aid the radiologist or physician with view selection. On patient charts and histories, automobile accident is usually abbreviated A/A.

This section includes descriptions of injuries seen with front-end, rear-end, side-impact, and rollover accidents. In each of these areas, the description moves from the head and neck to the thoracic and then abdominal regions, and finally to the extremities.

▨ FRONT-END COLLISIONS

Front-end collisions are very common, and the types of injuries are usually consistent. The severity of the injuries can vary greatly, depending on the patient's position at the time of the impact, the speed and force involved, the patient's physical strengths and weaknesses, and the use of seat belts or other restraining devices.

When all other factors are equal, the use of seat belts and airbags can make a great difference in the patient's injuries. The details are briefly presented here because the same mechanism explains injuries to the brain and heart. When a vehicle is moving forward, it has momentum. If not for friction or gravity, it would continue to move forward. Everything in the vehicle also has momentum. This factor is easily demonstrated by the way loose objects in a car fly forward during hard braking. Part of the problem in automobile accidents is that the car stops, but the occupants, because of their momentum, continue to move forward. Although they will all stop moving eventually, they may not stop at the same rate. Modern cars are designed to come to a stop in a collision gradually. If a person is wearing a seat belt, he or she will come to a gradual stop with the car (because the person is attached to it). If a seat belt (or seat bag and airbag) does not restrain a person, the car will stop but the person will continue to move forward until he or she hits a part of the car or passes through the windshield. As an example, in a moderate-speed collision with a concrete wall, the car may come to a stop in $\frac{1}{10}$ of a second. A belted occupant stops in the same time. However, an unbelted occupant can come to a stop in $\frac{1}{100}$ of a second—10 times more abruptly. The resulting injuries would, of course, be greater. As mentioned before, momentum and different rates of stopping affect the brain and heart also.

Figure 5–1 shows the patient in a seated position with the typical front-end collision impact points. The areas of greatest concern are the head, neck, anterior thorax, femur, and foot.

The patient's head may strike the windshield, dashboard, or steering wheel. The person could also pass through the windshield. Damage can occur to the brain, frontal bone, facial bones, and cervical spine.

Damage to the brain has three major causes. The brain is a gelatinous organ with momentum much like that of the unbelted driver described earlier. As the frontal bone comes to a halt, the brain continues to travel forward, striking the bone. To complicate matters, as the anterior cerebrum compresses on the frontal bone, the posterior cerebrum is pulled away from the occipital bone. This creates a slight suction that can damage the brain or the blood vessels. Damage occurring on the side opposite to an impact point is sometimes called a *contre-coup injury.*

When the skull strikes an object, the force is transmitted through the brain. This shock wave is another way that the brain can be damaged in an automobile accident. When the impact is at the frontal bone, the force passes

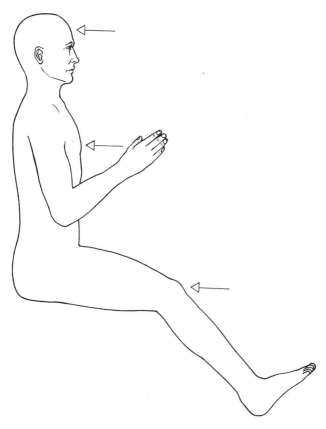

FIG. 5–1. Common impact points in front-end auto accidents.

through the brain and, as it reaches the narrow area of the occipital bone, can build, like a wave crashing on the beach. This force can cause damage to the areas of the brain that control the vital autonomic nervous functions.

A third way the brain can be damaged again deals with its moving within the skull. Arteries and veins run along the inner table of the cranium. Part of their diameter lies in a bony channel, and part lies in a depression in the brain. As the brain moves forward past the bony channels, the blood vessels are subjected to a shearing force. This shearing force can cause them to tear. Any resultant bleeding presses on the brain, inasmuch as it fills the entire cranium. This pressure can result in neurologic or consciousness changes, so the patient should be closely observed. If the bleeding is arterial (epidural hematoma), the changes occur quickly. If the bleeding is venous (subdural hematoma), the changes may not be noticed for 24 hours or more. Epidural hematomas often involve the middle meningeal artery, which is under the squamous portion of the temporal bone. Subdural hematomas are often seen at the vertex of the skull (from the superior sagittal sinus to the cerebral cortex). The symptoms of possible brain injury are unconsciousness, headache, blurred or double vision, hearing difficulties, vertigo, vomiting, and mood changes. There may or may not be skull fractures present with the types of brain damage just described. In addition, it is possible that the patient will suffer convulsions after a head injury. When fractures of the base of the skull are present, the patient may bleed from the nose (rhinorrhea) or ears (otorrhea). Rhinorrhea is a sign of a fractured cribriform plate. Otorrhea may result from a fracture of the petrous portion of the temporal bone. A physician should be notified especially if there is bleeding from the ears. Usually the physician will send a sample to the laboratory to test for cerebrospinal fluid (CSF). If bleeding is present, it indicates a serious cranial base injury. Because of all these serious complications, head injury patients should not be left alone.

The face is frequently injured in automobile accidents. The bleeding and disfigurement of some facial injuries can be quite alarming to the radiographer. Care must be taken not to convey this to the patient, either verbally or nonverbally. It is best to concentrate on performing the job. The major concern with facial injury bleeding is that it not interfere with the patient's breathing, as can be the case with maxillary and nasal bone fractures. If it does, the patient can be turned to a prone position or on to one side. If this is not possible because of suspected cervical spine fracture or other injury, then suctioning equipment must be used.

Other facial bone fracture concerns involve subcondylar fractures of the mandible and fractures of the mandibular symphysis. Such fractures can allow the tongue to obstruct the throat and block the airway. Fracture of the zygoma is also a concern, inasmuch as it is the main support between the cranium and the maxilla. A fracture here can also involve the inferior and the lateral portions of the orbital rim.

About half of all spinal column injuries are caused by traffic accidents. Movement of the patient is usually not permitted until radiography has revealed or ruled out injury to this vital area. Forced flexion is the usual method of injury in front-end collision. Tingling, numbness, and loss of motion in the extremities are symptoms of possible cervical spine damage. The more superior the symptoms, the closer the affected area is to C-1 and C-2. The presence of these symptoms does not necessarily mean that the spinal cord has been severed. Spinal injuries can include strained muscles, a hematoma pressing on the cord (spinal bruise or contusion), spinal fracture, spinal subluxation, and dislocation or fracture with displacement. With the milder injuries, loss of function and feeling may be temporary. Dislocations and displaced fractures usually do mean that the cord has been transected. Severe injuries to C-2 or C-1 typically result in death. The odontoid process is involved in about 10 percent of all spinal fractures and is sometimes seen with a displaced atlas. In the lower cervical area many subluxations and dislocations are at C-5 and C-6, which illustrates a primary rule for radiographers: Demonstrate all seven cervical vertebrae.

Thoracic injuries, except for single rib fractures, are very serious and have a high mortality. Automobile accidents account for approximately 60 percent of all thoracic injuries. These injuries can directly or indirectly affect vital organs such as the heart and lungs or vital structures like the great vessels. Direct injury to the heart, for example, can occur much in the same way as the momentum injuries occur to the brain. The heart is a large, heavy muscle. If the sternum and anterior chest strike the steering wheel or dashboard, the heart can continue to travel forward until it strikes the sternum. If there is enough force, the thoracic spine may then hit the posterior surface of the heart. If a great amount of force is present, as when a speeding car strikes a concrete barrier, the heart may shear off of the great vessels. The victim, of course, is dead on arrival (DOA). This is sometimes referred to as a sudden deceleration death.

Indirect injuries to the vital thoracic organs can be from fractured ribs, a fractured sternum, or fractured clavicles. Fractured ribs may puncture a lung, causing atelectasis, pneumothorax, hemopneumothorax, or hemothorax. In fact, pneumothorax is one of the most common thoracic injuries. A fractured sternum is almost always depressed and can damage the heart and great vessels. It may cause mediastinal widening or cardiac tamponade. Fractures of the clavicle (and upper ribs) may damage the underlying blood vessels of the arms and head. Of course, these injuries are quite painful by themselves, even if they do not damage the internal organs.

Note that damage to the thoracic spine itself has not been mentioned. Being well protected by the ribs, it does not usually suffer damage in front-end automobile accidents. The scapula is not usually injured in these types of accidents, either.

Abdominal trauma from front-end collisions can be caused by the steering wheel. Some injuries also may be produced by lap-type seat belts, which are sometimes found in the front seats of older cars. The spleen and liver can be involved, and a hematoma at the impact site can be a sign of significant damage. If the pelvis is fractured, there is always the possibility that the bladder is ruptured. Whether it is or not, the patient should be moved very carefully (if at all) to prevent damage to the internal organs. Because the pelvis forms a ring, it is usually fractured in two locations. If there is only one fracture, then there is usually a separation of the symphysis pubis or the sacroiliac joint.

Rear-seat passengers can be severely injured, even when the front-seat passenger or driver has minor injuries. The cause can be wearing the rear seat belt when only a lap belt is provided. When a passenger wears only a lap belt, the force of the momentum during a crash causes the patient to bend at the waist, flexing the lumbar (and thoracic) spines. This can mean spinal fractures and loss of function from damage to the spinal cord.

The lower extremity is more vulnerable in front-end accidents and may be injured directly or indirectly. Most of the injuries involve the femur, although one other common injury involves the foot. This foot injury is sometimes called *aviator's astragalus,* or an *aviator's fracture.* Its name came from a common World War I pilot's crash-landing injury. Today it results mostly from forces transmitted through the floorboard of the car. It forces the neck of the talus superiorly into the anterior tibia. The result is typically a fracture of the neck of the talus.

Lower extremity fractures involving the femur depend on the amount of force, position of the femur at the time of impact, and any weak areas of the bone. The impact of the knee on the dashboard may produce transverse or stellate fractures of the patella. Intercondylar or impacted fractures may be seen at the distal end of the femur. It is possible for the femur to break midshaft, or for the neck of the femur to fracture. Sometimes the femur does not break. Instead, the force is transmitted along its length, and the head of the femur breaks the posterior rim of the acetabulum, producing a posterior hip dislocation. This is sometimes called a *posterior rim,* or *dashboard, fracture.*

Femur fractures can damage the large thigh muscles, and it is possible for the patient to bleed enough into the thigh to produce hypovolemic shock. Patients with suspected femur fractures should be moved carefully, with adequate support both above and below the fracture site. It is also common for the thigh muscles to contract after a femur fracture along the shaft, causing the fragments to overlap (or bayonet).

▓ REAR-END COLLISIONS

The classic injury associated with rear-end collisions is *whiplash,* or forced extension of the cervical spine. But other injuries can be similar to those from a front-end impact. This is more often the case when the patient is not wearing a seat belt. Then the person is thrown forward into the front of the car, rather than the car stopping and the person's momentum carrying him or her forward to impact parts of the car's interior.

The brain can be injured in a rear-end impact by methods similar to those discussed in front-end impacts. The force can damage the posterior and anterior portions of the brain, and the same shearing of blood vessels can be present. As with other possibly brain-injured patients, these patients should be watched carefully for changes in consciousness or other signs of neurologic damage. If the patient's head strikes the steering wheel or windshield, the facial bone and frontal bone injuries mentioned for front-end impacts also may be present.

Whiplash injury to the cervical spine is quite common in these types of accidents. It can range from strained neck muscles to displaced fractures. As with all cervical spine injuries, the radiographer should assume that the patient has a fractured cervical spine until a physician has declared that the radiographs have proven otherwise. This patient will be wearing a cervical collar, and for medical and legal reasons, it is inadvisable for the radiographer to remove the cervical collar.

There may be damage to the vital thoracic area—heart, lungs, and great vessels—or ribs and sternum. Anterior damage would result from the patient being thrown forward into the front of the car. Posterior damage is increased as the force of the collision increases and as the size of the car decreases. In two-seat subcompact or sports cars, the back portion of the car or the engine (when mounted in back) can be forced forward into the patient. This also may result in damage to the kidneys.

The kidneys lie in the posterior third of the abdomen and do not bear trauma well. The types of kidney damage, ranging from less serious to more serious, include a contusion (or bruise), a laceration, a rupture, and fragmentation (the kidney broken into sections). Flank pain, tenderness, hematuria, flank mass, and abdominal rigidity are symptoms that suggest renal damage.

There are no extremity injuries that are notably common in rear-end impacts. Some patients sustain typically minor shoulder area injuries from seat belts as the force of the accident throws them against the belt and its inertia lock tightens it.

SIDE-IMPACT COLLISIONS

Figure 5–2 shows common impact points when a vehicle is hit from the side. These are sometimes called T-bone accidents because of the T formed when the front end of one car strikes the side of another. If the patient was wearing a seat belt, then most of the injuries will be on the side that was hit. If the patient was not wearing a seat belt, the person can be thrown across the car, sustaining injuries on both sides. The introduction of side-impact airbags should decrease the severity of some of the injuries described here.

If the head receives a direct blow, there can be fractures of the relatively thin temporal bone, zygomatic arch, mandible, and orbit. This is not common, however. Typically head and neck injuries from side impacts involve the cervical spine and, sometimes, the brain. When the brain is involved, the damage can be a concussion or the shearing and momentum injuries described earlier. In a driver's side impact, for example, the primary damage to the driver would be on the left side and the contrecoup injuries would be on the right. The force of a driver's side impact can force the driver's head to the right. This may decrease the intervertebral spaces on the right (as they are compressed) and strain the neck muscles on the left (as they are stretched).

Damage to the thoracic region can be severe in these accidents. The ribs are most commonly involved. Injuries can range from single rib fractures to flail chest or a punctured lung. Figure 5–3 represents a patient with flail chest. The injury occurs because of segmented fractures to adjacent ribs and results in paradoxical breathing. Single rib fractures are not usually serious; the adjacent, uninjured ribs, intercostal muscles, and remainder of the injured rib act as a splint and keep the fracture fragments in place. In *flail chest*, a section of the thorax has broken free. During breathing, it acts independently from, and in opposition to, normal respiration. As the diaphragm descends, it cre-

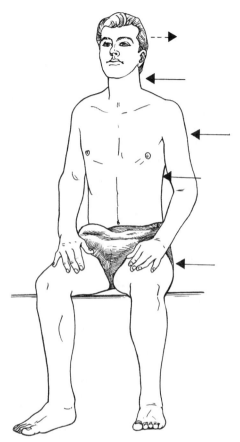

FIG. 5–2. Common impact points in side-impact auto accidents.

ates a vacuum and air rushes into the lungs. With a flail chest, instead of air rushing into the lungs, the free section of the ribs moves in when it should move out. During expiration the reverse happens, hence the use of the term *paradoxical breathing*. Thus, a section of the chest is working in opposition to the way it normally should. The pa-

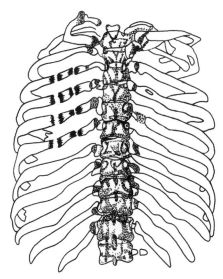

FIG. 5–3. Flail chest.

tient then suffers dyspnea. In addition to flail chest, the patient can have atelectasis, pneumothorax, hematopneumothorax, and hematothorax.

In the abdominal region, the spleen is frequently damaged. A small hemorrhage may produce tenderness in the left upper quadrant of the abdomen. A larger hemorrhage, or a ruptured spleen, produces left upper quadrant tenderness and abdominal pain. The kidneys also may have damage as described for rear-end impacts, but this may be limited to the side that was hit.

The upper extremity on the impact side is often injured. The type of injury depends on its location at the time of the collision. If the arm was at the patient's side, the injuries include fractures of the forearm, intercondylar fractures of the distal humerus, fracture of the midshaft and proximal humerus, and possibly fracture of the clavicle and scapula (especially from the humeral head being forced into, and fracturing, the glenoid fossa). If the window was rolled down and the arm was resting on the door, the injuries may include comminuted fractures of the elbow, impacted or intercondylar fractures of the distal humerus, impacted fractures of the humeral head, and damage to the glenoid fossa.

In the lower extremity, the hip and pelvis are major concerns. The force of a side impact can cause intertrochanteric fractures and impacted fractures on the femoral head, or it may force the head of the femur into the acetabulum, causing it to burst and send fragments internally. The force may also fracture the pelvis. This can result in damage to the urinary tract (especially the bladder), reproductive system, circulatory system, and lower abdominal organs, as well as fractures of the iliac wing. Of equal concern for the radiographer is the potential for additional damage from these injuries while the patient is being moved.

ROLLOVER ACCIDENTS

Accidents in which a vehicle rolls over or flips onto its roof can cause some special injuries for the patient. These are the results of axial loading—downward force applied along the axis of the body. Usually this involves trauma to the vertex of the head.

Of course, linear or depressed fractures of the vertex are possible, with or without damage to the brain. A bursting fracture of the atlas (C-1) is also possible. It results from pressure from the occipital condyles to the atlas. This pressure breaks the ring of the atlas and usually results in lateral and posterior displacement of the fragments. It does not necessarily include injury to the spinal cord. The radiographer should take extra care not to cause any, either.

Other injuries peculiar to rollover accidents tend to involve the spine. Compression fractures of the vertebral bodies are possible. When these fractures are present, they usually cause a decrease in the anterior (or ventral) height of the body. The intervertebral disks may herniate or sustain other damage. It is also possible for the force to shear off the transverse processes of the vertebra, especially those of the lumbar spine. This is not a serious condition, but it can be painful.

It is possible for the shoulder to sustain some axial-load damage. This could include separations of the A-C joint or shoulder joint, and fractures of the clavicle, scapula, or humerus.

■ ■ MOTORCYCLE ACCIDENTS

Few endeavors provide such vulnerability to critical physical injury as riding a motorcycle. If the patient does not wear a helmet, massive skull trauma and death are more than possible in the event of an accident. Beyond this, it is difficult to generalize about the injuries from these accidents. Anything is possible. Even if a helmet is worn, the patient may still suffer significant skull and brain damage. The rider may slide headfirst into some barrier (or a tree), and have axial-load type injuries to the spine or shoulder. If the rider slides across pavement, he or she may have "road rash"—an abrading away of their skin from the rough surface of the road. About the only broad statement that can be made about the injuries of motorcycle accident victims is that many of them have fractures at the midshaft of the femur. This seems to occur because of the way the gas tank crosses the femur. A fall to either side catches the thigh between the motorcycle (most of which weigh a few hundred pounds) and the unyielding road. In summation, the radiographer will have to rely on observation and a conservative approach to radiograph these patients adequately without causing further injury.

■ ■ INDUSTRIAL INJURIES

Although safety conditions have improved greatly for industrial and physical workers, there is still a large potential for serious injury. Many times, the injured area will be obvious: It will be at the site of the impact. But, just as with automobile accidents, knowing the patient's history can aid the radiographer in demonstrating the nonobvious injuries and in handling the patient.

▨ HEAD AND NECK

In the various types of industrial and work areas, traumatic force may come from any direction. From the front, the worker can be struck with projectiles large and small. A worker may walk into an object, may trip, or fall from a height landing on the face. A person may be struck from behind with a board, impact hammer, or rivet gun. Foreign bodies from a screw or nail gun may become imbedded in the skin. And, of course, someone could drop something onto the top of another person's head, or someone could fall from a height and land on the vertex. With the accidents that involve the transmission of force through the skull, the mechanisms of injury are similar to those in automobile accidents. Linear or depressed fractures at the impact point, with or without underlying brain damage, are possible. Contrecoup injuries may be present. The chance of this injury increases as the amount of force increases. Also, shearing forces to the blood vessels could produce subdural or epidural hematomas. The radiographer should keep in mind that the temporal bones are weaker than the rest of the cranium, that the occipital bone protects the vital autonomic nervous system, and that forces strong enough to damage the brain and cranium may also cause injury to the cervical spine.

Damage to the cervical spine can range from strained muscles to displaced fractures. However, the radiographer should assume the worst until it is proven otherwise. Damage can occur from compression, flexion, hyperextension, forced rotation, or indirect force. Compression of the cervical spine can result from a fall from a height in which the patient lands on the vertex, or from an object that is dropped on the head. Compression of the cervical spine is not always accompanied by a skull injury. If the patient was wearing a hard hat, the cranium may be spared, but the force can still damage the spine. The *Jefferson fracture*, a bursting of the atlas (C-1) with lateral displacement of the fragments, is produced by force to the top of the head. Damage to the spine from flexion can occur from a blow to the posterior cranium and often results in strained muscles—unless the force is great. Hyperextension, or whiplash, can be caused by force to the anterior cranium, which can also produce muscle strain. If greater trauma is involved, fractures are possible. Forced rotation injuries can be caused by trauma to the side of the face, head, neck, or the shoulder, causing the spine to rotate. This can result in subluxation of the cervical spine. Last, injury from indirect force is typified by the *shoveler's fracture.* The name originates from clay shovelers, whose spinous processes in the cervical spine would avulse from the force applied to the tendons by throwing the heavy clay.

With all cervical spine injuries, the patient's symptoms should be well documented for medical and legal reasons. The radiographer should remember that pain and numbness are felt in areas inferior to the actual spinal injury that could be causing them. Also, the more superior the numbness or tingling sensation, the more superior the cervical vertebra that is involved.

THORAX

Injuries to the thorax result from both direct trauma and indirect sources. The direct injuries may range from non-serious single rib fractures to life-threatening damage to the lungs and heart. The direct injuries are usually obvious, involving the area around the impact point. When multiple rib fractures are suspected, or with rib fractures that may be displaced internally, the radiographer should move the patient with extreme caution and avoid having the patient lie on the affected side. Direct trauma to the sternum may cause cardiac tamponade or widening of the mediastinum. Indirect injuries can result from a fall from a height in which the patient lands on the head, shoulder, feet, or coccyx. In these cases the force may cause the thoracic vertebral bodies to collapse, or it may cause damage to the intervertebral disk.

ABDOMEN

As with the thorax, injuries to the abdomen can come from direct and indirect forces. Again, the direct forces generally produce the more serious injuries. Damage is usually in the area of impact. Left anterior abdominal trauma often damages the spleen, producing left upper quadrant pain and tenderness. Right anterior blunt trauma may damage the liver. Force to the abdomen, especially anterior and lateral, could damage the bowel and may or may not produce free air in the abdomen. A blow to the back or falling onto the back may damage the kidneys, producing flank pain, tenderness, and hematuria (blood in the urine). Indirect injury to the abdominal region generally involves the lumbar spine and may result from falls from a height or objects falling onto the shoulders. For example, if an object was to fall on the patient's right shoulder, the force may be transmitted through the body and shear off the right transverse processes of the lumbar spine. Falling from a height may cause compression fractures of the lumbar vertebral bodies, or if the patient lands in a seated position, he or she may fracture the coccyx.

▨ EXTREMITIES

The extremities are the most frequently injured area of the body in work situations. Of the extremities, the hand is used most often, so it suffers the greatest amount of damage. Hand injuries range from imbedding of foreign bodies to crushing injuries from punch presses to traumatic amputation. With the more severe injuries, the hand is frequently wrapped in large amounts of gauze. Unattached, or barely attached, fingers also may be included in the bandage. Frequently the fingers are flexed. It is not advisable for the radiographer to remove these dressings, especially for the preliminary exposures.

If a worker falls on an outstretched arm, he or she may have a *Colles' fracture.* This is a fracture of the distal radius with posterior displacement. The ulnar styloid process may also be involved. The same fracture with anterior displacement is called a *Smith's fracture.* Other fractures of the forearm usually involve the radius and the ulna. If only one of the bones is fractured, there will usually be a disruption of the proximal or distal radioulnar articulation. For example, a fracture of the ulna (but not the radius) usually means that the radial head is dislocated (*Monteggia's fracture*). The wrist and forearm may also be involved in crushing injuries.

Injuries to the elbow may prevent the patient from fully extending it. When this occurs, the joint should *never* be forced. The elbow may be dislocated, usually with the ulna forced superiorly (or posteriorly). This can cause fractures of the coranoid process. The olecranon process is typically fractured by a direct blow—something striking it or the patient falling on it.

The humerus is injured primarily by direct trauma. If there is a fracture of the shaft at the distal third, then the radiographer should not rotate the humerus. Fragments in this area could sever the radial nerve if the arm is rotated. Fractures of the proximal end of the humerus are usually near the surgical neck. In these cases, the radiographer should not abduct the arm unless necessary, and then only enough to place a cassette between the humerus and the patient's body for a lateromedial projection (see Chapter 6).

Injuries to the shoulder area include fractures (primarily from direct trauma) and dislocations. Most shoulder dislocations are anterior; fewer than 5 percent are posterior. If the arm is extended above the patient's head or partially abducted when the patient falls on his or her side (a downward force is applied to the shoulder), a rare type of dislocation may be produced, called *luxatio erecta*. The arm is extended up and the head of the humerus is dislocated inferior to the glenold fossa. These patients are best radiographed in an upright position.

Most of the work-related injuries to the lower extremity involve the feet. Although the use of safety-toe work shoes and boots has reduced the number of injuries to the feet from dropped objects or from carts being driven over them, some are still seen. And not everyone wears safety-toe shoes. I once radiographed a fast-food restaurant worker who had dropped a box of frozen hamburger meat on his foot. It did a thorough job of breaking each metatarsal at midshaft.

The other major type of injury to the feet involves a person falling from a height and landing on the feet. Injuries from this may be traumatic flat feet, Lisfranc's dislocations, fractures of the calcaneus, and fractures or dislocations of the ankle. Traumatic flat feet are produced when the force flattens the arches of the feet. *Lisfranc's dislocations* involve dorsal displacement of the tarsometatarsal joints. If the patient lands on the heels, they may have comminuted fractures of the calcaneus. About 10 percent of these injuries are bilateral. Also, about 10 percent of these patients have compression fractures of the lumbar or thoracic spines. Landing flat on the feet may force the talus against the tibia and the fibula to produce bimalleolar or trimalleolar fractures. Bimalleolar fractures involve both the medial and lateral malleoli. Trimalleolar fractures are misnamed; they are actually bimalleolar fractures with a fracture of the posterior portion of the distal tibia. If a patient lands on the side of the foot, the ankle may dislocate so that the foot is on the side of the ankle. This can also cause a compound fracture of the ankle in which the tibia and fibula are driven through the skin (where the foot used to be).

The force of falling from a height also can be transmitted up through the body. Damage at the knee may occur to the tibial plateau, or there may be impacted fractures of the femoral condyles. If the force is great enough, it can cause a *Malgaigne fracture* of the pelvis. This involves fractures of the rami of the pubis and fracture of the ilium or sacrum or dislocation of the sacroiliac joint. Superior displacement of the pelvis may also be present. Other transmitted force injuries can involve the vertebral bodies (compression fractures) or the transverse processes of the lumbar spine.

Of course, there are always the unusual injuries. For instance, carpenters using pneumatic nail guns have nailed their feet to their work. One chef, wearing running shoes for comfort, stepped on the handle of a knife that promptly flipped up in the air only to embed itself in the top of his other foot. In another instance, a painter, wearing shorts and using a high-pressure paint gun, injected about 100 milliliters of latex paint into his thigh. Try as we might, we never demonstrated anything more than general swelling in this case, even when using xeroradiography.

While doing their best to demonstrate or rule out the nature of the patient's injuries, radiographers should also keep in mind that these cases are often involved in worker's compensation proceedings. The radiographs and radiographer's history may be evidence in a hearing or trial. Therefore, every effort should be made to record observations and the patient's history, including the date, time, and radiographer's initials. All radiographs should be properly marked. The patient's name, number, hospital or clinic name, the date, and time should be photographed or radiographed onto all films.

SPORTS INJURIES

Although injuries to other areas are seen, the majority of sports injuries involve the extremities. In these injuries to extremities, the hand is often involved because it is used in almost every sport, and the knee is frequently damaged because it is not a strong joint. Contributing to knee injuries is the fact that this joint can only flex and extend, whereas many sports require it to abduct and adduct.

Perhaps even more than automobile and work-related accidents, certain sports tend to produce certain injuries. Once again, it is to the radiographer's advantage to know how the patient was injured. This is important for the radiologist's history, for guidance in moving the patient or part, and for selecting methods of radiographing the part.

HEAD AND NECK

Concussion is always a possibility with the more violent sports. This information is helpful for observing the patient while radiographing other injuries, inasmuch as the damage from concussion is rarely serious enough to be radiographically demonstrable. The face can be damaged in contact sports (such as football or boxing), and tennis, racquetball, handball, or squash. Most obvious in boxing are fractures of the nasal bones. It is possible to break one or both of the nasals. Boxing also produces fractured zygomatic arches and sometimes, fractured mandibles. Although any sport might produce a broken nose, these injuries are more common in contact sports, such as football and basketball. Tennis and other sports that use a small, soft, hollow ball can produce very difficult fractures to radiograph. The orbit protects the eye. However, a small, hollow ball hitting the orbit can distort and strike the eyeball. This force presses the eyeball back into its fatpad. The pressure on the fatpad can cause the orbit to break at its weakest point—the floor of the orbit. These are called blowout fractures of the orbit and are difficult to radiograph. Because the floor of the orbit is the ceiling of the maxillary sinus, these fractures are sometimes diagnosed from an opacified antrum.

Damage to the neck and cervical spine can result from contact sports and diving. Contact sports can produce injuries to the anterior neck from blows by the elbow or forearm. Sports like football and hockey can produce cervical spine damage ranging from strained muscles to fractures and dislocations. Tackling or checking from the back can produce whiplash injuries. Pass receivers and defenders jumping up for a ball can have their feet knocked out from under them, spinning them around in midair and causing them to land on their head. Forced flexion and forced rotation are also possible. Also, diving into shallow water is still a major cause of cervical spine damage as the patient's head strikes bottom.

▨ THORAX

Injury to the thorax usually involves the ribs and contact sports. Many of these injuries are single rib fractures, but multiple rib fractures, atelectasis, and pneumothorax are possible. Skydivers who land incorrectly or with great force may have compression fractures of the thoracic spine. Sternoclavicular separations, or separations of the sternum, clavicle, and first rib are possible from football helmets applied to the chest. Also, golfers may have stress fractures of the ribs. All stress fractures are difficult to demonstrate radiographically, especially this type. Stress fractures of the thoracic first ribs are sometimes seen in campers or hikers who carry a heavy backpack.

▦ ABDOMEN

Blunt trauma to the abdomen can produce spleen, liver, kidney, and bowel damage, and contact sports are most likely to cause these injuries. The symptoms of these injuries are the same as those in automobile accidents. Skydivers may have compression fractures in the lumbar spine, in addition to those of the thoracic spine.

▦ EXTREMITIES

As mentioned earlier, many sports can injure the hand. Baseball and softball produce dislocated fingers and avulsion fractures of the phalanges. The term *baseball finger* (also called *mallet finger* or *dropped finger*) refers to injuries of the distal phalanx from a baseball striking the end of the extended finger. *Boxer's fracture* involves the fourth and fifth metacarpals. The most common injury from snow skiing is to the thumb. Although not usually reported at the time of injury, the damage is caused by a fall or force to the thumb that presses it against the ski pole. The ski pole handle acts as a fulcrum and can damage the interphalangeal joint and the first metacarpophalangeal joint.

Wrist and forearm sports injuries are not common or typical, but a Colles' fracture could result from a sport when the patient falls on the outstretched hand. Gymnasts sometimes suffer dislocated elbows. If these cannot be fully extended, they should *not* be forced. If they are posterior dislocations, there also may be a fractured coranoid process. *Little League elbow* is usually seen in young baseball players, especially pitchers, from the throwing motion. It causes an epiphyseal fracture involving the medial epicondyle. The humerus has no typical sports injuries, but fractures are possible from direct trauma.

The shoulder is often involved in sports injuries, usually with dislocation damage leading the list. Most are anterior dislocations. They are caused by contact sports such as football and ice hockey. Fractures are also possible. Little League pitchers can have epiphyseal fractures of the proximal humerus and shoulder, besides the medial epicondyle. Trapshooters may have fractures of the coracoid process caused by the recoil of the gun.

The feet sustain injuries from sky diving, basketball, hiking, marching, and from running. Sky divers and parachutists can damage their feet by an improper or too hard landing. They may have traumatic flat feet or fractures of the calcaneus, or both. These injuries can be combined with compression and transverse process fractures of the thoracic and lumbar spines. Basketball players may have dislocations of the talonavicular or talocalcaneal joints from jumping up and then landing on a foot that is inverted. Stress fractures of the midshaft of the metatarsals or of the calcaneal tuberosity can result from hiking, marching, and sometimes from running. These fractures are more common in people who are just starting these activities, or in those unconditioned for them, rather than in long-time participants.

The ankle is susceptible to sprains, or more serious damage, from any running or jumping sport. Football and soccer can place medial or lateral stress on the ankle joint. In basketball, volleyball, or sky diving the patient may land on an inverted foot or ankle. These are some of the more obvious ways of injuring the ankle. It can also be damaged by hiking (especially over uneven or rocky ground) or from a rough dismount in gymnastics from the rings, balance beam, or parallel or uneven bars.

The lower leg receives some common injuries from running or jogging, sky diving, ballet dancing, and downhill skiing. Running or jogging may produce stress fractures at midshaft or at the distal ⅓ of the tibia. These are sometimes called "shin splints," although not all shin splints (or anterior lower leg pains) are stress fractures. Sky divers who land hard may have fractures of the proximal fibula. These fractures may or may not accompany the other sky diving injuries mentioned earlier, and include damage to the tibial plateau from impact on the femoral condyles. Ballet dancers may have stress fractures of the midtibia. Downhill skiers may have *ski-boot fractures,* which receive this name because they tend to happen at the top of the ski boot. They usually result from a fall in which the ski bindings do not release and the patient rolls downhill. The rotational force causes a spiral fracture of the lower leg rather than damage to the ankle (the ankle is held rigid by the ski boot). Although most of these fractures occur at the top of the boot (distal ⅓ to midshaft of the lower leg), there are sometimes associated fractures at the proximal end of the lower leg. This illustrates the importance of including both joints on both projections of long bone examinations.

The knee has been described as "two bones balanced on top of one another and held together by rubberbands." Because of its inherent weakness and its lack of medial or lateral movement, it sustains many injuries. Probably the most notorious sport for producing damaged knees is football. However, soccer, hockey, basketball, and others make their contributions, too. Knee damage usually involves the ligaments or menisci. It is possible for the contractions of the quadraceps muscles to avulse the tibial tuberosity or for a direct blow to fracture the patella or femur, but this is not as common as the soft tissue injuries.

Last, the pelvis may be involved in sports injuries from running (especially sprinting), hurdling, gymnastics, and cheerleading. Runners, particularly sprinters, may avulse one or both anterior superior iliac spines (ASISs). The young are more susceptible, in which case, these also would be epiphyseal fractures. Hurdlers (and sometimes cheerleaders) may have avulsion, epiphyseal fractures of one or both ischial tuberosities. This is caused by contraction of the hamstrings (the biceps femoris, semimembranosus, and semitendinosus muscles). The hamstrings adduct and extend the thigh and flex the leg. The stretching required to clear hurdles, and the kicking (or doing the "splits") in cheerleading, can cause this injury.

INJURIES IN THE HOME

Trauma to the head and neck in the home is usually either minor or severe, with few falling between these extremes. Falling off a ladder, out of a tree, or off a roof can produce the same head and neck injuries in the homeowner as those described for industrial workers. However, people seem to land on their back or coccyx just as often as on their head. And each year a few shade-tree mechanics working with only a bumper jack for support have a car, or parts thereof, fall on their heads. Once again, radiographers should take a conservative approach: Assume a fractured cervical spine until it is ruled out, and watch for changes in consciousness.

Although it is sometimes painful, a less serious injury to the cervical spine is *clay shoveler's* fracture. Described earlier in the discussion on work injuries, this injury can happen at home from gardening or from shoveling snow. It is more common when the snow is heavy and wet. Although these fractures are typically seen in the cervical spine, they are sometimes present in the thoracic spine as well.

Most home injuries requiring radiography involve the extremities. Again, because it is used so often, the hand is injured the most. Two of the biggest sources of severe hand injury in the home are lawn mowers and snow throwers. It is difficult to understand what might possess someone to put his or her fingers or hand inside a running lawn mower or snow thrower, but every year quite a few people do it. Others will hit their fingers and hands with hammers, or severe them with power tools. Usually they arrive in the radiography department with the entire end of the arm wrapped in gauze. It is often left to the initial radiographs to determine what is inside.

In addition to people slicing, dicing, smashing, and bashing their hands, other upper extremity injuries include falls on the outstretched arm. They may slip on ice or in the tub, or trip over toys and tools. The classic result of these mishaps is the Colles' fracture (distal radius with posterior displacement, with or without a fractured uinar styloid). Other injuries result from a weakness in a bone or an unusual fall. They include a fractured navicular or lunate, midshaft fracture of the radius and ulna, fracture of the radial head, fracture of the shaft or neck of the humerus, shoulder dislocations, or clavicle fractures. In addition, these falls may produce supracondylar humerus fractures in children.

Home injuries to the lower extremity usually involve the shaft and neck of the metatarsals and phalanges from objects being dropped on the foot. Severe injuries to the foot can occur when people mow the lawn downhill without shoes or wearing only lightweight shoes. Sometimes they slip, and their feet slide under the mower. In these cases they usually present with the foot wrapped in gauze, much as the hands when they are involved in a similar accident. Of a less serious nature is a *midnight fracture.* This is a fracture of the fifth toe. It typically happens when someone walks around the house at night with no lights on and hits a toe against a corner or piece of furniture.

■ ■ INJURIES FROM OTHER SOURCES

Few compilations would be complete without a category for things that do not fit into other categories. Trauma pertinent to the radiographer is no exception.

In the thorax, chronic coughing can cause stress fractures of the lower ribs. In the first rib, stress fractures can be caused by dyspnea.

A great amount of damage can be caused to the thorax and abdomen from gunshot and knife wounds. Gunshot wounds can be difficult to demonstrate because the bullet may enter at one location but not travel in a straight line. For example, it may enter the anterior right lower quadrant and exit the patient's side or the posterior left upper quadrant. Other injuries to the abdomen can be caused in fights, with the kidneys particularly susceptible to a fist or board applied to the lower back.

Gamekeeper's thumb is a term used to describe a chronic injury suffered by people in this profession. It involves the collateral ligament of the metacarpophalangeal joint of the thumb. It results from wringing the necks of wounded game.

Nursemaid's elbow, or *jerked elbow,* is an injury to children caused by an impatient adult pulling the arm or hand. Usually the child begins to cry while holding the arm. The hand is usually semipronated. The exact injury is most often dislocation of the radial head, which may not have ossified yet. The child is often "cured" when the radiographer supinates the hand for an AP forearm radiograph. Supination relocates the radial head, and no further problems are noticed.

Other injuries to the shoulder include epiphyseal shoulder fractures in newborns occurring during childbirth and luxatio erecta dislocations. Luxatio erecta injuries are rare and can happen from a fall if the arm is abducted, in which case the acromion process is a fulcrum for the humerus. The head of the humerus is forced out of, and inferior to, the glenold fossa.

In the lower extremity, the previously described Lisfranc injury can result from falling down stairs or from stepping off a curb. Ankle sprains and dislocations can result from inversion injuries caused by high-heeled shoes, slipping off a curb, or a combination of the two.

Bumper fractures result from a person being caught between the bumpers of two cars. These are usually severe, crushing injuries just below the knees, often requiring amputation. They can happen when a person is jaywalking, standing between two cars, and one car is struck from behind. Another possibility is when a car breaks down along the road and another car is parked behind or facing it. This commonly happens at night, when the intention is to position the car so that the headlights can shine on the broken car. If one car is struck from behind, anyone standing between the cars will have their lower legs caught between the bumpers of the two cars. One of the authors radiographed one man with a bumper fracture who was lying supine on the cart, but his feet pointed to the floor.

Finally, stress fractures of the pelvic rami are occasionally produced during the third trimester of pregnancy.

▪ ▪ FRACTURES WITH EPONYMS

Many fractures and injuries have acquired names over the years. Usually they are named after the type of accident that produces them or a person who identified or classified them. This list can help the radiographer identify the anatomical area in question should a physician refer to an injury by its eponym.

aviator's fracture or **aviator's astragalus:** a vertical fracture of the neck of the talus, sometimes expanded to include fractures of the body and other talar fractures with dislocations.

backfire fracture: *see* chauffeur's fracture.

Barton's fracture: intra-articular fracture of the distal radius, usually involving the posterior surface.

baseball finger: hyperflexion of the distal interphalangeal joint, sometimes with an avulsion fracture. Also called mallet finger or dropped finger fracture.

basketball foot: a subtalar dislocation of the foot.

Bennett's fracture: avulsion fracture of the base of the first metacarpal with subluxation of the first carpometacarpal joint.

boxer's fracture: fracture of the neck of the fifth metacarpal, but sometimes used to describe fractures of the fourth and fifth metacarpals, especially if they were caused by a fist fight.

bumper fracture: fracture of the tibia, and fibula, just distal to the knee; caused by being struck by a car bumper.

chauffeur's fracture: fracture of the radial styloid or of the distal radius. Name originates from the time when cars were started by a hand crank. Sometimes the engine would backfire, and the crank would strike the medial side of the distal forearm. Also called a backfire or Hutchinson fracture.

clay shoveler's fracture: *see* shoveler's fracture.

Colles' fracture: transverse fracture of the distal radius with posterior displacement of the distal fragment. In addition, the ulnar styloid process may, or may not, be fractured.

contrecoup injury: injury on the side opposite to the impact point.

dashboard fracture: fracture of the posterior rim of the acetabulum. Also called posterior rim fracture. Typically results from impact of the knee on the dashboard of a car in a front-end impact. May be seen with midshaft femur and patellar fractures.

dome fracture: a fracture of the acetabulum or of the talus. In the acetabulum, the weight-bearing surface is involved. In the talus, the superior articulating surface is involved.

dropped finger: *see* baseball finger.

drawer syndrome: a severing of the anterior or posterior cruciate ligaments of the knee. This can be radiographically documented with stress views of the knee. If the anterior cruciate is torn, then the tibia will slide forward, as when opening a drawer. If the posterior cruciate is torn, the tibia will slide back.

flail chest: produced when a number of adjacent ribs are broken in two places. This section of the chest now functions independently, and in opposition to the rest of the chest and to normal breathing. Also called paradoxical breathing.

Galeazzi fracture: a fracture of the distal third of the radius with posterior dislocation of the ulna; also called a reverse Monteggia's fracture. It is a rare injury.

gamekeeper's thumb: injury to the ulnar collateral ligament at the first metacarpophalangeal joint. May also have an avulsion fracture of the proximal phalanx.

hangman's fracture: fracture of the axis (second cervical vertebra). The fracture may be through the pedicles or the lamina. It received its name because C-2 is fractured if a person is properly hanged by the neck.

hip pointer: an impacted fracture of the superior wing of the ilium. Found in football players.

horseback rider's knee: dislocation of the head of the fibula. Occurs when a rider's knee strikes a gatepost.

Hutchinson's fracture: *see* chauffeur's fracture.

Jefferson fracture: a bursting apart of the atlas (C-1) with lateral displacement of the fragments.

jerked elbow: *see* nursemaid's elbow.

LeFort fracture: a method for classifying fractures of the face involving the maxilla, or maxilla and zygoma. There are three possible levels. (There is also a LeFort fracture of the fibula. It is an avulsion fracture involving the tibiofibular ligament.)

Lisfranc's fracture: fracture or dorsal dislocation or both, involving the tarsometatarsal joints.

Little League elbow: an avulsion fracture of the medial epicondyle.

Malgaigne fracture: double fracture of the pelvis with superior displacement. The pubic rami are fractured, along with a fracture of the ilium or scarum or dislocation of the S-I joint. The pelvis is left very unstable, especially the smaller segment.

mallet finger: *see* baseball finger.

marching fracture: stress fracture of the metatarsals, usually at midshaft, due to hiking or marching.

mechanical bull thumb: fracture of the base of the first metacarpal.

midnight fracture: fracture of the fifth toe.

Monteggia's fracture: fracture of the proximal third of the ulna with dislocation of the radial head.

nightstick or **parry fracture:** fracture of the ulnar shaft without dislocation of the proximal or distal radius or fracture of the radius. Results from a direct blow. Typically caused by raising the forearm for protection from a nightstick or baton, which then strikes the ulna.

nursemaid's elbow: dislocation of the radial head in a toddler. Common cause is pulling of the hand or wrist by an adult. Also called jerked elbow. In many cases the radial head has not ossified yet and cannot be demonstrated radiographically. Radiography is often the cure, however; as the arm is supinated for the AP forearm or elbow examination, the radial head is relocated.

parachute jumper injury: dislocation of the head of the fibula.

paradoxical breathing: *see* flail chest.

paratrooper fracture: fracture of the distal tibia and fibula.

posterior rim fracture: *see* dashboard fracture.

Rolando fracture: a comminuted Bennett's fracture.

Salter-Harris fracture: classification system (from 1 through 4) of epiphyseal fractures.

seat-belt fracture: compression fracture of the vertebral bodies. Also called lap seat-belt fracture. Can be caused by a lap belt stopping the forward momentum of the body, but without a shoulder belt, the spine undergoes forced flexion.

shoveler's fracture: avulsion fracture of the spinous processes of the cervical, and sometimes dorsal, spines. Also called clay shoveler's fracture.

sideswipe fracture: fracture of the distal humerus, usually comminuted. May also include fractures of the proximal radius and ulna. This can happen when the patient's car is hit a glancing blow while the patient has an arm resting out an open window.

ski-boot fracture: fracture of the lower leg from a fall during snow skiing. It is usually a spiral fracture at the top of the boot but may have associated fractures just below the knee.

ski-pole fracture: fracture at the base of the first metacarpal.

Smith's fracture: a reverse Colles' fracture; a fracture of the distal radius with anterior displacement.

straddle fracture: fracture or fractures of the ischial rami, the pubic rami, or both.

toddler fracture: spiral fracture of the tibia (usually in a 2- or 3-year-old child).

turf toe: injury of the first metatarsophalangeal joint from hyperextension; common to football players.

whiplash: injury to the cervical spine from force applied from behind the patient. Force striking the dorsal spine sends a wave up to the cervical spine and skull. In the cervical spine, the force resembles the end of a whip being cracked. Injuries can range from strained muscles to fractures.

SUMMARY

This chapter identified common injuries from common trauma. Although almost any injury is often *possible*, it is important for the radiographer to know those that are more *probable*. Knowing which injuries are more probable aids the radiographer in selecting methods less likely to cause additional injury and avoiding those that might harm the patient. Knowing common injuries also helps guide the radiographer in assessing the patient's condition, in observing the patient for complications or medical emergencies, in moving the patient, and in deciding whether or not to include additional radiographs.

■ ▓   **SELF-ASSESSMENT TEST 1**

1. List the common injuries to each of these areas that result from front-end impact automobile accidents.
   a. The head and neck
   b. The thoracic region
   c. The abdominal region
   d. The extremities
2. List the common injuries to each of these areas that result from rear-end impact automobile accidents.
   a. The head and neck
   b. The thoracic region
   c. The abdominal region
   d. The extremities
3. List the common injuries to each of these areas that result from side-impact automobile accidents.
   a. The head and neck
   b. The thoracic region
   c. The abdominal region
   d. The extremities
4. List the injuries that are unique to automobile accidents in which the car rolled over.
5. List injuries to each of these areas that are common to industrial or work environments.
   a. The head and neck
   b. The thoracic region
   c. The abdominal region
   d. The upper extremity
   e. The lower extremity
6. List the sports that typically produce injuries in each of these areas. List the part usually injured in each.
   a. The head and neck
   b. The thoracic region

c. The abdominal region
d. The upper extremity
e. The lower extremity

▓ ▓ SELF-ASSESSMENT TEST 2

1. Your patient was involved in an automobile accident but is unable to give you a history. You do know that he was driving. You have just radiographed his knee, and he has a stellate fracture of the patella. What type of impact do you think he was involved in, and what other injuries might he have sustained?
2. An elderly patient has slipped on an ice-covered sidewalk. As he was falling, he stuck his arm out to break his fall. What type of injury is most common in these situations? What other injuries are possible?
3. Your patient was involved in a head-on collision in which her forehead hit the windshield. You have taken a portable lateral cervical spine and lateral skull. The posterior cranium is not included on your film. Is there any reason to include it, and if so, what is it?
4. Explain how a person who falls off a scaffold or ladder and lands on the feet could have fractures of the transverse processes of the lumbar spine.

▓ ▓ BIBLIOGRAPHY

Drafke, R: Personal communication, May 1988.
Felson, B (ed): Roentgenology of Fractures and Dislocations. Grune & Stratton, New York, 1978.
Huckstep, RL: A Simple Guide to Trauma, ed 3. Churchill Livingstone, New York, 1995.
Thomas, CL (ed): Taber's Cyclopedic Medical Dictionary, ed 18. FA Davis, Philadelphia, 1997.

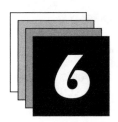

6

RADIOGRAPHING TRAUMA

OUTLINE

▒ ▒ INTRODUCTION

This chapter lists the procedures for radiographing trauma victims. It explains the general considerations of trauma radiography before describing specific procedures. The positions are described in a unique way. Although they are not totally unlike common radiographic positioning descriptions, these descriptions make no assumptions about the position the patient or the body part may be in. Therefore, they are applicable, as written, to any situation. Finally, it is not possible to describe a radiographic position or method for every traumatic possibility, so the last section of this chapter describes the factors radiographers need to consider when they must create their own position to fit a certain situation.

▨ ▨ GENERAL PRINCIPLES OF TRAUMA RADIOGRAPHY

Trauma radiography covers a wide range of possibilities. It includes everything from amputations to zygomatic arch fractures. For many injuries, the standard department routine is sufficient. Others require adaptations of the routine positions, like obtaining a Towne projection radiograph in a slightly different way. For a few, the radiographer will have to create his or her own positions. This chapter, therefore, has three goals: to be an easy reference for traditional methods that can be used in trauma radiography, to show how positions or the basic positioning principles can be altered for various circumstances, and to show the radiographer how to make his or her own adaptations.

It is not possible to cover every situation in trauma radiography. It is possible, however, to provide radiographers with the tools they need for different trauma situations. The first part of this chapter covers the basic tools—general principles of trauma radiography and basic positioning principles. The middle section contains established and adapted positions that can be used in trauma. In describing these positions no assumptions have been made regarding the patient's position. The positions are described by how the film and central ray (CR) are positioned in relation to the body part. The positions work whether the patient is supine, prone, lateral recumbent, upright, or immobile. Many are well-known, routine positions but are described in this new way; knowing positions in this way will free the radiographer to adapt them to any situation more accurately and more efficiently. The last section of this chapter covers advanced principles in creating new positions.

▨ TWO RULES FOR TRAUMA RADIOGRAPHY

The first rule of trauma radiography is if there is *any* chance of injury to the cervical spine, *do not* move the patient's head and neck until a horizontal beam lateral cervical spine radiograph has been interpreted by a physician. There is too great a chance of paralysis, or even death, from moving a patient with cervical spine damage. The lateral cervical spine radiograph should be performed while the patient is still on the emergency room (ER) cart. All seven vertebrae must be demonstrated. A radiologist or other physician must review the radiograph and give permission for the patient to be moved. It should be noted that it is *possible* for other radiographs to be taken before a lateral cervical spine *if* they do not involve moving the patient. For example, if the patient is being examined in the ER and an anteroposterior (AP) chest examination is needed immediately, it might be possible to obtain one without lifting the patient (see the section on radiography of the thorax, later in this chapter). These decisions, however, are the physician's, not the radiographer's.

The second rule of trauma radiography is do not panic. To avoid panic, the radiographer should be prepared and should concentrate. Preparation should occur long before any active involvement in a trauma situation. The preparation should include reading this book, observation of other radiographers in trauma circumstances, and review and analysis of trauma cases.

If the radiographer is called to a trauma case before he or she is needed, the radiographer should use those minutes to analyze the situation, solve any problems, plan which methods to use and in what order to perform them, and to record technics for each. In this way the patient can be examined quickly and efficiently, with no wasted time or motion.

Concentration is also important in trauma radiography. The radiographer must focus on the task at hand. He or she must not react to the patient's appearance or condition. This detracts from the performance of the job. Completing the examination correctly and quickly is the best way to serve the patient. In addition, many injuries—especially with the face—appear much worse than they are. Besides distracting the radiographer from the job, verbal or non-verbal responses can upset the patient unnecessarily.

▦ BASIC PRINCIPLES OF RADIOGRAPHIC POSITIONING

The basics of radiographic positioning must be examined in order to understand why the established radiographic positions are the way they are, to be able to adapt them to new situations, and to enable the radiographer to create his or her own positions. The basic principles are:

1. Obtain two projections, 90 degrees apart.
2. Whenever possible these projections should be an anteroposterior (AP) or posteroanterior (PA) projection and a lateral projection.
3. Angle the part, the CR, or the film to avoid any interfering objects.
4. The only thing that matters is the relationship between the part, the CR, and the film.
5. Include the entire structure, or area, in the examination.

The first principle is necessary because people are three dimensional and the film is only two dimensional. A PA projection radiograph shows height and width but no depth. If a lateral projection is taken with the CR 90 degrees from the PA, the height is repeated, but the depth is also included.

The second principle calls for an AP or PA projection and lateral projection. These projections are best because the physicians are most familiar with viewing the body from these aspects. If it is not possible to obtain these projections, then the radiographer should attempt two other projections, 90 degrees apart—possibly two obliques. If it is not possible to obtain two 90-degree projections, then two projections as close to 90 degrees apart as possible should be taken. Only as a last resort should the radiographer obtain one projection (except for those rare occasions when only one projection is routinely made, as with an AP abdomen or KUB [kidney, ureters, and bladder]). It is also helpful to the radiologist to explain what was done on the history sheet if it was not the routine.

The third principle concerns angulation of the x-ray beam, the patient, or the film. In general, angulation should be avoided. The optimum situation would have the x-ray beam perpendicular to the film, with no rotation of the patient. Of course, this is not always possible. Principle 3 is used when superimposition of structures is a problem. In radiography of the thorax and abdomen, the unwanted object is often the spine. In radiography of the skull, the petrous portion of the temporal bone is often a problem. Other interfering objects include fracture fragments, bowel patterns, and foreign bodies. When something must be angled, it is usually better to rotate the part or put the patient in an oblique position rather than angle the CR. In trauma cases, however, the patient is often immobile. Then the CR must be angled or the film tilted, or both. For many situations, the best methods have been established and are listed in the middle section of this chapter. The last section of this chapter explains how to calculate angles for new situations.

Principle 4 is the key to adapting positions to nonroutine conditions. As long as the CR, the part, and the film maintain their relationships, the position will produce the desired results. In routine radiography, the CR is usually vertical and the film is horizontal (either in the Bucky tray or on top of the radiographic table). When first trying to radiograph immobile or semimobile patients, many radiographers try to make them conform to this vertical beam method. Some do not readily understand that a film resting on the patient's cart is in the same position as one resting on the radiographic table. It does not occur to them, for example, that Figures 6–1, 6–2, and 6–3 are identical. The beam-part-film alignment is maintained in all three figures, so the radiographs will be identical. To be able to adapt positions well requires that the positions must be thought of in a new way. Instead of describing how the patient or part is positioned on the table and to the CR, the relationships of the film to the part and the CR to the film are described. An example of the Towne method for semiaxial projection of the skull illustrates the different viewpoints.

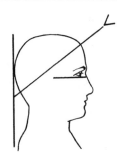

FIG. 6–1. Semiaxial skull position with patient upright. (Compare with Figs. 6–2 and 6–3.)

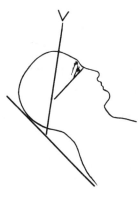

FIG. 6–2. Semiaxial skull position with patient semiupright. (Compare with Figs. 6–1 and 6–3.)

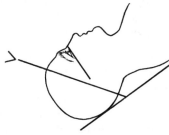

FIG. 6–3. Semiaxial skull position with patient in the Trendelenburg position. Although this situation would probably never occur, it illustrates that patient position is unimportant to the final radiograph as long as the part-film-central ray relationship is maintained. (Compare with Figs. 6–1 and 6–2.)

Conventional Description

Film–In the Bucky.

Patient–Supine or upright facing the tube.

Part–Midsagittal plane (MSP) perpendicular and centered to the table. Orbitomeatal line (OML) or infraorbitomeatal line (IOML) perpendicular to the table. Place top of film at top of head.

CR–If the OML is perpendicular, angle 30 degrees caudal. If the IOML is perpendicular, angle 37 degrees caudal. The CR enters at the MSP, 3 inches superior to the superciliary ridges.

Adaptive Description

Grid–Required.

Film–Placed in contact with posterior skull, perpendicular and centered to the MSP, perpendicular to the OML or IOML, with the top of the film at the top of the head.

CR–If the film is perpendicular to the OML, angle 30 degrees caudal as measured from the OML (60 degrees from the film). If the film is perpendicular to the IOML, angle 37 degrees caudal as measured from the IOML (53 degrees from the film). The CR enters at the MSP 3 inches superior to the superciliary ridges.

The differences between the two descriptions may appear subtle, but they are important. The adaptive description applies to any patient position. By learning the adaptive description, the radiographer is prepared for the routine patient and any other situation that arises. By knowing only the conventional description, the radiographer is prepared for the routine patient but can be hampered when faced with extraordinary conditions. The radiographer may try to make the patient conform to the methods used on routine patients, make substandard variations on the routine methods, or create his or her own positions. Each of these actions reduces the standard of care given to the patient and reduces the efficiency of the radiographer. All of the positions in this chapter are presented as adaptive descriptions. This may require some radiographers to think of their methods in new terms, but it will save them time and effort in an emergency situation (when it counts the most) and will make them more flexible in their approach to all situations.

The fifth principle is designed to ensure that no injuries are missed. For structures, it means that both joints must be included with a bone; for example, the knee and ankle must be included in an examination of the lower leg, and the shoulder and the elbow must be included for a humerus examination. The two joints do not have to be on the same film, however, but they must be included in the examination. If, for example, a lower leg was too long for a 14 × 17 inch (35 × 43 cm) film, then the joint closest to the point of injury should be included on the 14 × 17 inch (35 × 43 cm) radiograph. Separate films of the opposite joint should then be taken to complete the procedure. Also, both joints must appear in all projections. It is not permissible to include the knee on an AP projection and the ankle on a lateral projection, and claim that both joints have been included.

Applying Principle 5 to areas of the body means, for example, that the entire abdomen is included in the examination. For some patients this may require two films. Including the entire area also applies to the chest. Both lungs must be included from their apices to both lateral borders and both costophrenic angles. For patients with gunshot wounds, including the entire area may mean the chest and abdomen. Some bullets may enter the anterior chest and exit, or lodge in, the posterior abdomen. Bullet fragments may also enter the chest or abdomen, exit, and finally stop in an extremity, so "entire area" can also mean "until all the fragments are located." Including the entire structure or area also means that the entire length of a prosthesis, metal fixation rod, plate, or foreign body (such as a knife) must be included.

■ **GENERAL CONCERNS OF
TRAUMA RADIOGRAPHY**

The latter sections of this chapter involve specific trauma
radiography methods. Some general problems should
be examined first. These include problems with AP and
lateral projections with an immobile, supine patient;
problems with cassette and CR placement; moving the
patient or the limbs; application of the heel effect; immobilization; radiation protection; body fluid isolation; and
planning.

Many trauma patients are supine and may be strapped
to a backboard for immobilization. This presents problems
for the AP and lateral projections. The problems with the
AP projections are placement of the cassette under the patient and making the exposure through the backboard. Solutions include:

• Making the exposure through the backboard and the
  ER cart.
• Placing the cassette under the backboard.
• Placing the patient and the backboard on a radiographic
  table.
• Placing the patient on the radiographic table.
• Lifting the patient and placing the film beneath him
  or her.

Initial radiographs should be made without moving the
patient. They can be made through most backboards and
some ER carts. Plastic and aluminum backboards atten-
uate the x-ray beam the least and require little or no increase in kilovoltage (KV). Ventilated or patterned backboards impart that pattern to the radiograph, and this is
permissible for the first films to provide a general survey
for gross damage. Wood backboards can be penetrated
with an increase of about 5 KV. Some wood backboards
are sectioned and the parts joined with metal rods. If the
rods interfere with a structure, then Principle 3 must be
used (angling the CR), or the patient must be removed
from the backboard. Some ER carts have a second bottom,
or shelf, which allows the cassette to be placed under the

patient without moving the patient. The exposure is made through the backboard and the cart. This method also requires a radiolucent pad on the cart. When possible, this method should be used because the patient does not have to be lifted onto a radiographic table or lifted for the placement of a cassette. If a patient is to be removed from a backboard for initial or follow-up radiographs, the radiographer must have a physician's approval.

When the patient must be lifted, the radiographer should ensure that there is adequate help to move the patient slowly and smoothly. If the patient is to be lifted and a cassette placed beneath him or her, the radiographer should not help with the lifting; other people should lift the patient, and the radiographer should place the cassette according to the needs of the radiographic position being performed. These rules also apply when a limb is being moved. Adequate lifting help for a limb requires a minimum of two people. One person lifts the limb, giving support above and below the injury (Fig. 6–4), while the other person positions the cassette. When multiple AP projections are being performed on the same limb, then the limb should be lifted, the cassettes exchanged, and the limb laid down again. This procedure is preferable to lifting the limb, removing the old cassette, lowering the limb, getting a new

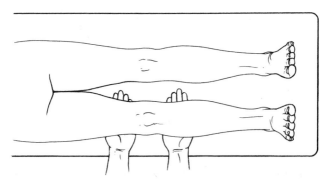

FIG. 6–4. Proper support for lifting or moving the leg when the injury is at the knee (top view).

cassette, raising the limb, positioning the new cassette, and then laying the limb down again.

Lateral projections that are performed on a supine, immobile patient will be horizontal beam projections (HBPs). These projections present a problem with the cassette and film. As illustrated in Figure 6–5, when a cassette rests on a radiographic table or backboard, the film inside the cassette is about ½ inch (1.25 cm) above the table. Extreme posterior structures, like the occipital bone in the skull, will not be included on the radiograph. This problem is compounded by the divergence of the x-ray beam

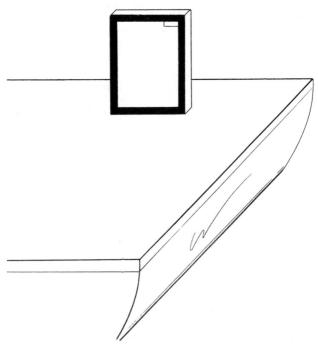

FIG. 6–5. Even when a cassette is vertical, directly on the tabletop, the edge of the film inside it is about ½ inch above the table. Structures close to the tabletop will not be demonstrated.

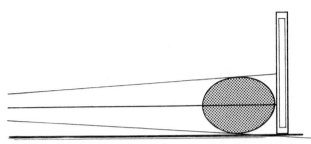

FIG. 6–6. Divergence of the x-ray beam projects structures on, or close to, the tabletop below the film (view from end of table).

(Fig. 6–6). In normal radiography, the patient would be placed on a radiolucent pad for HBPs. Because this is not possible with the immobile patient, the radiographer must position the cassette edge below the radiographic table or backboard. This may be accomplished by using a film holder, with its base placed under the backboard or ER cart pad (Fig. 6–7). Some radiographic or fluoroscopic tables have troughs, or gutters, on the side of the table opposite to the Bucky tray slot, and a flat area that supports the

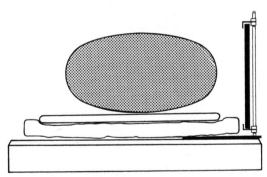

FIG. 6–7. A method for positioning the edge of the film below the patient for a horizontal beam projection (view from end of table).

image intensifier. The bottom of the cassette can be placed in the gutter, and the top can be held with a standard cassette holder (Fig. 6–8). Another method for placing the bottom of a cassette lower than the bottom of a cart is shown in Figure 6–9. Here, the cart is placed next to an upright Bucky tray. This also can be achieved by using a chest unit, head unit, upright or cassette holder, or by turning a fluoroscopy table upright. The least desirable method is to have someone hold the cassette in place, pressing it into the cart pad so that its edge is below the posterior border of the part. If this is the only way the radiograph can be made, then proper radiation protection methods must be used.

If crucial structures resting on the table are not being demonstrated, and the patient cannot be moved, there is another approach that works in some circumstances. In normal radiography, the CR is usually centered in the middle of the part. As the x-ray beam diverges, angled

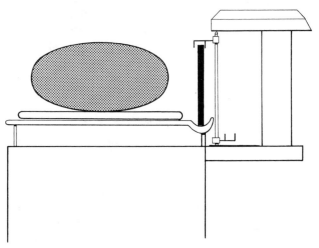

FIG. 6–8. A method for positioning the edge of the film below the patient for a horizontal beam projection (view from end of table).

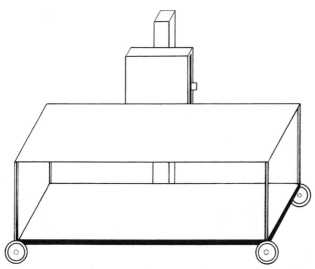

FIG. 6–9. A method for positioning the edge of the film below the patient for a horizontal beam projection (view from end of table).

rays strike the edges of the part. This projects them away from their anatomic location and causes magnification. In an HBP, the angled rays may project the edge of a part below the edge of the film (the same problem illustrated in Fig. 6–6). If the edge of the cassette cannot be placed below the patient and the edge of the table, it may help to have the perpendicular central rays strike the posterior edge of the part. This can be done by placing the CR at the most posterior part of the patient, just above the tabletop (Fig. 6–10). It should be noted that the collimation will have to be almost twice as wide as normal, but the wasted half of the beam will strike, or pass under, the table and should not affect patient radiation dose. Two additional points are important: First, this will gain about ½ inch compared with normal centering for an HBP lateral skull, and about 1 inch for an HBP lateral dorsal or lumbar spine. Second, angling the CR ante-

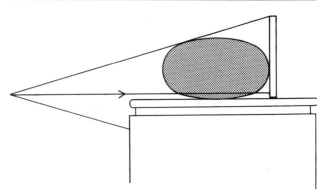

FIG. 6–10. Centering the beam closer to the tabletop can help overcome the problem of divergent x-rays projecting structures (view from end of table). (See Figs. 6–5 and 6–6.)

riorly (Fig. 6–11) will not improve the projection if, as is usually the case, the beam must pass through the cart or x-ray table closest to the tube.

When a grid cassette is used for an HBP, the relationship between the cassette and the x-ray beam is more restricted than in nongrid work. With a grid, the x-ray beam can be angled only along the long axis of the grid (Fig. 6–12) (except for cross-hatch grids, which allow no angulation of the beam and are not suited for this work). Angling the CR along the short axis of the grid will cause grid cutoff (Fig. 6–13). Deliberate angulation of the CR along the short axis of a grid is rare. However, in HBPs it is common for the grid cassette to be tilted, producing the same effect (Fig. 6–14). Sometimes it is possible to place the grid cassette so that any slippage would be along the long axis of the grid. This would produce a slightly distorted radiograph, but one that would, it is hoped, be adequate considering the circumstances. In the cases in which this is not possible, the radiographer should use whatever cassette-holding devices, such as sponges, folded sheets, and (especially) sandbags, that are required to support the cassette firmly. The radiogra-

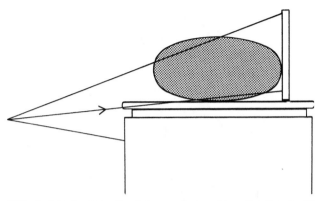

FIG. 6–11. Angling the tube up (away from the floor) will not overcome the problem of divergent x-rays projecting structures near the tabletop below the film. Instead, it will project the edge of the table (which is often metal) or the edge of a patient cart onto the film (view from end of table).

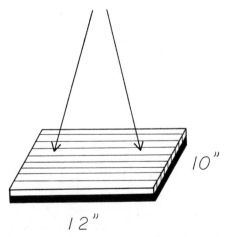

$10''$

$12''$

FIG. 6–12. Permissible central ray angles when using a grid.

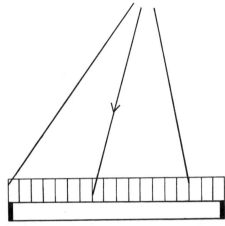

FIG. 6–13. Incorrect central ray angulation (or grid angulation) will result in grid cutoff.

pher must also watch the grid cassette before and during the exposure. These measures may take a few extra seconds initially, but that is less time than it would take to repeat the entire position.

The anode heel effect should be used in trauma radiography just as in normal radiography. Whenever possible, the increased radiation at the cathode end of the tube should be placed at the thickest end of the part. Also, the heel effect is most noticeable with short source-to-image-

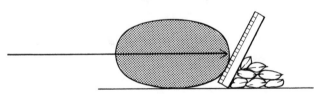

FIG. 6–14. Grid tilt that will result in grid cutoff (view from end of table).

receptor distances (SIDs) and large films. Long SID exposures and small films use the more homogeneous center portion of the beam. Examinations in which the heel effect is most useful and placement of the tube are summarized in Table 6–1.

In the urgency of many trauma radiography situations, radiation protection is often neglected. It should not be. Protection for the trauma patient should still include collimation, shielding, and a minimum number of repeat exposures. Collimation should be to the film size or smaller. This includes HBPs. Shielding of radiosensitive areas should also be done. However, the three criteria for shielding the reproductive organs must be examined, with extra attention to the third one. The reproductive organs must be shielded:

- For everyone with reasonable child-bearing capabilities (generally up to age 45 for women and age 55 for men),

TABLE 6–1. HEEL EFFECT AND TUBE PLACEMENT

Projection	Placement of Cathode
AP thoracic spine	Caudal
Lateral thoracic spine	Cephalic
AP lumbar spine	Caudal
Lateral lumbar spine	Caudal
AP or PA ribs	Caudal
Oblique ribs	Caudal
AP forearm	Near elbow
Lateral forearm	Near elbow
AP humerus	Near shoulder
Lateral humerus	Near shoulder
AP lower leg	Near knee
Lateral lower leg	Near knee
AP femur	Near hip
Lateral femur	Near hip

- When the primary beam is within 2 inches (5 cm) of the reproductive organs, and
- When shielding will not interfere with the clinical objectives of the examination.

Last, patient radiation dose can be held to a minimum by reducing repeat exposures. Repeat exposures can be reduced by using high-KV technics (which have wider exposure latitude), by using automatic exposure controls or technic charts (technic charts should be available for HBPs and portables, too), and by ensuring that the part, film, and CR are properly positioned for the initial exposures.

Personnel radiation protection in trauma radiography is also important. The basic methods of radiation protection—time, distance, and shielding—must be applied to all hospital personnel, other patients, and visitors. Using immobilization methods that include sandbags, sponges, and film holders rather than having people hold the cassette minimizes the time. Another way to use time to reduce radiation exposure is to rotate radiographers through high-exposure areas. If it is absolutely necessary for someone to hold the patient or a cassette, then the radiation dosage should be spread among as many people as possible. This generally means that radiographers should be the last ones to hold a cassette or patient. Having nonradiographers assist in holding items is not always practical, but when it is, the person must be given explicit instructions on how to hold the patient or film. Additionally, anyone holding an object must be given proper protection.

Because holding a patient or cassette means that the person doing the holding must be close to the radiation source and scatter, distance as a radiation protection measure is of little value. When it is possible to hold the patient or cassette effectively and move away from the primary beam or the patient (the source of scatter), this must be done. It should be kept in mind that doubling the distance between the source and the person holding can decrease the dose that person receives by 4 times. Also, whenever anyone holds a patient or cassette, he or she must stand out of the path of the primary beam (off to the side) and be properly shielded.

Shielding should include a lead apron (preferably with 0.5-mm lead equivalent), lead gloves, and lead glasses. Protection for people not holding the patient or cassette who must remain in the area (as in a portable examination in the ER) includes a mandatory warning to all of them that an x-ray exposure is about to be made, and adequate time must be allowed for them to leave the area. The x-ray beam should be aimed away from everyone, preferably toward a wall. If other health personnel must remain with the patient during an exposure (the physician or respiratory therapist, for example), they must be given a lead apron and other protective shielding, depending on their distance from the primary beam. The radiographer should remember that he or she is the expert in radiography and radiation protection, and it is his or her ethical responsibility to ensure that all precautions have been taken.

Remember also that there is a concern for communicable diseases, especially acquired immunodeficiency syndrome (AIDS). The safest approach is total body fluid isolation for all patients. In trauma radiography, there is a very great chance that the radiographer or the equipment, or both, may come into contact with body fluids. The prudent radiographer should take all safety precautions for all patients for all body fluids, especially blood. The radiographer should wear protective isolation gloves for all patients. If the patient's blood may come in contact with the radiographer's clothing, the radiographer should also wear a protective gown. The radiographer's equipment also should be protected. Grids, cassettes, sponges, sandbags, and other radiographic or immobilization devices that come in contact with the patient, or that could become contaminated, should be protected with a barrier drape or pillowcase. The radiographer must then follow the department's disposal procedure carefully, as well as decontaminate the radiographic table and equipment.

▪ ▪ TRAUMA RADIOGRAPHY POSITIONS

These descriptions make no assumptions about the patient's position. They can be applied to the immobile supine patient or the mobile upright patient. For each position, the technical name is given, along with any eponym that is commonly used. Grid usage, meaning a grid cassette or Bucky, is given as required, recommended, or not required. The position of the grid lines is also listed. Grid lines parallel to the MSP mean that the long side of the grid is placed parallel to the MSP (as would be the case if the patient were to be supine and the Bucky's grid lines were being described). If the grid lines are to be perpendicular to the MSP, then the short side of the grid is parallel to the MSP. Part position is given as the film's position in relation to a radiographic baseline or body surface (in these descriptions the term *film* is synonymous with cassette, grid cassette, and Bucky); for example, the film is perpendicular to the MSP, or the film is in contact with the anterior surface of the hand. References to the film being placed lengthwise mean that the long axis of the film is aligned with the long axis of the part. Placing the film crosswise means that the long axis of the film is perpendicular to the long axis of the part. The CR angle or placement is given in relation to the film or part, whichever is more appropriate. Any special notes on a position follow the description. When the reverse projection of a position could be useful, it is listed immediately after the original.

Figures 6–15, 6–16, and 6–17 review the body and skull baselines, planes, and points used to describe radio-

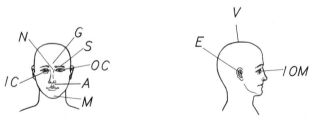

FIG. 6–15. Topography of the skull. IC: inner canthus of the eye. N: nasion. G: glabella. S: superciliary arch and ridge. OC: outer canthus of the eye. A: acanthion. M: mental point. E: EAM, external auditory meatus. V: vertex (apex). IOM: inferior orbital margin.

FIG. 6–16. *Baselines and planes of the skull. IPC: interpupillary line. MSP: midsagittal plane. G: GML, glabellomeatal line. O: OML, orbitomeatal line. I: IOML, infraorbitomeatal line. A: AML, acanthomeatal line. M: MML, mentomeatal line.*

graphic positions. Abbreviations and descriptions of the positioning planes and lines are listed below.

■ TOPOGRAPHIC POINTS OF THE SKULL

Mental point: chin
Acanthion: base of the nose (nasal spine)
Nasion: between the eyes
Inner canthus: inner corner of the eye
Outer canthus: outer corner of the eye
Superciliary ridges: bony ridge above the eyebrow
Glabella: middle of the forehead
Vertex (or apex): top of the head
Inion: external occipital protuberance
EAM: external auditory meatus

■ POSITIONING PLANES AND LINES OF THE HEAD AND BODY

MSP: Midsagittal plane (divides the body into equal right and left halves)

MCP: Midcoronal plane (divides the body into anterior and posterior halves)

MAL: Midaxillary line (runs along the sides of the body through the middle of the axilla [the armpit])

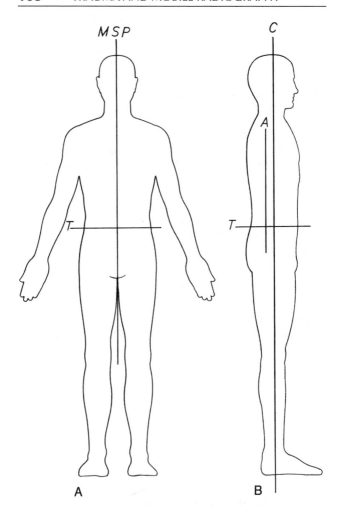

FIG. 6–17. Positioning planes and lines of the body. (A) Anterior view. (B) Lateral view. MSP: midsagittal plane. T: transverse plane. C: midcoronal plane. A: midaxillary line.

GML: Glabellomeatal line (connects the glabella with the external auditory meatus [EAM])

OML: Orbitomeatal line (connects the outer canthus of the eye to the EAM. Also referred to as the radiographic baseline)

IOML: Infraorbitomeatal line (connects the inferior margin, or ridge, of the orbit to the EAM. Also referred to as Reid's baseline)

AML: Acanthomeatal line (connects the acanthion to the EAM)

NNL: Mentomeatal line (connects the mental point of the mandible to the EAM)

IPL: Interpupillary line (connects the pupils of the eyes when the patient is looking straight ahead)

TRAUMA RADIOGRAPHY OF THE HEAD AND NECK

 THE HEAD

 ## LATERAL PROJECTION SKULL
(FIG. 6–18)

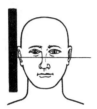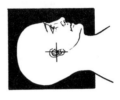

FIG. 6–18. Lateral skull.

Grid–Required, grid lines perpendicular to the MCP.

Film–Placed so the long axis is parallel to the top of the head. The film is perpendicular to the IPL. It should be centered to the sella turcica—¾ inch anterior and superior to the EAM, or positioned to include the cranium from the nasion to the foramen magnum. The name blocker and markers should be placed toward the face.

CR–Perpendicular to the film. It should enter ¾ inch anterior and superior to the EAM (see Fig. 6–10 for HBPs).

Note–Both lateral skull projections should be made. In situations in which only the minimum number of radiographs can be made, at least one lateral projection must be included. When only one lateral projection is possible, it should be of the side suffering the impact or the most damage.

AP PROJECTION SKULL
(FIG. 6–19)

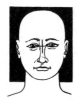 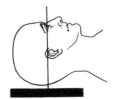

FIG. 6–19. *AP skull.*

Grid–Required. Grid lines parallel to the MSP.

Film–The film is placed behind the patient, with the short side at the top of the head. It is perpendicular to the MSP and perpendicular to the OML. The film is centered to the nasion. The name blockers and markers should be at the bottom of the film.

CR–Perpendicular to the film, entering the nasion.

Note–An AP or PA skull should be part of every routine, even if only the minimum number of radiographs can be made.

 # PA PROJECTION SKULL
(FIG. 6–20)

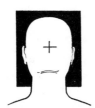 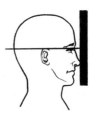

FIG. 6–20. *PA skull.*

Grid–Required. Grid lines parallel to the MSP.

Film–Placed in front of the patient with the short side parallel to the top of the head. It is perpendicular to the MSP and the OML, centered to the nasion. The name blockers and markers should be at the bottom of the film.

CR–Perpendicular to the film, exiting the nasion.

Note–An AP or PA skull should be a part of even minimal radiograph routines of the head, and the name blocker and markers should be at the bottom of the film.

 ## SEMIAXIAL AP SKULL (TOWNE, GRASHEY, OR CHAMBERLAIN METHOD) **(FIG. 6–21)**

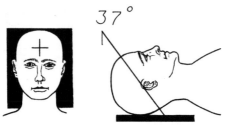

FIG. 6–21. Semiaxial AP skull, IOML perpendicular to the film.

Grid–Required. Grid lines parallel to the MSP.

Film–Placed behind the patient, with the short side parallel to the top of the head. It is perpendicular to the MSP and OML, or IOML. The top of the film should be at the top of the head, and the name blocker and markers should be at the bottom of the film.

CR–Angled 30 degrees caudal if the film is perpendicular to the OML; 37 degrees caudal if the film is perpendicular to the IOML. It enters 3 inches superior to superciliary ridges (the eyebrows).

Note–This projection is vital to every skull routine for assessment of the occipital bone. It can also be used for mandibular condyles or zygomatic arches.

SEMIAXIAL PA SKULL (REVERSE TOWNE AND HAAS METHODS)
(FIG. 6–22)

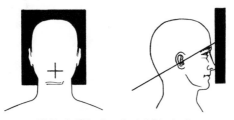

FIG. 6–22. Semiaxial PA skull.

Grid–Required. Grid lines parallel to the MSP.

Film–Placed in front of the patient, with the short side parallel to the top of the head. It is perpendicular to the MSP and the OML, or IOML for a reverse Towne projection; perpendicular to the MSP and OML for a Haas projection. The film is centered to the glabella.

CR–For a reverse Towne projection, angle 30 degrees cephalic if the film is perpendicular to the OML; 37 degrees cephalic if the film is perpendicular to the IOML. Angle 25 degrees cephalic for a Haas method. The CR enters at the base of the skull and exits the glabella.

LATERAL FACIAL BONES
(FIG. 6–23)

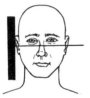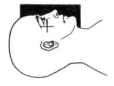

FIG. 6–23. Lateral facial bones.

Grid–Required. Grid lines parallel to the MCP.

Film–The film is placed lengthwise, parallel to the MSP and perpendicular to the IPL. It is centered to the middle of the zygomatic arch.

CR–Perpendicular to the film, it enters the middle of the zygomatic arch.

PARIETOACANTHIAL PROJECTION FOR FACIAL BONES (WATERS METHOD)
(FIG. 6–24)

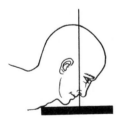

FIG. 6–24. Parietoacanthial projection for facial bones (Waters method).

Grid–Required. Grid lines parallel to the MSP.

Film–The film is placed lengthwise touching the chin. It is perpendicular to the MSP (and roughly perpendicular to the MML). It should be 40 degrees from the OML and centered to the acanthion.

CR–Perpendicular to the film entering the posterior parietal region and exiting the acanthion.

ACANTHOPARIETAL PROJECTION FOR FACIAL BONES (REVERSE WATERS)
(FIG. 6–25)

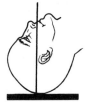

FIG. 6–25. Acanthoparietal projection for facial bones (reverse Waters method).

Grid–Required. Grid lines parallel to the MSP.

Film–In contact with the posterior parietal region of the skull (near the lambda), perpendicular to the MSP and 40 degrees from the OML.

CR–Perpendicular to the film entering the acanthion.

AXIAL PROJECTION FOR ZYGOMATIC ARCHES (MAY METHOD)
(FIG. 6–26)

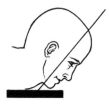

FIG. 6–26. Axial projection for zygomatic arch (May method).

Grid–Not required.

Film–In contact with the chin, parallel to the IOML (or as close to parallel to the IOML as possible). Initially the film is placed perpendicular to the MSP, then the head is tilted away from the side being examined 15 degrees from perpendicular, 75 degrees from the film.

CR–Perpendicular to the IOML (even if the IOML is not parallel to the film), passing through the middle of the arch.

SUBMENTOVERTICAL (SMV) PROJECTION FOR ZYGOMATIC ARCHES
(FIG. 6–27)

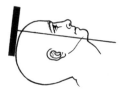

FIG. 6–27. SMV projection for bilateral zygomatic arches.

Grid–Not required.

Film–In contact with the vertex, perpendicular and centered to the MSP and parallel to the IOML.

CR–Perpendicular to the IOML through the middle of the arch.

 ## MODIFIED SMV PROJECTION FOR ZYGOMATIC ARCHES (SUPINE, IMMOBILE PATIENTS) **(FIG. 6–28)**

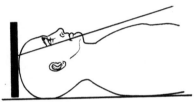

FIG. 6–28. Modified SMV projection for bilateral zygomatic arches.

Grid–Not required.

Film–In contact with the vertex, perpendicular and centered to the MSP, parallel to the IOML.

CR–As close to perpendicular to the IOML as possible, passing through the middle of the arch.

OBLIQUE FACIAL BONES
(FIG. 6–29)

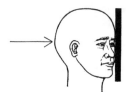

FIG. 6–29. Oblique facial bones.

Grid–Recommended, grid lines parallel to the MSP.

Film–In contact with the side of the face being examined, 53 degrees from the MSP, perpendicular to the AML. The orbit of the side being examined centered.

CR–Perpendicular to the film.

Note–This will also demonstrate the optic foramen, as in the Rhese method.

 # REVERSE OBLIQUE
FACIAL BONES
(FIG. 6–30)

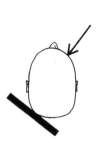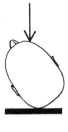

FIG. 6–30. Reverse oblique facial bones (view from end of table).

Grid–Recommended, grid lines parallel to the MSP.

Film–In contact with the posterior portion of the skull opposite the side being examined. It is 53 degrees from the MSP and perpendicular to the AML.

CR–Perpendicular to the film, entering the orbit of the side being examined.

 ## SUBSTITUTE OBLIQUE FACIAL BONES (SUPINE, IMMOBILE PATIENTS)
(FIG. 6–31)

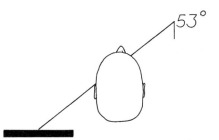

FIG. 6–31. Substitute oblique facial bones (view from end of table).

Grid–Recommended. If a grid is used, the grid lines must be perpendicular to the MSP.

Film–On the table, or cart, the edge touching the skull opposite of the side being examined.

CR–Angled lateral-to-medial 53 degrees from the MSP (53 degrees from vertical), enters the orbit of the side being examined. (For a similar but less distorted projection, angle 37 degrees from the MSP.)

AXIOLATERAL MANDIBLE
(FIG. 6–32)

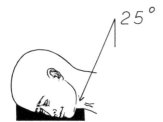

FIG. 6–32. Axiolateral projection for the mandibular body.

Grid–Recommended. If a grid is used, the grid lines should be placed superoinferiorly to allow a cephalic CR angle.

Film–Initially parallel to the MSP, then, if possible, in contact with the side of the mandible being demonstrated. Center the side being examined.

CR–Angled cephalic, 65 degrees from the film (25 degrees from perpendicular to the film), enters the side closest to the film halfway between the chin and the mandibular ramus.

PA MANDIBLE
(FIG. 6–33)

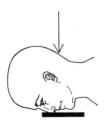

FIG. 6–33. PA mandible.

Grid–Required. Grid lines parallel to the MSP.

Film–In front of the patient, perpendicular to the MSP and OML. Centered to the mouth.

CR–Perpendicular to the film, exiting the mouth.

✳ AP MANDIBLE
(FIG. 6–34)

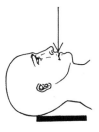

FIG. 6–34. AP mandible.

Grid–Required. Grid lines parallel to the MSP.

Film–Behind the patient, perpendicular to the MSP and OML. Centered to the mouth.

CR–Perpendicular to the film, enters at the mouth.

THE NECK

 ## LATERAL CERVICAL SPINE
(FIG. 6–35)

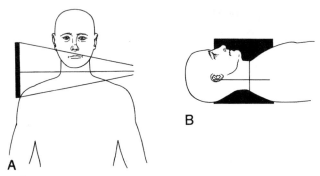

FIG. 6–35. Lateral cervical spine. (A) Top view. (B) Side view.

Grid–Not required.

Film–Parallel to the MSP, bottom edge touching the lateral border of the shoulder.

CR–Perpendicular to the film, entering at a level of C4.

Note–The shoulders should be depressed to ensure that C7 is included on the radiograph. If the patient is upright (seated or standing), weights may be placed in each hand. If the patient is recumbent, straps may be placed in each hand with weights hanging off the end of the cart or table. The last alternative is for someone to apply slow, gentle traction to both arms during the exposure. All radiation safety precautions must be followed if this is done. If the shoulders cannot be depressed or are only partially depressed, the radiographer should consider centering at C7 so that the divergence of the beam does not project C7 into the shoulder. Also, the SID should be 72 inches (180 cm) to reduce magnification.

AP CERVICAL SPINE
(FIG. 6–36)

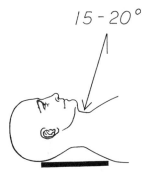

FIG. 6–36. AP cervical spine.

Grid–Required. Grid lines parallel to the MSP.

Film–Behind the patient, perpendicular to the MSP. Centered to the MSP and C-4 (thyroid cartilage).

CR–Angled 15 to 20 degrees cephalic, enters the thyroid cartilage.

 # C1 AND C2
(OPEN-MOUTH METHOD)
(FIG. 6–37)

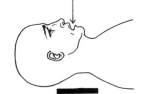

FIG. 6–37. Open-mouth AP cervical spine.

Grid–Recommended, grid lines parallel to the MSP.

Film–Behind the patient, perpendicular to the MSP and perpendicular to a line connecting the inferior border of the upper teeth and the mastoid processes. Centered to the mouth. The mouth is open as wide as possible.

CR–Perpendicular to the film through the open mouth.

SUBSTITUTE C1 AND C2 (IMMOBILE, SUPINE PATIENTS) (FIG. 6–38)

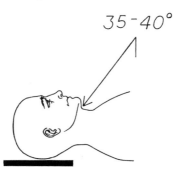

FIG. 6–38. Substitute position to demonstrate C1 and C2 on immobile, supine patients.

Grid–Required. Grid lines parallel with the MSP.

Film–Behind the patient, perpendicular and centered to the MSP. The bottom of the film is placed at the base of the skull.

CR–Angled 35 to 40 degrees cephalic; it enters at the thyroid cartilage.

OBLIQUE CERVICAL SPINE
(FIG. 6–39)

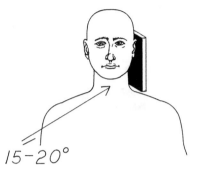

15–20°

FIG. 6–39. Oblique cervical spine (top view).

Grid–Required. Grid lines parallel to the MSP.

Film–45 degrees from the MSP. Centered to C4.

CR–If the film is behind the patient, angle 15 to 20 degrees cephalic; if the film is in front of the patient, angle 15 to 20 degrees caudal.

Note–Two posterior or two anterior obliques should be taken.

SUBSTITUTE OBLIQUE CERVICAL SPINE
(FIG.6–40)

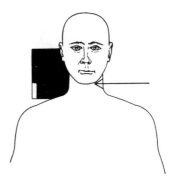

FIG. 6–40. Substitute oblique cervical spine. Note that the short side of the cassette is against the patient's neck so that the grid strips are parallel to the CR (top view).

Grid–Not required.

Film–Behind the patient, perpendicular to the MSP or against the side of the patient's neck. Centered to C4.

CR–Angled 45 degrees lateromedially and 15 to 20 degrees cephalic. Enters C4.

LATERAL DISTAL CERVICAL AND PROXIMAL THORACIC SPINES (SWIMMER'S METHOD)
(FIG. 6–41)

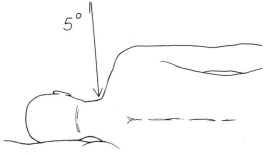

FIG. 6–41. Lateral distal cervical and proximal thoracic spines (swimmer's method).

Grid–Required Grid lines to parallel the MSP.

Film–With one shoulder depressed and the opposite shoulder and arm extended, the film is placed next to the extended arm, parallel to the MSP. If possible, also position one shoulder anterior and the opposite shoulder posterior to the spine.

CR–Angled 3 to 5 degrees caudally, passing through C7 and T1. (C7 is easily palpated because of its long spinous process.)

REVERSE SWIMMER'S METHOD (SUPINE, IMMOBILE PATIENTS) (FIG. 6–42)

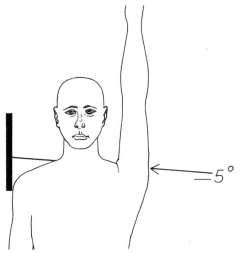

FIG. 6–42. Reverse swimmer's method for supine, immobile patients (top view).

Grid–Required. Grid lines parallel to the MSP.

Film–With one shoulder depressed and the opposite shoulder and arm extended, the film is placed next to the depressed shoulder, parallel to the MSP. If possible, also position one shoulder anterior and the opposite shoulder posterior to the spine.

CR–Angled 3 to 5 degrees cephalic, passing through C7 and T1. (C7 is easily palpated because of its long spinous process.)

Note–By reversing this projection (which is only feasible with an HBP), the humeral head of the extended arm is magnified and interferes less with the spine than in the previous position.

TRAUMA RADIOGRAPHY OF THE THORAX

General Note–Because of the chance of a fractured rib perforating a lung, each patient must be carefully evaluated. The patient should not lie on the injured area if there is a possibility of multiple rib fractures or displaced rib fractures.

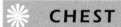 CHEST

 PA CHEST
(FIG. 6–43)

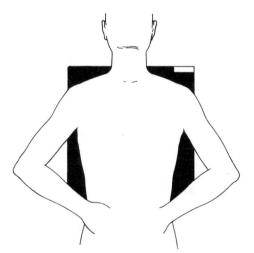

FIG. 6–43. PA chest.

Grid–Recommended (required when the KV exceeds 90). Grid lines parallel to MSP.

Film–In front of the patient, perpendicular to the MSP. The top of the film should be 1½ to 2 inches above the shoulders. The shoulders should be rolled forward and depressed.

CR–Perpendicular to the film, 72 inches from the film (if possible), and centered to the film.

Note–Respiration is suspended after the second full inspiration.

This position is used when the patient can stand or sit upright without assistance. The PA projection, seated position can also be used in portable radiography with the patient sitting on the side of the bed.

✳ AP CHEST
(FIGS. 6–44 AND 6–45)

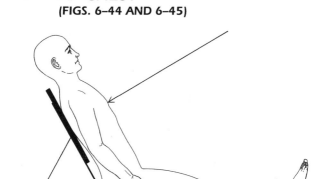

FIG. 6–44. *AP chest, patient semiupright.*

Grid–Recommended (required when the KV exceeds 90). Grid lines parallel to MSP.

Film–Behind the patient, perpendicular to the MSP. The top of the film should be 1½ to 2 inches above the shoulders. The shoulders should be rolled forward and depressed.

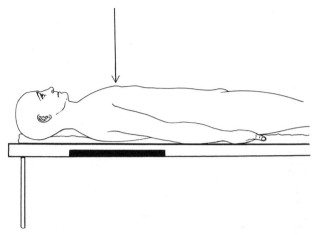

FIG. 6–45. AP chest, patient recumbent.

CR–Perpendicular to the film, 72 inches from the film (if possible), and centered to the film.

Note–Respiration is suspended after the second full inspiration.

To demonstrate possible air-fluid levels, the patient should be upright (the MCP 90 degrees to the floor). If the patient cannot sit fully upright, he or she should be placed as upright as possible and the degree of angulation between the MCP and the floor recorded for the radiologist (see Fig. 6–44). If the examination is specifically for air-fluid levels, then the CR should be horizontal even if the patient is not upright. This will result in distortion of the heart and lungs.

Some patient carts have a tray or second bottom immediately under the supine patient. A cassette can be placed on this tray, under the patient, without moving the patient in severe trauma cases or when there is a suspected cervical spine fracture (see Fig. 6–45).

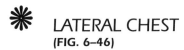

LATERAL CHEST
(FIG. 6–46)

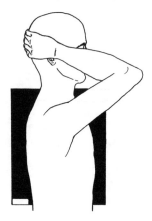

FIG. 6–46. Lateral chest.

Grid–Recommended (required when the KV exceeds 90). Grid lines parallel to the MSP.

Film–Against the patient's side, parallel to the MSP, the top 1½ to 2 inches above the shoulder. Both arms are extended at least 90 degrees from the body.

CR–Perpendicular to the film, 72 inches from the film (if possible), centered to the film.

Note–Respiration is suspended after the second full inspiration.

DORSAL DECUBITUS LATERAL CHEST
(FIG. 6–47)

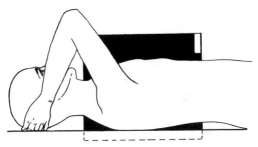

FIG. 6–47. Dorsal decubitus chest.

Grid–Recommended (required when the KV exceeds 90). Grid lines parallel to the MSP.

Film–With the patient supine on a radiolucent pad, the film is placed against the patient's side, parallel to the MSP. The top of the film is placed 1½ to 2 inches above the shoulder. Both arms are extended at least 90 degrees from the body, preferably 180 degrees.

CR–Perpendicular to the film (horizontal), 72 inches from the film (if possible), centered to the film.

Note–Respiration is suspended after the second full inspiration.

RIBS

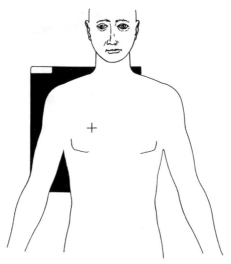

UPPER RIBS
(FIG. 6–48)

FIG. 6–48. Upper ribs.

Grid–Required. Grid lines parallel to the MSP.

Film–Placed in contact with the injured area, perpendicular to the MSP. The top of the film should be 1½ to 2 inches above the shoulder.

CR–Perpendicular to the film; centered to the film.

Note–Respiration is suspended on full inspiration. This projection may be PA or AP—depending on the injury— and may be bilateral or unilateral. Short-scale contrast technic should be used, especially when trying to demonstrate stress fractures of the ribs.

LOWER RIBS
(FIG. 6–49)

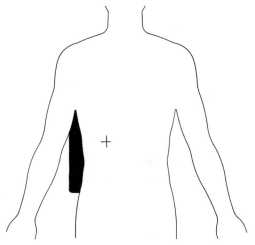

FIG. 6–49. Lower ribs.

Grid–Required. Grid lines parallel to the MSP.

Film–Placed in contact with the injured area, perpendicular to the MSP. Centered to T12.

CR–Perpendicular to the film; centered to the film.

Note–Respiration is suspended on full expiration. This projection is usually AP (for the lower 2 to 4 ribs) but is occasionally PA for the anteromedial portion of the 9th and 10th ribs. This projection may be bilateral or unilateral, depending on the injury.

OBLIQUE RIBS
(FIGS. 6–50 AND 6–51)

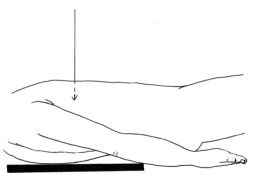

FIG. 6–50. Oblique ribs for posterior injuries.

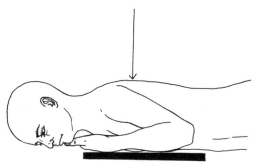

FIG. 6–51. Oblique ribs for anterior injuries.

Grid–Required. Grid lines parallel to the MSP.

Film–For posterior rib injuries the film is in contact with the injured area, 45 degrees from the MSP (see Fig. 6–50). For anterior injuries the film is placed 45 degrees from the MSP but is not in contact with the injured area (see Fig. 6–51). These positions prevent the spine from being superimposed on the area being examined. The top of the film is placed 1½ to 2 inches above the shoulder.

CR–Perpendicular to the film; centered to the film.

Note–Respiration is suspended on inspiration when the injury is above the diaphragm, and on expiration when the injury is below the diaphragm.

SUBSTITUTE OBLIQUE RIBS (SUPINE, IMMOBILE PATIENTS) (FIG. 6–52)

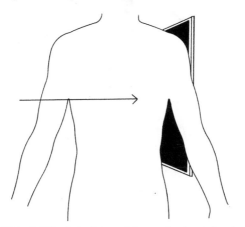

FIG. 6–52. Substitute oblique ribs (top view).

Grid–Required. Grid lines perpendicular to the MSP.

Film–Behind the patient, under the side being examined. The film is parallel to the MCP, the top of the film is 1 inch above the shoulder.

CR–Angled 45 degrees mediolaterally; centered to the film.

Note–Respiration is suspended on inspiration for injuries above the diaphragm, and on expiration for injuries below the diaphragm. This projection is for axillary rib injuries.

THORACIC SPINE

AP THORACIC SPINE
(FIG. 6–53)

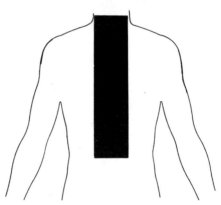

FIG. 6–53. AP thoracic spine.

Grid–Required. Grid lines parallel to the MSP.

Film–Behind the patient, perpendicular to the MSP with top 1½ to 2 inches above the shoulder. Center the film to the MSP.

CR–Perpendicular to the film; centered on the film.

Note–Respiration should be suspended.

LATERAL THORACIC SPINE
(FIG. 6–54)

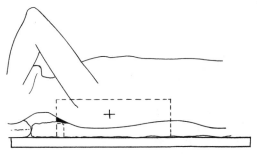

FIG. 6–54. Lateral thoracic spine, patient recumbent.

Grid–Required. Grid lines parallel to the MSP.

Film–Against the patient's side, parallel to the MSP with the top 1½ to 2 inches above the shoulder. Both arms are extended at least 90 degrees from the body. Center the film to the MAL.

CR–Perpendicular to the film; centered to the film.

Note–Respiration may be suspended on expiration, or a breathing technique may be used. To use the breathing technique, the patient must be breathing normally and a long exposure time must be set.

 # LATERAL PROXIMAL THORACIC SPINE

The reader is referred to Lateral Distal Cervical and Proximal Thoracic Spines, under The Neck section in Trauma Radiography of the Head and Neck.

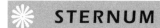

STERNUM

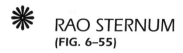

RAO STERNUM
(FIG. 6–55)

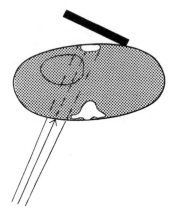

FIG. 6–55. RAO sternum.

Grid–Required. Grid line parallel to the MSP.

Film–In contact with the right anterior portion of the chest with the film or patient rotated just enough to prevent the spine from being superimposed on the sternum. The film is centered halfway between the xiphoid process and the manubrium.

CR–Perpendicular to the film; centered to the film.

Note–This position projects the heart on the sternum. Short-scale contrast technic should be used. Respiration may be suspended on expiration, or a breathing technique (normal respiration and long exposure time) may be used.

SUBSTITUTE OBLIQUE STERNUM (SUPINE, IMMOBILE PATIENTS) (FIG. 6–56)

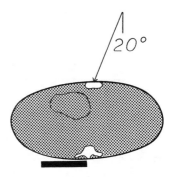

FIG. 6–56. Substitute oblique sternum for supine, immobile patients.

Grid–Required. Grid lines perpendicular to the MSP.

Film–Behind the patient, one edge at the MSP, centered halfway between the xiphoid and manubrium.

CR–Angled 15 to 20 degrees mediolaterally; centered to the film. The CR enters the sternum and exits the left posterior side of the patient.

Note–Respiration is suspended on expiration.

LATERAL STERNUM
(FIG. 6–57)

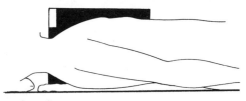

FIG. 6–57. Lateral sternum, patient supine.

Grid–Required.

Film–Against the patient's side, parallel to the MSP, centered halfway between the xiphoid and the manubrium. If possible, the patient's arms should be placed behind the back.

CR–Perpendicular to the film; centered to the film.

Note–Respiration should be suspended on full inspiration.

TRAUMA RADIOGRAPHY OF THE ABDOMEN

 ABDOMINAL ORGANS

 ## KUB (AP ABDOMEN, FLATPLATE ABDOMEN)
(FIGS. 6–58 AND 6–59)

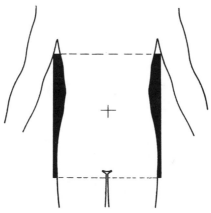

FIG. 6–58. KUB (top view).

Grid–Required. Grid lines parallel to MSP.

Film–Behind the patient, perpendicular to the MSP, centered to the iliac crest. Respiration is suspended for the exposure.

CR–Perpendicular to the film.

Note–When using a grid cassette, the patient's weight must be equally distributed on the right and left sides. (The right and left sides of the film must be the same distance from the tube.) If they are not, there will be grid cut off on the film (and possibly no image).

203

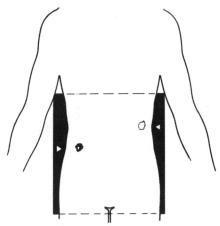

FIG. 6–59. KUB for gunshot wounds showing proper marking of entry and exit sites (top view).

If the patient is radiographed upright (e.g., for a free-air series), the radiograph should be marked "upright."

If the examination is for a gunshot wound, the level of the entry point or the exit point or both should be marked. The marker must not be mistaken for a bullet fragment. It should be distinctive and at the edge of the film (Fig. 6–59). If there is only an entry wound, the radiographer's right or left marker can be placed at the same level as the wound.

LEFT LATERAL DECUBITUS ABDOMEN
(FIG. 6–60)

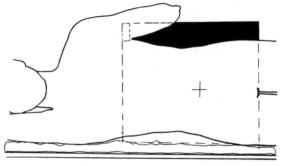

FIG. 6–60. Left lateral decubitus abdomen.

Grid–Required. Grid lines parallel to the MSP.

Film–Perpendicular to the MSP, centered to the crest. The film may be in front of, or behind, the patient (an AP or PA projection can be used). The patient must lie on the left side, and the film must be vertical. Respiration is suspended.

CR–An HBP, perpendicular to the film.

Note–The left lateral decubitus position is used to avoid confusing free-air in the abdomen with air in the stomach.

LUMBAR SPINE

 ## AP LUMBAR SPINE
(FIG. 6–61)

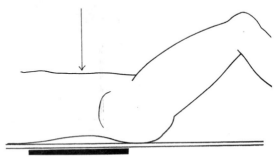

FIG. 6–61. AP lumbar spine.

Grid–Required. Grid lines parallel to the MSP.

Film–Behind the patient, perpendicular to the MSP. The film is centered to L3. Respiration is suspended.

CR–Perpendicular to the film.

AP L5-S1
(FIG. 6–62)

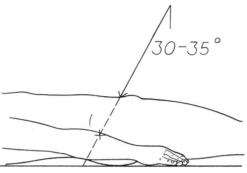

FIG. 6–62. AP L5-S1 and AP S-I joints.

Grid–Required. Grid lines parallel to the MSP.

Film–Behind the patient, perpendicular to the MSP, centered to the MSP.

CR–Angled cephalic, 30 degrees for men, 35 degrees for women. The CR must pass through the space between L5 and S1. The space is halfway between the iliac crest and the anterior superior iliac spine (ASIS) and 1½ inches posterior to the midaxillary line. (One method of placing the CR is to open the collimators as widely as possible—so the light field and CR shadow lie across the patient and down his or her side. Find the level of L5-S1 on the patient's side. Keep one finger at the localization point and move the tube until the CR shadow is at that point. Collimate to the film size or smaller and make the exposure.)

Note–This position will also demonstrate AP sacroiliac joints.

LATERAL LUMBAR SPINE
(FIG. 6–63)

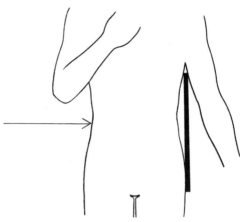

FIG. 6–63. Lateral lumbar spine, patient recumbent (top view).

Grid–Required (preferably high ratio). Grid lines parallel to the MSP.

Film–At the patient's side, parallel to the MSP. Centered to the MAL and L3.

CR–Perpendicular to the film. Respiration should be suspended.

Note–When not using an HBP, place a piece of lead behind the patient to absorb scatter radiation.

LATERAL L5-S1
(FIG. 6–64)

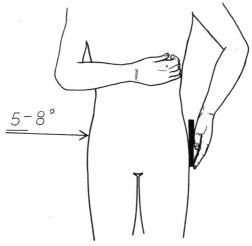

5 – 8 °

FIG. 6–64. Lateral L5-S1, patient recumbent (top view).

Grid–Required (preferably high ratio). Grid lines parallel to the MSP.

Film–At the patient's side, parallel to the MSP, centered to the CR.

CR–Angled caudal, 5 degrees for men, 8 degrees for women. The CR enters halfway between the crest and the ASIS, 1½ inches posterior to the MAL.

OBLIQUE LUMBAR SPINE
(FIG. 6–65)

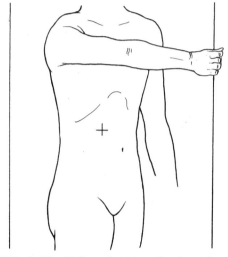

FIG. 6–65. Oblique lumbar spine (top view).

Grid–Required. Grid lines parallel to the MSP.

Film–Behind the patient, 45 degrees from the MSP (the patient may be rotated 45 degrees [see Note] or the film may be angled 45 degrees.)

CR–Perpendicular to the film, entering the patient about 2 inches lateral to the MSP, at the level of L3.

Note–Both obliques (an RPO and LPO) are normally done. Trauma to the upper abdomen may fracture the lower ribs. Rotating the patient for oblique lumbar spine positions may lacerate the liver, spleen, or other abdominal organs. If the patient has upper abdomen trauma, especially posteriorly, review the need for these positions with the radiologist or physician and consider alternatives.

SUBSTITUTE OBLIQUE LUMBAR SPINE
(FIG. 6–66)

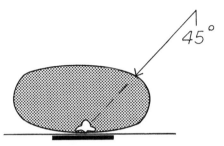

FIG. 6–66. Oblique lumbar spine on an immobile patient (view from head of table).

Grid–Required. Grid lines are *perpendicular* to the MSP.

Film–Behind the patient, perpendicular to the MSP. It is centered halfway between the spine and the patient's side, at the level of L3. Both sides are normally taken.

CR–Angled 45 degrees from lateral to medial. It enters 2 inches lateral to the MSP away from the side the film is centered to (i.e., if the film is centered to the patient's left side, the tube will be over the patient's right side, angled 45 degrees lateromedially, and entering 2 inches to the right of the MSP).

Note–For less distortion, a 30-degree CR angle may be used.

SACRUM AND COCCYX

 AP SACRUM
(FIG. 6–67)

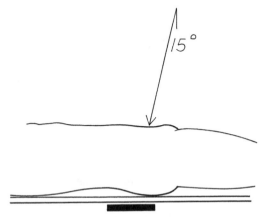

FIG. 6–67. AP sacrum.

Grid–Required. Grid lines parallel to the MSP.

Film–Behind the patient, perpendicular to the MSP, centered to the CR.

CR–Angled 15 degrees cephalic, entering the patient at the MSP and halfway between the ASIS and the symphysis pubis.

AP COCCYX
(FIG. 6–68)

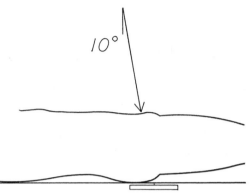

FIG. 6–68. AP coccyx.

Grid–Required. Grid lines parallel to the MSP.

Film–Behind the patient, perpendicular to the MSP, centered to the CR.

CR–Angled 10 degrees caudal, entering the patient at the MSP and 2 inches superior to the symphysis pubis.

 LATERAL SACRUM AND COCCYX
(FIG. 6–69)

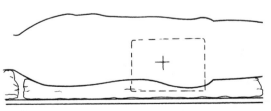

FIG. 6–69. Lateral sacrum and coccyx, patient recumbent.

Grid–Required. Grid lines parallel to the MSP.

Film–At the patient's side, parallel to the MSP. It is centered 3 to 4 inches posterior to the MAL and halfway between the crest and distal end of the coccyx (or halfway between the crest and symphysis pubis).

CR–Perpendicular to the film.

✳ AP SACROILIAC JOINTS

The reader is referred to AP L5-S1, earlier.

✳ OBLIQUE SACROILIAC JOINTS
(FIG. 6–70)

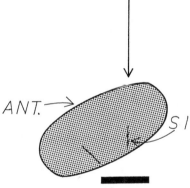

FIG. 6–70. Oblique sacroiliac joints (view from head of table).

Grid–Required. Grid lines parallel to the MSP.

Film–Behind the patient, 25 to 30 degrees from the MSP. It is centered 2 inches medial to the ASIS of the side farther from the film.

CR–Perpendicular to the film, entering the patient 2 inches medial to the ASIS of the side farther from the film.

Note–Both obliques (LPO and RPO) must be done.

TRAUMA RADIOGRAPHY OF THE UPPER EXTREMITIES

 HAND

 PA HAND

Grid–Not required.

Film–In contact with the anterior (palmar) side of the hand. Centered to the third metacarpophalangeal (MCP) joint. The fingers should be fully extended.

CR–Perpendicular to the film, entering at the third MCP joint.

 OBLIQUE HAND

Grid–Not required.

Film–Angled 45 degrees from the hand. The anterior (palmar) side of the hand faces the film. The medial (little finger) side of the hand is in contact with the film. The film is centered to the third MCP joint. To demonstrate interphalangeal (IP) joint spaces, the fingers should be extended (parallel) to the film.

CR–Perpendicular to the film, entering at the third MCP joint.

 LATERAL HAND (LATEROMEDIAL PROJECTION)

Grid–Not required.

Film–In contact with the medial side of the hand, perpendicular to the hand. The film is centered to the fifth MCP joint. The fingers may be separated and parallel to the film or extended (and superimposed). The thumb should be parallel to the film and not superimposed on the hand or fingers.

CR–Perpendicular to the film, entering at the second MCP joint.

Note–If a lateromedial projection cannot be used, a mediolateral projection will obtain similar results.

 ## PA FINGER

Grid–Not required.

Film–In contact with the anterior side of the finger, centered to the proximal IP joint. The finger should be extended and separated slightly from the other fingers and thumb.

CR–Perpendicular to the film, entering at the proximal IP joint.

 ## OBLIQUE FINGER

Grid–Not required.

Film–Positioned as for an oblique hand. The film is angled 45 degrees from the hand. The anterior side of the hand faces the film with the medial (little finger) edge touching the film. The finger should be parallel to the film, with the proximal IP joint centered. The finger should be separated slightly from the other finger and the thumb.

CR–Perpendicular to the film, entering at the proximal IP joint.

✳ LATERAL FINGER
(FIG. 6–71 MEDIOLATERAL PROJECTION)

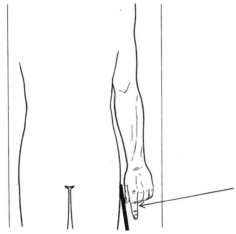

FIG. 6–71. Lateral index finger on an immobile patient (top view).

Grid–Not required.

Film–Perpendicular to the hand as close to the finger being examined as possible. The index and middle fingers will be mediolateral projections. The ring and little fingers will be lateromedial projections. The finger being examined should be extended and parallel to the film; the fingers not being examined should be flexed (the ring finger will probably need to be immobilized for it to remain extended). The proximal IP joint is centered.

CR–Perpendicular to the film entering at the proximal IP joint.

AP THUMB

Grid–Not required.

Film–In contact with the posterior side of the thumb (the hand is usually placed in extreme internal rotation). The thumb should be extended and the fingers should not be superimposed on it. The film is centered to the first MCP joint.

CR–Perpendicular to the film, entering at the first MCP joint.

OBLIQUE THUMB

Grid–Not required.

Film–In contact with the anterior side of the hand. The fingers should be extended and the hand positioned for a PA hand (the thumb will usually be positioned in a 45-degree oblique angle). Center to the first MCP joint.

CR–Perpendicular to the film, entering at the first MCP joint.

LATERAL THUMB (MEDIOLATERAL PROJECTION)

Grid–Not required.

Film–In contact with the anterior side of the hand. The fingers should be extended, and the hand should be positioned for a PA projection. The hand is rolled toward its lateral side until the lateral side of the thumb is touching the film. The film is centered to the first MCP joint.

CR–Perpendicular to the film, entering at the first MCP joint.

AP HAND AND FINGERS
(FIGS. 6-72, 6-73, AND 6-74)

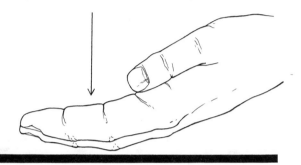

FIG. 6-72. AP hand for distal and middle phalanges.

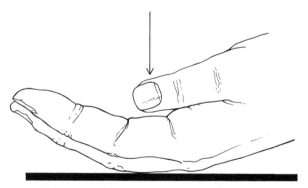

FIG. 6-73. AP hand for proximal phalanges.

Grid–Not required.

Film–Multiple projections may be needed when the fingers cannot be extended because of injury or bandages. The film is placed parallel to and centered on the area being examined.

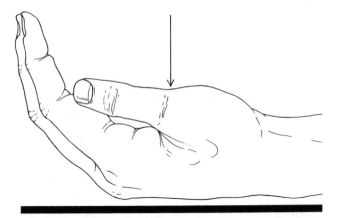

FIG. 6–74. AP hand to demonstrate metacarpals.

CR–Perpendicular to the film, entering the middle of the area being examined.

Note–These projections can serve as an initial, general survey of crushing injuries to the fingers and hand, especially when they are wrapped in large amounts of bandaging.

   If there is only a slight amount of flexion (less than 5 degrees), a single projection may be sufficient, inasmuch as the diverging beam will compensate for the angle.

PA HAND AND FINGERS (WITH A CURVED CASSETTE)
(FIG. 6–75)

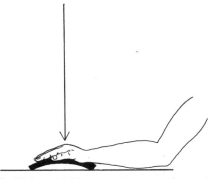

FIG. 6–75. PA hand with curved cassette for patients who cannot extend fingers or hand.

Grid–Not required.

Film–If a curved cassette is available and the patient's fingers cannot be extended, this position can be used instead of the usual PA hand or the AP hand and fingers position described earlier. The curved cassette is placed in contact with the anterior side of the hand, and the fingers are allowed to remain flexed. The film is centered to the third MCP joint.

CR–Perpendicular to film, entering at the third MCP joint.

Note–The curved cassette should be reloaded just before it is used. Curved cassettes are not used often and are sometimes left unloaded or have old, fogged film in them.

WRIST

 PA WRIST

Grid–Not required.

Film–In contact with the anterior side of the wrist centered to the middle of the wrist. The fingers may be flexed to reduce the object-to-image-receptor distance (OID).

CR–Perpendicular to the film, entering at the middle of the wrist.

 AP WRIST

Grid–Not required.

Film–In contact with the posterior side of the wrist, centered to the middle of the wrist. The wrist should not be flexed or extended.

CR–Perpendicular to the film, entering at the middle of the wrist.

Note–The AP projection is usually just a replacement for the PA projection when it cannot be obtained.

 OBLIQUE WRIST (SEMIPRONE)

Grid–Not required.

Film–Angled 45 degrees from the wrist. The anterior side of the wrist faces the film with the medial (little finger) side touching the film. The film is centered to the middle of the wrist.

CR–Perpendicular to the film, entering at the middle of the wrist.

OBLIQUE WRIST (SEMISUPINE)

Grid–Not required.

Film–Angled 45 degrees from the wrist. The posterior side of the wrist faces the film, usually with the medial (little finger) side touching the film. The film is centered to the middle of the wrist.

CR–Perpendicular to the film, entering at the middle of the wrist.

LATERAL WRIST (LATEROMEDIAL PROJECTION)

Grid–Not required.

Film–Perpendicular to the wrist, touching the medial side of the wrist. The film is centered to the middle of the wrist. The wrist should not be flexed or extended but form a continuous extension of the forearm.

CR–Perpendicular to the film, entering at the middle of the wrist.

Note–A mediolateral projection will produce similar results and can be used when a lateromedial projection cannot be obtained.

CARPAL NAVICULAR (STECHER METHOD)

Grid–Not required.

Film–In contact with the anterior side of the wrist (as if positioning for a PA wrist). It is centered to the carpal navicular (proximal row, lateral side).

CR–Angled 20 degrees toward the elbow entering at the carpal navicular.

Note–Some radiologists prefer this position to be done with the wrist in ulnar (medial) flexion.

LATERAL CARPAL BONES AND INTERSPACES (ULNAR OR MEDIAL FLEXION)

Grid–Not required.

Film–In contact with the anterior side of the wrist (as if positioning for a PA wrist). The wrist is placed in ulnar, or medial, flexion by the radiographer by holding the patient's forearm and hand and flexing the medial (little finger) side of the patient's hand toward the forearm. The wrist should not be flexed so much that it becomes oblique. The film is centered to the middle of the wrist.

CR–Perpendicular to the film, entering at the middle of the wrist.

MEDIAL CARPAL BONES AND INTERSPACES (RADIAL OR LATERAL FLEXION)

Grid–Not required.

Film–In contact with the anterior side of the wrist (as if positioning for a PA wrist). The wrist is placed in radial, or lateral, flexion by the radiographer by holding the patient's forearm and hand and flexing the lateral (thumb) side of the patient's hand toward the forearm. The film is centered to the middle of the wrist.

CR–Perpendicular to the film, entering at the middle of the wrist.

✳ FOREARM

✳ AP FOREARM

Grid–Not required.

Film–In contact with the posterior side of the forearm. The hand should be supinated so that the radius and ulna are not crossed. The film is centered halfway between the wrist and elbow (both of which should be included on the radiograph). To take advantage of the heel effect, the anode should be placed at the wrist.

CR–Perpendicular to the film, entering at the midshaft of the radius and ulna.

✳ LATERAL FOREARM
(FIG. 6–76)

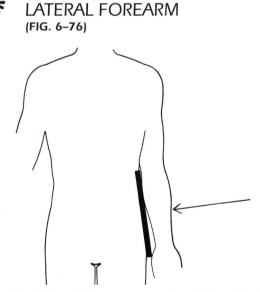

FIG. 6–76. Lateral forearm on an immobile patient (top view).

Grid–Not required.

Film–In contact with the medial side of the forearm. The film is centered halfway between the wrist and the elbow (both of which should be included on the radiograph). The hand should be extended and perpendicular to the film. The elbow should be flexed 90 degrees and in the same plane as the shoulder (so the humeral epicondyles are superimposed). To take advantage of heel effect, the anode should be placed at the wrist.

CR–Perpendicular to the film, entering at the midshaft of the radius and ulna.

Note–Figure 6–76 shows a HBP lateral forearm on a supine, immobile patient.

 ELBOW

 AP ELBOW

Grid–Not required.

Film–In contact with the posterior side of the elbow. The elbow should be fully extended (if it cannot be, see Substitute AP Elbow position and PA Elbow with Curved Cassette). The film should be the same distance from each humeral epicondyle to ensure a true AP elbow position. The film is centered to the middle of the elbow joint.

CR–Perpendicular to the film, entering at the middle of the elbow joint.

INTERNAL (MEDIAL) OBLIQUE ELBOW

Grid–Not required.

Film–In contact with the posterior and medial sides of the elbow. The elbow should be extended, and the humeral epicondyles should be 45 degrees from the film. The hand should be supinated. The film is centered to the middle of the elbow joint.

CR–Perpendicular to the film, entering at the middle of the elbow joint.

Note–Some radiologists may prefer the hand in pronation.

 ## EXTERNAL (LATERAL) OBLIQUE ELBOW

Grid–Not required.

Film–In contact with the posterior and lateral sides of the elbow. The elbow should be extended, and the humeral epicondyles should be 45 degrees from the film. The hand should be supinated. The film is centered to the middle of the elbow joint.

CR–Perpendicular to the film, entering at the middle of the elbow joint.

LATERAL ELBOW (LATEROMEDIAL PROJECTION)
(FIG. 6–77 MEDIOLATERAL PROJECTION)

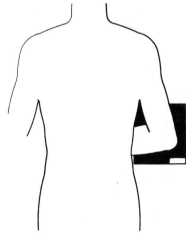

FIG. 6–77. Lateral elbow, patient upright facing the film.

Grid–Not required.

Film–In contact with the medial side of the elbow. The elbow should be flexed 90 degrees, and the film should be perpendicular to the humeral epicondyles. The film is centered to the middle of the elbow joint.

CR–Perpendicular to the film, entering at the middle of the elbow joint.

Note–Figure 6–77 shows a mediolateral projection on a standing patient unable to move the elbow or shoulder.

PROXIMAL FOREARM WITH ELBOW IN COMPLETE (ACUTE) FLEXION

Grid–Not required.

Film–In contact with the posterior side of the humerus. The elbow is completely flexed. The film is equidistant from (or parallel to) the humeral epicondyles. The film is also centered to the epicondyles. The hand should be supinated.

CR–Perpendicular to the forearm (not the film), entering at the epicondyles.

 # DISTAL HUMERUS WITH ELBOW IN COMPLETE FLEXION

Grid–Not required.

Film–In contact with the posterior side of the humerus. The elbow is completely flexed. The film is equidistant from (or parallel to) the humeral epicondyles. The film is also centered to the epicondyles.

CR–Perpendicular to the film, entering at the epicondyles.

NOTE–This position also demonstrates the olecranon process.

SUBSTITUTE AP ELBOW

This is to be used when the elbow cannot be fully extended (partial flexion elbow positions).

Note–The next two projections with the elbow partially flexed are needed to replace AP projection with the elbow fully extended.

 # SUBSTITUTE AP ELBOW FOR PROXIMAL FOREARM
(FIG. 6–78)

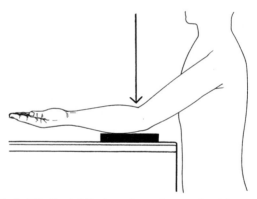

FIG. 6–78. Partial flexion elbow for proximal forearm.

Grid–Not required.

Film–In contact with the posterior forearm, centered to the elbow joint. The hand should be supinated.

CR–Perpendicular to the film, entering at the elbow joint.

SUBSTITUTE AP ELBOW FOR DISTAL HUMERUS
(FIG. 6–79)

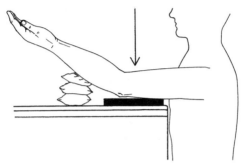

FIG. 6–79. Partial flexion elbow for distal humerus.

Grid–Not required.

Film–In contact with the posterior humerus, centered to the elbow joint. The forearm should be supported, if necessary. The hand should be supinated.

CR–Perpendicular to the film, entering at the elbow joint.

PA ELBOW WITH CURVED CASSETTE
(FIG. 6–80)

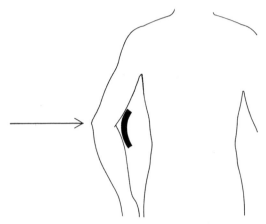

FIG. 6–80. PA elbow with curved cassette (top view).

This is a substitute AP elbow when the elbow cannot be fully extended.

Grid–Not required.

Film–A curved cassette is placed in contact with the anterior side of the elbow, centered to the elbow joint. The hand should be supinated.

CR–Perpendicular to the midpoint of the film, entering at the olecranon process.

Note–Curved cassettes are used infrequently and may be left unloaded or loaded with outdated film. To help reduce the need for repeat radiographs, it should be reloaded just before use.

HUMERUS

 ## AP HUMERUS

Grid–Not required unless arm is unusually large.

Film–In contact with the posterior side of the humerus. The film is equidistant from (or parallel to) the humeral epicondyles and centered halfway between the elbow and the shoulder. Both the elbow and the shoulder should be included in this projection; both must be included in the examination.

CR–Perpendicular to the film, entering at the midshaft of the humerus.

Note–Rotation of the arm with a suspected fracture of the distal third of the humerus is best done by a physician because of the danger of severing the radial nerve.

A PA projection of the humerus will yield similar results.

 ## LATERAL HUMERUS (LATEROMEDIAL PROJECTION)

Grid–Not required unless the arm is unusually large.

Film–In contact with the medial side of the humerus. This is usually accomplished by internal rotation of the humerus. When there is a suspected fracture of the distal third of the humerus, any rotation of the arm is best done by a physician, or the position for substitute lateral humerus for immobile patients (see below) may be used. The humeral epicondyles are superimposed (perpendicular to the film). The film is centered halfway between the elbow and the shoulder. Both the elbow and the shoulder should be included in this projection; both must be included in the examination.

CR–Perpendicular to the film, entering at the midshaft of the humerus.

✳ ## SUBSTITUTE LATERAL HUMERUS FOR IMMOBILE PATIENTS (LATEROMEDIAL PROJECTION) (FIG. 6–81)

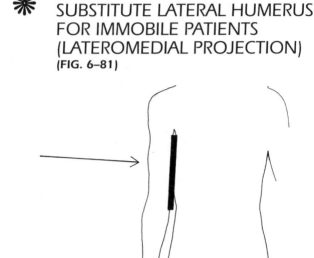

FIG. 6–81. Lateral humerus, distal end, on an immobile patient (top view).

Grid–Not required unless the arm is unusually large.

Film–The film is inserted between the patient's side and the humerus being examined until the top of the film is touching the axilla. The tube side of the cassette touches the medial side of the humerus. The film is positioned so that the humeral epicondyles will be superimposed (so that they are perpendicular to the film).

CR–Perpendicular to the film, entering at the midshaft of the humerus or to include the distal end of the humerus and the elbow joint.

Note–This position can be used to demonstrate the distal two thirds of the humerus when the patient is unable to rotate the arm or is otherwise immobile. This position may be submitted with a lateral proximal humerus. (Transthoracic mediolateral projection or a Y view of the shoulder for a complete demonstration of the humerus.)

 LATERAL PROXIMAL HUMERUS (TRANSTHORACIC, MEDIOLATERAL PROJECTION) (FIG. 6–82)

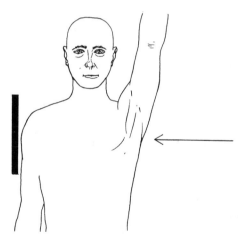

FIG. 6–82. Transthoracic lateral humerus.

Grid–Required. Grid lines parallel to the MSP.

Film–In contact with the side being examined, parallel to the MSP. It is centered to the surgical neck of the humerus. The arm of the side not being examined is fully abducted to prevent superimposition. If the patient is upright, the elbow may be flexed to rest the forearm on the top of the head. Respiration may be suspended, or a breathing technique may be used. Breathing technique requires that the patient breathes normally and uses a long exposure time.

CR–Perpendicular to the film, entering the axilla of the side not being examined and exiting the surgical neck of the humerus.

Note–This position may be submitted with a substitute lateral humerus for immobile patients to complete the demonstration of the upper arm, or it may be used alone to show shoulder dislocations.

SHOULDER

✳ AP SHOULDER, INTERNAL ROTATION

Grid–Required. Grid lines parallel to the MSP.

Film–With its long axis perpendicular to the MSP, it is in contact with the posterior side of the shoulder, parallel to the midcoronal plane. It is centered to the coracoid process. The humerus is placed in a lateral position (epicondyles superimposed). Respiration is suspended.

CR–Perpendicular to the film, entering the coracoid process.

AP SHOULDER, EXTERNAL ROTATION

Grid–Required. Grid lines parallel to the MSP.

Film–With its long axis perpendicular to the MSP, it is in contact with the posterior side of the shoulder, parallel to the midcoronal plane. It is centered to the coracoid process. The humerus is placed in an AP (or anatomic) position (epicondyles equidistant from the film). Respiration is suspended.

CR–Perpendicular to the film, entering the coracoid process.

Y VIEW OF THE SHOULDER

Grid–Required. Grid lines parallel to the MSP.

Film–With its long axis parallel to the MSP, it is in contact with the anterior or lateral side of the humerus, perpendicular to the body of the scapula, and is centered to the middle of the scapula. If the patient is upright, he or she is facing the film in an oblique position, with the side being examined touching the film and the MSP 30 degrees from the film (or the MCP 60 degrees from the film). The humerus is allowed to rest at the patient's side.

CR–Perpendicular to the film, entering at the medial border of the scapula.

Note–This position is a good substitute for the transthoracic lateral humerus position. The ribs are not superimposed on the humerus, and it gives an excellent demonstration of humeral dislocations.

This position should be used to demonstrate the proximal humeri when both are injured and cannot be rotated for a conventional lateral or raised for a transthoracic lateral humerus.

When used with a substitute lateral humerus for immobile patients, it provides a complete demonstration of the part.

This position may be reversed but will result in magnification unless the SID and, consequently, the MAS are increased. The side being examined is away from the film when the position is reversed.

 ## SCAPULA

 ## AP SCAPULA

Grid–Required. Grid lines parallel to the MSP.

Film–In contact with the posterior side of the patient, parallel to the midcoronal plane. It is centered to middle of the scapula. The arm of the side being examined is abducted until it is 90 degrees from the body (the elbow is usually flexed for patient comfort). Respiration is suspended.

CR–Perpendicular to the film, entering approximately at the coracoid process.

 ## OBLIQUE SCAPULA

Grid–Required. Grid lines parallel to the MSP.

Film–At the anterior or posterior side of the patient, 30 degrees from the midcoronal plane. It is centered to the middle of the scapula. The arm or the side being examined is abducted and the elbow flexed so that the forearm is touching the forehead. Respiration is suspended.

CR–Perpendicular to the film, centered to the middle of the film.

LATERAL SCAPULA
(MEDIOLATERAL PROJECTION)

Grid–Required. Grid lines parallel to the MSP.

Film–Perpendicular to the body of the scapula, centered to the scapula. The arm of the side being examined is brought across the chest, and the hand grasps the opposite shoulder. Respiration is suspended.

CR–Perpendicular to the film, entering at the middle of the scapula between the medial border at the thoracic spine.

CLAVICLE

PA CLAVICLE

Grid–Recommended, grid lines perpendicular to the MSP.

Film–With the long axis of the film parallel to the long axis of the clavicle, it is placed in contact with the anterior side of the patient. It is centered to the clavicle and placed parallel to the midcoronal plane. Respiration is suspended.

CR–Perpendicular to the film and centered to the film.

AP CLAVICLE

Grid–Recommended, grid lines perpendicular to the MSP.

Film–With the long axis of the film parallel to the long axis of the clavicle, it is placed in contact with the posterior side of the patient. It is centered to the clavicle and placed parallel to the midcoronal plane. Respiration is suspended.

CR–Perpendicular to the film, entering at the midshaft of the clavicle.

 ## PA SEMIAXIAL CLAVICLE

Grid–Recommended, grid lines parallel to the MSP.

Film–In contact with the anterior side of the patient, centered to the midshaft of the clavicle. It is parallel to the midcoronal plane. Respiration is suspended.

CR–Angled 25 to 30 degrees caudal, entering at the midshaft of the clavicle. The film is adjusted so that it is centered to the exiting CR.

 ## AP SEMIAXIAL CLAVICLE

Grid–Recommended, grid lines parallel to the MSP.

Film–In contact with the posterior side of the patient, centered to the midshaft of the clavicle. It is parallel to the midcoronal plane. Respiration is suspended.

CR–Angled 25 to 30 degrees cephalic, entering at the midshaft of the clavicle. The film is adjusted so that it is centered to the exiting CR.

TRAUMA RADIOGRAPHY OF THE LOWER EXTREMITIES

 FOOT

 ## AP TOES

Grid–Not required.

Film–In contact with the plantar surface of the foot, centered to the middle of the toes (usually the second metatarsal phalangeal joint).

CR–Perpendicular to the film.

 ## AP TOES FOR INTERPHALANGEAL JOINT SPACES

Grid–Not required.

Film–In contact with the plantar surface of the foot, centered to the middle of the toes (usually the second metatarsal phalangeal joint).

CR–Angled 15 degrees from perpendicular (75 degrees from the film) toward the heel (cephalad).

OBLIQUE TOES
(FIG. 6–83)

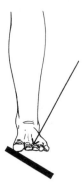

FIG. 6–83. Oblique foot on an immobile patient (top view).

Grid–Not required.

Film–Initially, touching the plantar surface of the foot. With the medial (great toe) side of the foot touching the film, it is placed 30 degrees from the plantar surface of the foot.

CR–Perpendicular to the film.

LATERAL TOE (MEDIOLATERAL OR LATEROMEDIAL PROJECTION)

Grid–Not required.

Film–Perpendicular to the plantar surface of the foot in contact with the medial or lateral side of the foot (similar to Fig. 6–85). For the great toe and second toe, the film is in contact with the medial side of the foot. For the fourth and fifth toes, the film touches the lateral side of the foot. For the third toe, the film should be placed closest to the toe. If possible, separate the toe being examined from the others.

CR–Perpendicular to the film.

✳ AP FOOT
(FIG. 6–84)

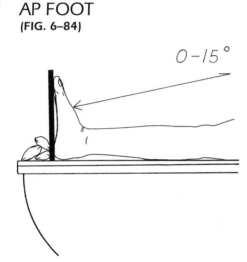

$O - 15°$

FIG. 6–84. *AP foot on an immobile patient.*

Grid–Not required.

Film–In contact with the plantar surface of the foot, centered to the base (proximal end) of the third metatarsal.

CR–Perpendicular to the film, or angled up to 15 degrees toward the heel (cephalad), according to the physician's preference. The CR enters at the base (proximal end) of the third metatarsal.

OBLIQUE FOOT

Grid–Not required.

Film–Initially, touching the plantar surface of the foot. The film is then placed at a 30-degree angle to the plantar surface of the foot (similar to Fig. 6–83). The film is centered to the middle of the foot at a level of the base of the fifth metatarsal (located by palpating to tuberosity at the base of the fifth metatarsal).

CR–Perpendicular to the film, entering at a level of the base of the fifth metatarsal, halfway between the medial and lateral sides of the foot.

 # LATERAL FOOT (LATEROMEDIAL AND MEDIOLATERAL PROJECTIONS) (FIG. 6–85)

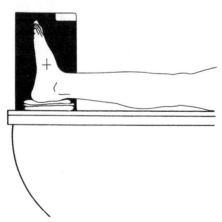

FIG. 6–85. Lateral foot on an immobile patient.

Grid–Not required.

Film–Perpendicular to the plantar surface of the foot, centered halfway between the toes and the heel and halfway between the dorsal (anterior) and plantar (posterior) sides of the foot. The film touches the medial side of the foot for a lateromedial projection, or the lateral side for a mediolateral projection. If possible, flex the ankle 90 degrees.

CR–Perpendicular to the film, entering the middle of the foot.

✳ STANDING (WEIGHT-BEARING)
HBP LATERAL FOOT
(LATEROMEDIAL PROJECTION)
(FIG. 6–86)

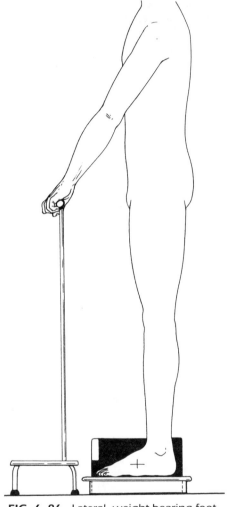

FIG. 6–86. Lateral, weight-bearing foot.

Grid–Not required.

Film–Positioned as for a lateral foot (see previous position) except that the patient is standing with his or her weight equally distributed on both feet. The patient must stand on a flat, rigid surface that allows the bottom of the cassette to be placed lower than the bottom of the foot. Also, many radiography tubes cannot be lowered to the floor. The patient may have to stand on a stool or the radiographic table. In these cases, the patient must be given secure support (e.g., a long-handled stool placed on the radiographic table).

CR–Horizontal and perpendicular to the film, entering the middle of the foot.

 ## LATERAL CALCANEUS (MEDIOLATERAL AND LATEROMEDIAL PROJECTIONS)

Grid–Not required.

Film–In contact with the lateral side of the foot for a mediolateral projection; in contact with the medial side of the foot for an anteromedial projection (on immobile patients and HBPs the lateromedial projection is usually used). The film is perpendicular to the plantar side of the foot, centered 1½ inches inferior to the malleoli. The ankle should be flexed 90 degrees.

CR–Perpendicular to the film, entering 1½ inches inferior to the malleoli.

Note–If the ankle cannot be flexed 90 degrees, similar results can be obtained by maintaining the 40-degree angle between the plantar surface of the foot and the CR (but ignoring the usual 50-degree angle between the CR and the film).

AXIAL CALCANEUS
(FIG. 6–87)

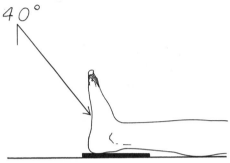

FIG. 6–87. Axial calcaneus.

Grid–Not required.

Film–In contact with the posterior side of the ankle, centered to the ankle joint (halfway between the malleoli). The ankle should be flexed 90 degrees. The film is then perpendicular to the plantar side of the foot and the medial and lateral sides of the foot.

CR–Angled 40 degrees cephalic from the plantar surface of the film (or 50 degrees from the film). The CR enters the middle of the calcaneus at a level of the base of the fifth metatarsal (located by palpating the tuberosity of the fifth metatarsal).

 ## ANKLE

 ## AP ANKLE

Grid–Not required.

Film–In contact with the posterior side of the ankle, centered to the ankle joint (halfway between the malleoli). The ankle is flexed 90 degrees to prevent the ankle joint from being projected onto the calcaneus. The film is then perpendicular to the plantar side of the foot, and the medial and lateral sides of the foot.

CR–Perpendicular to the film, entering halfway between the malleoli.

 ## OBLIQUE ANKLE

Grid–Not required.

Film–In contact with the posterior or medial portion of the ankle, centered to the middle of the ankle joint (halfway between the malleoli). The ankle is flexed 90 degrees, and the film is about 45 degrees from the foot (a plane passing through the malleoli should be parallel to the film).

CR–Perpendicular to the film, entering at the middle of the ankle joint.

 ## LATERAL ANKLE (MEDIOLATERAL PROJECTION)
(FIG. 6–88 LATEROMEDIAL PROJECTION)

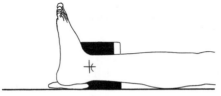

FIG. 6–88. Lateral ankle on an immobile patient.

Grid–Not required.

Film–In contact with the lateral side of the ankle, centered to the ankle joint. The ankle is flexed 90 degrees, and the film is perpendicular to the plantar surface of the foot. The film is also perpendicular to the patella.

CR–Perpendicular to the film, entering at the middle of the ankle joint.

Note–For immobile patients, a lateromedial HBP is used (Fig. 6–88).

AP ANKLE FOR
THE ANKLE MORTICE

Grid–Not required.

Film–In contact with the posterior side of the ankle, centered halfway between the malleoli. The ankle is flexed 90 degrees, and the film is then perpendicular to the plantar surface of the film. The foot is inverted 5 to 15 degrees to show the tibial-talar articulation unobstructed.

CR–Perpendicular to the film.

LOWER LEG

AP LOWER LEG

Grid–Not required.

Film–In contact with the posterior side of the lower leg, centered to the middle of the lower leg and halfway between the knee and the ankle (both of which must be included in the examination). The ankle is flexed 90 degrees. The film is perpendicular to the foot. The knee is fully extended.

CR–Perpendicular to the film, entering midshaft of the lower leg.

LATERAL LOWER LEG (MEDIOLATERAL PROJECTION)

Grid–Not required.

Film–In contact with the lateral side of the lower leg, centered to the middle of the leg and halfway between the knee and the ankle (both of which must be included in the examination). The film is perpendicular to the patella. The ankle is flexed 90 degrees, and the knee is fully extended.

CR–Perpendicular to the film, entering midshaft of the lower leg.

Note–For immobile patients a lateromedial HBP is used.

 KNEE

 # AP KNEE

Grid–Not required for knees smaller than 10 cm (4 inches). Recommended for knees larger than 10 cm.

Film–In contact with the posterior side of the knee, centered to the knee joint (½ inch inferior to the apex of the patella). The film is perpendicular to the foot (because lower extremity rotation occurs in the hip joint, if the film is perpendicular to the foot, the extremity is positioned for an AP projection). The knee should be fully extended. If the knee is flexed, a curved cassette may be used, and a PA knee, or partial flexion knee position may be substituted (see later).

CR–Perpendicular to the film, entering ½ inch inferior to the apex of the patella. For demonstration of the knee joint space, the CR may be angled 5 degrees cephalic.

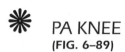

PA KNEE
(FIG. 6–89)

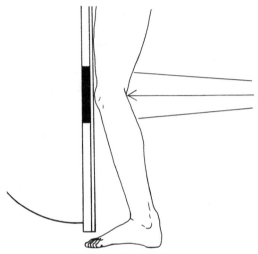

FIG. 6–89. PA knee.

Grid–Not required for knees smaller than 10 cm (4 inches). Recommended for knees larger than 10 cm.

Film–In contact with anterior surface of the knee, centered to the knee joint (½ inch inferior to the patellar apex). The film is parallel to a plane passing through the femoral condyles.

CR–Perpendicular to the film, entering the back of the knee and exiting ½ inch inferior to the patellar apex.

Note–This position is mainly used when the patient's knee cannot be fully extended and a curved cassette is not available. The divergence of the CR makes knees with 7 to 8 degrees of flexion appear similar to a fully extended AP knee. Knees flexed more than 8 degrees will demonstrate progressively more distortion.

Partial flexion knee positions may be substituted for a PA knee.

✳ PARTIAL FLEXION PA KNEE POSITIONS
(FIGS. 6–90 AND 6–91)

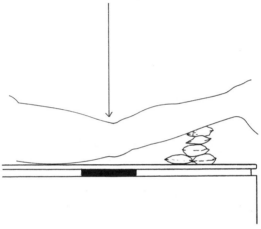

FIG. 6–90. Partial flexion knee for distal femur.

Grid–Not required for knees smaller than 10 cm (4 inches). Recommended for knees larger than 10 cm.

Film–Two exposures are required to replace the AP knee when the patient's knee is partially flexed (and cannot be extended). The knee must be flexed less than 90 degrees for complete demonstration of the distal femur and proximal lower leg. The patient is best examined in a lateral recumbent or prone position. The first exposure is made with the film in contact with anterior side of the thigh, parallel to the femoral condyles and centered to the knee joint (½ inch inferior to the patellar apex) (Fig. 6–90). The second exposure is made with the film in contact with the anterior side of the lower

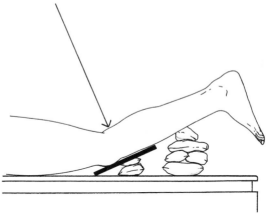

FIG. 6–91. Partial flexion knee for proximal lower leg.

leg, parallel to the femoral condyles and centered to the knee joint. This may require that the femur be supported on sponges (Fig. 6–91).

CR–For both exposures the CR is perpendicular to the film.

 ## INTERNAL (MEDIAL) OBLIQUE KNEE

Grid–Not required for knees smaller than 10 cm (4 inches). Recommended for knees larger than 10 cm.

Film–In contact with the posteromedial aspect of the knee, centered to the knee joint (½ inch inferior to the apex of the patella). The film is at a 45-degree angle to a plane passing through both femoral condyles. The knee should be extended.

CR–Perpendicular to the film, entering at the knee joint.

Note–This position is important in the demonstration of intra-articular fractures and tibial plateau fractures.

EXTERNAL (LATERAL) OBLIQUE KNEE

Grid–Not required for knees smaller than 10 cm (4 inches). Recommended for knees larger than 10 cm.

Film–In contact with the posterolateral aspect of the knee, centered to the knee joint (½ inch inferior to the apex of the patella). The film is at a 45-degree angle to a plane passing through both femoral condyles. The knee should be extended.

CR–Perpendicular to the film, entering at the knee joint.

Note–This position is important in the demonstration of intra-articular fractures and tibial plateau fractures.

 # LATERAL KNEE (MEDIOLATERAL PROJECTION)
(FIG. 6–92 LATEROMEDIAL PROJECTION)

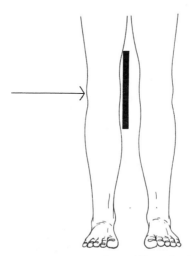

FIG. 6–92. Lateral knee on an immobile patient (top view).

Grid–Not required for knees smaller than 10 cm (4 inches). Recommended for knees larger than 10 cm.

Film–In contact with the lateral side of the knee, perpendicular to the patella, centered to the knee joint (½ inch inferior to the apex of the patella). The knee is usually flexed up to 45 degrees, unless there is a possibility of a transverse fracture of the patella.

CR–Perpendicular to the film, entering at the knee joint.

Note–HBP lateral knees are usually lateromedial projections (Fig. 6–92).

✳ PA PATELLA
(FIG. 6–93)

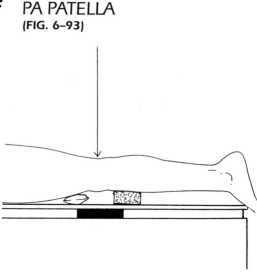

FIG. 6–93. PA patella.

Grid–Recommended if knee is larger than 10 cm.

Film–In contact with the anterior side of the knee, parallel to the patella and centered to the middle of the patella. The knee is extended.

CR–Perpendicular to the film, exiting the middle of the patella.

Note–If the patient is prone, it may be too painful for the patella to touch the film. If this is the case, supports should be placed above and below the patella.

An AP patella may be substituted for the PA on immobile patients.

 ## LATERAL PATELLA (MEDIOLATERAL PROJECTION)

Grid–Not required.

Film–In contact with the lateral side of the knee, centered to the patella and perpendicular to the patella. The knee must *not* be flexed until the possibility of a transverse fracture of the patella has been ruled out.

CR–Perpendicular to the film, entering at the center of the patella.

Note–HBP lateral patellas are usually lateromedial projections (similar to Fig. 6–92).

AXIAL PATELLA (SETTEGAST METHOD)
(FIG. 6–94)

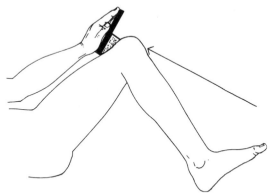

FIG. 6–94. Inferosuperior projection, axial patella.

Note–This position requires the knee to be flexed. Do *not* flex the knee until the possibility of a transverse fracture of the patella has been ruled out from a PA (or AP) patella, or a lateral patella, or both.

Grid–Not required.

Film–In contact with the anterior side of the thigh, centered to the patella. The knee is flexed as much as possible, or until the patella is perpendicular to the film. If the knee can be only slightly flexed, the film is supported perpendicular to the patella.

CR–Parallel to the patella (which should also mean perpendicular to the film), entering the retropatellar space (the space between the posterior side of the patella and the femur).

FEMUR

 AP FEMUR

Grid–Required. Grid strips parallel to the femur.

Film–In contact with the posterior side of the thigh, centered to the midshaft of the femur. If possible, the foot should be inverted 15 degrees to place the femoral neck parallel to the film.

CR–Perpendicular to the film, entering halfway between the knee and the hip joints, both of which must be included in the examination.

Note–If the femur is too long to be included on one film, include the joint nearest to the point of interest on the long film and make a separate exposure of the other joint.

 LATERAL FEMUR (MEDIOLATERAL PROJECTION)

Grid–Required. Grid strips parallel to the femur.

Film–In contact with the lateral side of the femur. Center the film to the midshaft of the femur or, because it is rare to be able to include both joints on a lateral femur, place the bottom of the film 2 inches below the knee joint. The film is perpendicular to the patella.

CR–Perpendicular to the film.

Note–The proximal femur is not usually seen on the lateral femur projection, so an inferosuperior hip projection may be needed.

BP radiographs on immobile patients are usually lateromedial projections.

HIP AND PELVIS

 AP HIP

Grid–Required. Grid strips parallel to the MSP.

Film–In contact with the posterior side of the hip, parallel to the midcoronal plane. The film is centered 2 inches medial to the ASIS of the side being examined and at the level of the greater trochanter. If possible, invert the toes 15 degrees to place the femoral neck parallel to the film.

CR–Perpendicular to the film, entering 2 inches medial to the ASIS of the side being examined at the level of the greater trochanter.

INFEROSUPERIOR PROJECTION OF THE FEMORAL NECK FOR TRAUMA PATIENTS (DANELIUS-MILLER MODIFICATION OF THE LORENZ METHOD)
(FIG. 6–95)

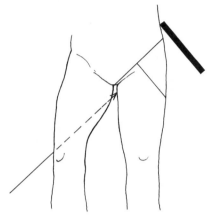

FIG. 6–95. Danelius-Miller modification of the Lorenz method for femoral neck on a trauma patient (top view).

Grid–Required. Grid strips are horizontal.

Film–The top of the film touches the patient at the iliac crest and is parallel to the femoral neck. Instructions for placing the film follow:

1. Carefully place support under the pelvis so that the patient is about 2 inches above the table top.
2. Draw an imaginary line from the ASIS of the side being examined to the symphysis pubis.
3. Find the midpoint of this line.
4. Draw a second imaginary line from the midpoint of the first line to a point 1 inch inferior to the greater

trochanter of the side being examined. This is the angle of the femoral neck.

5. Place the film perpendicular to the table, parallel to the second line.

CR–Perpendicular to film through the femoral neck. The knee and hip of the side *not* being examined must be flexed so that the leg does not interfere with the x-ray beam.

Note–Because of the required flexion of the uninjured leg, this position cannot be used when the patient has bilateral femoral neck injuries or problems. See the following position.

 ## INFEROSUPERIOR PROJECTION OF THE FEMORAL NECKS (CLEMENTS-NAKAYAMA MODIFICATION)
(FIG. 6–96)

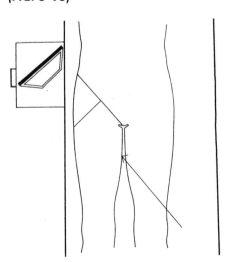

FIG. 6–96. Clements-Nakayama method for femoral neck on a trauma patient.

This is a modification of the Danelius-Miller modification of the Lorenz method.

Grid–Required. Grid strips are horizontal.

Film–The patient must be near the side of the table. The film should be placed vertically in the Bucky tray (or on the image intensifier ledge). It is then placed parallel to the femoral necks, using the 5-step method from the inferosuperior projection of the femoral necks listed earlier. Then the top of the film is tilted away from the patient until it is 75 degrees from the Bucky tray.

CR–Perpendicular to the film, passing through the femoral neck (this will require the CR to be placed first horizontal, then angled 15 degrees toward the floor, and then placed perpendicular to the film).

 # AP PELVIS

Grid–Required. Grid strips are perpendicular to the MSP.

Film–In contact with the posterior side of the patient. The top of the film is placed 1½ inches above the crest, parallel to the midcoronal plane. The feet should be inverted 15 degrees to place the femoral necks parallel to the film.

CR–Perpendicular to the film, centered to the middle of the film.

Note–Pelvis fracture fragments can easily damage the internal organs of the lower abdomen, especially the urinary bladder. Extra caution should be taken when moving these patients.

OBLIQUE PELVIS FOR ANTERIOR ACETABULAR COLUMN

Note–This position demonstrates the ilium and anterior (or iliopubic) column of the acetabulum. It may not be suitable for severely injured patients.

Grid–Required. Grid lines are perpendicular to the MSP.

Film–In contact with the posterior side of the pelvis that is being examined. It is angled 40 to 55 degrees from the MSP, or until it is perpendicular to the ilium of the side *not* being examined. The film is centered halfway between the crest and the greater trochanter (which is at the same level as the symphysis pubis) of the side touching the film.

CR–Perpendicular to the film, entering the anterior side of the pelvis halfway between the crest and the greater trochanter of the side touching the film.

OBLIQUE PELVIS FOR POSTERIOR ACETABULAR COLUMN

Note–This position demonstrates the ilium perpendicular to the film and the posterior (or ilioischial) column of the acetabulum. It may not be suitable for severely injured patients.

Grid–Required. Grid lines are perpendicular to the MSP.

Film–In contact with the posterior side of the pelvis. It is angled 40 to 55 degrees from the MSP, or until the ilium of the side being examined is perpendicular to the film. The film is centered on the ileum that is perpendicular (and farthest) from the film.

CR–Perpendicular to the film, entering the anterior side of the pelvis at the ASIS of the side farthest from the film.

 ## AP SEMIAXIAL ISCHIAL AND PUBIC RAMI (TAYLOR METHOD)

Grid–Required. Grid lines are parallel to the MSP.

Film–In contact with the posterior side of the pelvis, perpendicular to the MSP. The film is centered to the crest.

CR–Angled 25 degrees cephalic for men and 40 degrees cephalic for women. It enters 2 inches inferior to the most anterior part of the symphysis pubis (which is at the same level as the greater trochanter).

▨ ▨ IMPROVISING

In trauma, anything can happen. Therefore, it is impossible to list a radiographic position to cover every situation. This brings the chapter full circle; it began with basic principles, and it also ends with them.

A trauma situation that does not conform to traditional positions is simply a problem in need of a solution. To solve the problem, radiographers should start with the five basic principles of positioning explained at the beginning of this chapter. These principles not only provide insight into how positions were established but also form the basis for creating new ones. A method for solving problems and advanced considerations in forming new positions will also be needed.

▨ PROBLEM SOLVING

When trying to solve a problem (such as how to position a patient in a unique situation), it is better to have a system rather than to try random solutions. The general system presented here could be applied to any situation.

1. Define the problem. What are the constraints or limitations? Why did the usual solutions not work?
2. List alternatives. List all the possibilities without judging them. List the opposite for each—many problems that cannot be solved in one way can be solved by turning them 180 degrees.
3. Evaluate each. Look for things that would make a solution work or would prevent it from working.
4. Select the best one and try it.
5. Critique the results. If it worked, make a note of it. If it did not work, find out why, re-evaluate the method or the remaining alternatives, and try again.

When solving a radiographic positioning problem, the radiographer's knowledge of anatomy plays a key role. The radiographer should be able to visualize the structures in their normal and traumatically altered positions. There may be times when this is impossible, and a couple of scout radiographs may be needed to help define the problem. Other general considerations for developing new positions are the relationships between the part, film, and CR. Will part rotation solve the problem? (Then ask, can the patient move?) Will CR angulation demonstrate the area? Is tilting the film a possibility? And, of course, will a combination of these ideas work? Beyond these generalities there are many specific factors to be concerned with.

■ CONSIDERATIONS

The number of factors to consider when improvising a position may seem overwhelming. However, ignoring them can doom the radiographer's efforts to failure, waste valuable time, and expose the patient to needless radiation and stress. The best way to manage this task is to take each factor into account and to standardize as many of them as possible. For example, unless the situation prevents it, keep the SID to one of the common amounts—40 inches or 72 inches. Another example is the OID. Keep this to a minimum by having the film in contact with the part, and thus magnification can be eliminated as a problem. This process—of standardizing or eliminating as many factors as the problem allows—reduces the variables to a reasonable number and also helps define the problem. With practice and experience, improvisations can be made quickly and accurately.

The specific positioning considerations have been divided into factors concerning the x-ray tube, factors affecting the part, factors affecting the film, and technic and miscellaneous factors. Along with standardizing as many factors as possible, dividing the factors into four groups should improve their manageability.

TUBE FACTORS

Central Ray (CR) Angle

Any angle between the CR and the part or film will create some distortion. This is often offset by the ability of the CR angulation to avoid projecting objects on the area of interest. The optimum projection is obtained when the CR is perpendicular to the part and film. The projection becomes progressively more distorted as the CR is angled away from perpendicular to the film. Figure 6–97 shows how to calculate the needed CR angle to avoid superimposition of an unwanted structure (in this case it is the spine).

Source-to-Image-Receptor Distance (SID)

The shorter the SID, the greater the amount of magnification and density. SID should be standardized to 40 inches (100 cm) or 72 inches (180 cm). When the OID (see later section on film factors) is unusually large, an increase in SID can reduce the magnification. Magnification can be calculated by the following formula:

$$\frac{\text{SID}}{\text{SOD}} = \text{magnification}$$

where:

SOD = Source-to-Object Distance.

This can be calculated by SID − OID = SOD. The optimum magnification value is 1. The greater the answer is above 1, the greater the magnification.

Centering

The beam should be centered to the middle of the part, halfway between two joints, or on the area of interest or injury.

Edge Rays

The farther a part is from the CR, the greater the distortion, because the beam diverges (spreads out in a cone) from the source. When the CR is perpendicular to the film, only the rays at the center of the beam are perpendicular to the film. The farther from the CR the rays are, the greater their angle. Table 6–2 shows the angle of the rays from the perpendicular CR to the edge of the film when the SID is 40 inches.

TABLE 6–2. RAY ANGLE FROM PERPENDICULAR CR WHEN SID IS 40 INCHES

Film Size	Inches from CR	Degrees Angled
8 × 10	4	5.7
	5	7.1
10 × 12	5	7.1
	6	8.5
11 × 14	5.5	7.8
	7	9.9
14 × 17	7	9.9
	8.5	12

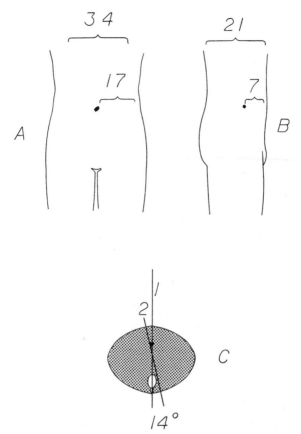

FIG. 6–97. (A) An object lies in the midline 17 cm from the patient's side and (B) 7 cm from the patient's anterior surface. (C) The situation is drawn to scale in a cross-sectional view in order to calculate the CR angle, or amount or part rotation, needed to avoid superimposition. If the spine is 5 cm wide, a 14-degree angle or rotation is needed. This is determined by measuring the angle between the MSP (1) and a line from the object past the width of the spine (2).

Minimum and Maximum Effective Focal Spot Sizes

The shorter the SID, the larger the effective focal spot size appears. Therefore, unsharpness will increase. Also, the effective focal spot will appear larger on the cathode side of the tube than on the anode side. Effective focal spot sizes can be considered normal when the SID is near 40 inches.

Anode and Cathode Placement

Because of the heel effect, there is more radiation at the cathode end of the tube than at the anode end. If one side of the part is thicker or denser than the other, the cathode should be placed at the thicker end. However, the heel effect is reduced as the SID increases and as the film size decreases.

Collimation

Reducing the area being exposed reduces patient dose, reduces the amount of scatter generated, reduces density, and produces higher contrast (shorter scale). Collimation should be to the film size or smaller.

▓ PART FACTORS

Patient Position

Determine whether the patient is mobile or immobile (through observation and the patient's history). Determine whether he or she must be supine, or can turn to prone or lateral recumbent. Determine whether the patient can sit or stand, with or without support.

Part Movement

Determine whether or not the patient can move the part to be examined. Can the patient flex, abduct, or rotate the part so that 2 projections, 90 degrees apart, can be made?

Length

Determine the size of the area to be radiographed. Long bones must include both joints on all projections in the examination but not necessarily on the same film. For example, the lower leg is being examined. The injury is near the ankle, and the leg is too long to fit on a 14 × 17 (35 × 43) even if it is placed diagonally. An AP and lateral lower leg to include the ankle should be done on a 14 × 17 (35 × 43), and separate AP and lateral knee projections should be made on 8 × 10s (18 × 24).

Shape

If the part has been distorted by the injury, modifications may be needed.

Interfering Objects

Are there any anatomic structures or medical support devices that will be superimposed on the area of interest? Determine whether the part can be rotated or moved away from the object or structure. If the part or patient cannot be moved, determine whether or not angling the CR will help. If so, use the smallest angle necessary. If the object is still superimposed, determine whether tilting the film will help.

Part Thickness and Tissue Density

If the projection is atypical, or if the part is swollen or distorted, standard technics may not work. Approximate the required MAS and KV by comparing the size and density of the new projection with the size and density of standard projections. For example, if the thickness the beam must traverse for a broken, swollen, and distorted elbow is about the same as an AP knee, use the knee technic. If that size knee would normally require the use of grid, a grid should also be employed for the elbow (increasing the part thickness and density creates more scatter and requires more KV for penetration, which also creates more scatter—hence the need for a grid).

▓ FILM FACTORS

Object-to-Image-Receptor Distance (OID)

This should be kept to a minimum. The greater the OID, the greater the magnification (see SID under Tube Factors).

Cassette Edge

The film does not extend to the cassette edge. It stops about ½ to 1 inch before the edge. If a part is at the edge of the cassette, it will not be recorded on the film. The edge of the cassette must be beyond or below the edge of the area being examined.

Film Angle in Relation to the Part and CR

Any angle between the film and part, or the film and CR, will create distortion. At times, such as obtaining (oblique projections), this is unavoidable. Film angle may be used to compensate for an immobile part or to avoid interfering objects.

ID Blockers and Markers

The film should be positioned so that the ID blockers do not interfere with the area of interest. Lead markers should not be placed where they will interfere with any structures.

Grid

The larger and denser the part, and the higher the KV, the greater the amount of scatter generated. If a grid is to be used, it must be carefully positioned. If the long edges are not equidistant from the tube, grid cutoff at the edges of the film will result. The CR can be angled toward only the short ends of the grid. Also, the higher the grid ratio, the better it will absorb scatter, but it will also tolerate less tilting of the long edges (it will also need more MAS and give more patient dose than a lower ratio grid). If the grid ratio remains constant, increasing the grid frequency (the number of lead strips per inch or centimeter) will reduce its ability to absorb scatter. Grid ratio is actually a measure of the *space* between grid strips. If the space and grid ratio remains the same but more strips are added per inch, the only choice is to make each one thinner. With thinner strips, there is less scatter removed. However, if more strips of the same width are added, then the space must get smaller and the grid ratio must increase.

▦ TECHNIC AND OTHER FACTORS

Density

Estimate the required density by comparing technics for standard projections to the new projection. Increasing MA (milliamperage), time, KV, screen speed, field size, and grid frequency (with constant grid ratio) will result in increased radiographic density. Increasing SID, part thickness, tissue density, grid frequency (with a changing grid ratio), and OID, and decreasing field size will decrease radiographic density.

Contrast

Most radiographs should have a medium scale of contrast (i.e., contrast that demonstrates structures in all areas of the part). Some soft tissue should be seen as well as bone details. The chest (for lungs) should have a long scale of contrast. Ribs, zygomatic arches, oblique sternums, KUBs, and foreign body studies should have a shorter scale of contrast. Increasing KV, scatter, and field size gives a longer scale of contrast. Using a grid and increasing OID and grid ratio gives a shorter scale of contrast.

MA and Time

Select the highest MA and shortest time possible to reduce motion unsharpness.

KV

Increasing KV increases penetration and density, creates more scatter, and gives longer scale contrast. When using a grid, the higher the KV, the higher the grid ratio should be. Also, increasing KV reduces patient skin dose and dose within the x-ray field, but it increases the dose to organs just outside the field because of additional scatter. If the organs in the field are more radio resistant than those outside the field, then raising the KV solely to affect patient dose may be counterproductive.

Scatter

If the KV cannot be reduced to decrease scatter, a higher ratio grid, smaller field size, lead absorbers placed just outside the x-ray field, and increasing the OID can be used. However, using a higher ratio grid will require an increase in MAS, which will increase patient dose. The field size can be reduced only so much, and increasing the OID will cause magnification or require an increase in SID (which will reduce density, requiring an increase in MAS, which might lengthen the time and cause more motion unsharpness).

Compensation Filters

If there is a large difference between the tissue density or thickness of a part, a compensating filter may be placed so that the thicker end of the filter is over the thinner end of the part.

Immobilization

Immobilize the patient, part, and film to reduce motion unsharpness and to support the part and film. Use only radiolucent objects. Avoid pillows, because many have metal zippers and stuffing that is radiopaque. Sandbags and folded sheets and pillowcases can be used for support but should not be placed over the area being examined.

Respiration

Suspend respiration when radiographing the chest and abdomen or when the patient's breathing will produce motion on the radiograph.

Shielding

Even in urgent situations the patient (and anyone else in the area) should be shielded. Especially shield the patient when he or she has reasonable reproductive capability, when the primary beam comes within 2 inches (5.0 cm) of the reproductive organs, and when the shielding will not interfere with the examination.

Documentation

When creating a new position, the methods used should be documented for the radiologist and for future reference.

▨ ▨ SUMMARY

The general guidelines for trauma radiography have been presented, along with specific procedures, some familiar and some new, in a format that can be used in any situation. The descriptions can be used to obtain the highest quality radiographs consistently for trauma patients and others. As will be seen in the next chapter, these methods are applicable to mobile radiography also. When the day comes that no previously conceived positions will work, the radiographer may use the information at the end of this chapter to devise a new position, thus practicing the highest form of the art.

▨ ▨ SELF-ASSESSMENT TEST

DIRECTIONS: For each of the situations below:

a. Select positions that will demonstrate the injured areas.

    b. Place the positions in the order in which they should be performed.

    c. List any accessory devices that will be needed e.g., "if the cassette must be perpendicular to the table, a cassette holder (or sandbags and so forth) will be needed."

    d. Describe any special arrangements that will have to be made, for example, "you will have to support the film perpendicular to the table."

1. A man has a dislocated right hip, comminuted fractures of the distal femurs (just proximal to the knees), bumper fractures of the lower legs, and possible fractures of the right foot.

2. A child is guarding her right elbow, which is held in partial flexion.

3. A woman was in an A/A. Her cervical spine was injured (she is strapped to a backboard and is wearing a cervical collar), along with her sternum and anterior right ribs.

4. A man was playing basketball when he fell on his outstretched left arm. He now complains of pain in his left wrist and shoulder and is unable to move his arm.

5. A woman was involved in an airplane crash. She is strapped to a backboard and is wearing a cervical collar. She complains of pain in her cervical, dorsal, and lumbar spines. The left side of her face and left side of her frontal bone are also injured. She can move her left shoulder and wrist, but not her left elbow. She is complaining of chest pain also.

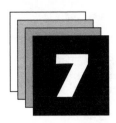

7

PORTABLE RADIOGRAPHY

PREREQUISITE

Knowledge of basic radiographic procedures, principles of image production, and basic principles of radiation protection should be acquired before studying this chapter. Also, the reader should be familiar with life-support and other medical equipment that includes nasogastric tubes, chest tubes, tracheostomy tubes, intravenous delivery systems, urinary tubing, electrocardiogram leads, respirators, and nursery isolettes.

OUTLINE

277

▪ ▪ INTRODUCTION

Portable radiography, which is often trauma radiography, is presented in this chapter. The general procedure to use before, during, and after the portable examination is covered, along with radiation protection and the importance of producing radiographs with consistent quality. Concerns for technical factors include constraints placed on radiographic equipment. The final section covers guidelines for specific anatomic areas.

Portable radiography is the term commonly used for mobile radiography. Portable refers to something that can be carried. Mobile means movable. A long time ago, there were portable (hand-carried) x-ray units, and a few can still be found today. The vast majority of units called *portable* are actually *mobile*. However, portable is the term used by most radiographers, and it is used here.

▪ ▪ RADIOGRAPHIC EQUIPMENT

Although it is still possible to find some of the small, 15-MAS portables and some 110-volt, plug-in models, most portables are self-propelled and battery operated, some even capable of computed (digital) radiography. The key to operating any portable x-ray unit is to know its capabilities. To know the capability and flexibility of a particular unit, the radiographer should start by learning the locks.

The control and release of the tube and supporting arm locks determine many of the limits for portable radiography. Some units have one lock. When it is released, the tube is moved into position and it is set. Others have nearly a dozen locks. It is to the radiographer's and the patient's advantage if time is spent exploring the possibilities.

Portable radiography is usually performed far from the main department. The radiographer needs to bring all of his or her equipment to avoid wasted trips to and from the patient's room. If a battery-operated portable is being used, the first step will be to check the battery level. It is good practice for the radiographer returning from an examination to recharge the portable unit so that it is fully charged for the next time.

Before leaving the department, the radiographer should be sure all equipment is obtained and stored in, or on, the unit. The radiographer will need some means of measuring the source-to-image-receptor distance (SID). Some portables have a tape measure or laser SID mounted to the collimator. If these items are not available, the radiographer should carry a small tape measure, or one should be with the portable unit. If nothing else is available, it is possible to estimate the SID with the collimator light. To do this, the radiographer must collimate to the exact film size. The tube is then moved closer to or farther away from the patient until the light field matches the size of the film. When the light field matches the film size, the tube is at the selected SID.

The radiographer will also need to bring the films needed for the examination, lead aprons, and any accessory devices (e.g., sponges, lead markers) that might be needed. Most of the larger portable units have a film storage compartment. The radiographer should be cautioned against using films that have been left in the portable—they may have been there quite some time and could be fogged. Also, during the examination, the radiographer must devise some method of separating exposed and unexposed films. One method is to have exposed film face one way and unexposed film face the opposite way. Another method is to attach the patient's flashcard to the cassette after the exposure has been made.

■ ■ THE CENTRAL RAY

Another concern of portable radiography is alignment of the central ray (CR) to the film. If the SID is known, the CR can be aligned with the film by collimating to the exact film size and then ensuring that the sides of the light field, and the top or bottom of the light field match the sides and top or bottom of the film. If the beam size (light field) is the same as the film size, and the sides match, and the top or bottom matches, then the CR will coincide with the center of the film.

Many radiographs require that the CR be perpendicular to the film. This can be difficult to obtain outside the controlled environment of the x-ray department. One way to position the CR perpendicular to the film is to stand back from the side of the unit and adjust the tube until the bottom of the collimator is *parallel* to the film. Because the CR is perpendicular to the bottom of the collimator, if the bottom of the collimator is *parallel* to the film, then the CR will be perpendicular to the film. Another method, which is more accurate but also takes more time, is to measure the distance from three corners of the collimator to their three corresponding corners of the film (Fig. 7–1). If the measurements are equal, then the bottom of the collimator is parallel to the film and the CR is perpendicular to the film. Three corners must be used, however. If two opposite corners or two adjacent corners are used, it is possible for the two measurements

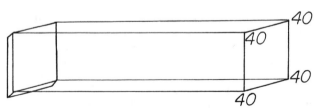

FIG. 7–1. Three of the four corners of the cassette and collimator must be measured to ensure that the cassette and collimator are parallel and the CR and cassette perpendicular.

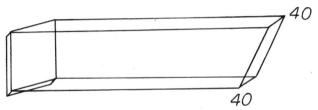

FIG. 7–2. Measuring two opposite corners of the collimator and cassette may yield equal distances but an angled cassette or CR.

to be equal and the CR not to be perpendicular to the film (Figs. 7–2 and 7–3).

■ ■ LIFE-SUPPORT AND OTHER MEDICAL EQUIPMENT

The patient, or the patient's room, may contain items that require the radiographer's attention. Tracheostomy tubes, nasogastric tubes, chest tubes, intravenous (IV) tubing, electrocardiogram (ECG) leads, and other apparatus may be present. The radiographer will have to work around these obstacles carefully with the portable unit and the cassette. It is important for the tracheostomy tube to remain in the patient's throat. However, when the tracheostomy tube is attached to a respirator, it is usually

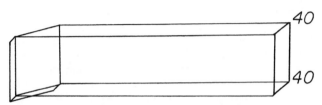

FIG. 7–3. Measuring two adjacent corners of the collimator and cassette may yield equal distances but an angled cassette or CR.

a loose fit (in which case if tension is placed on the respirator hose, it disconnects rather than pulls the tracheostomy tube from the patient's throat). If the respirator hose does become disconnected, the radiographer should slip it back onto the tracheostomy tube.

Nasogastric, chest, and IV tubing should never have tension placed on them. The radiographer must check for these tubes and not accidentally place stress on them when positioning the patient or when placing a film behind them. Pulling any of these tubes from the patient is a serious situation, which, at the least, will cause much discomfort to the patient as they are reinserted, and at the worst can gravely affect the patient's condition. The radiographer also should not dislodge ECG leads, but if they are dislodged, they can be easily repositioned.

The radiographer must also check for objects in the patient's bed or cart that may be projected onto the radiograph. Some patients have heating pads or blankets in their beds. The thermostat and wires in these items will interfere with the desired structures if they are superimposed on the film. The radiographer should also be cautioned against performing an x-ray study through too many sheets or blankets. Even wet or matted hair can be demonstrated. If the exposure must be made through a sheet (ideally there should be only one), the sheet should be flat and smooth to reduce the chance of a fold being demonstrated on the radiograph.

■ ■ CHECKING CHARTS

Although customs vary from hospital to hospital, it is a good idea for the radiographer to check the patient's chart before performing a portable examination. Orders for the examination can be reviewed, along with the condition of the patient. The chart should be checked to determine whether there are any restrictions on the patient's being placed in an upright position. Sometimes, the patient may be elevated only 45 degrees. This should then be noted in the history so that the radiologist is aware that air-fluid levels may not be demonstrated accurately. Any medications that the patient is receiving should also be checked to determine whether they may impair the patient's ability to cooperate (this may be done by checking the drug lists in Chapter 3). The patient's weight and mobility also may need to be checked in case the radiographer will need lifting assistance.

PRE-EXAMINATION ROOM PROCEDURES

On arriving at the patient's room, the radiographer should enter without the portable unit. An analysis of the situation should be performed and a mental plan of action formed instead of barging into a room with a large machine. First, the radiographer must verify the patient's name and introduce herself or himself. Verifying the patient's name can be accomplished by checking the patient's identification (ID) bracelet, by asking the patient for his or her name, or both. Visitors should be asked to leave. If the patient is in a double room and the patient's roommate can be moved, he or she should be taken out of the room. If the roommate cannot be removed, a lead apron must be provided. If hospital personnel are present but will not be assisting the radiographer, they should be asked to leave the room. If they must stay, they, too, must have lead aprons.

Before bringing the portable x-ray unit into the patient's room, the radiographer should enter and clear a path for the machine. Chairs, Mayo stands, and so forth should be moved. The room should be examined for objects close to the floor because the bumpers of the portable unit may hit them. Also, the walls should be examined for objects that the top of the unit might strike. In particular, the radiographer should watch for:

- Chest tube bottles on the floor.
- Urinary catheter drainage bags hanging from the sides of the beds.
- A bed elevated on blocks (for traction therapy or to place the patient in the Trendelenburg position).
- Traction therapy weights hanging at the ends of the bed.
- Wall-mounted oxygen and suction outlets.

- Oxygen tanks.
- Televisions (especially wall-mounted units, which are often at the same height as the top of the x-ray unit. Also, some hospitals rent the televisions, and if they are damaged, the radiographer could be personally liable for the cost of repairs or a replacement).

The radiographer must also watch for medical equipment on wheels. Because the portable unit outweighs almost all other movable hospital equipment, a small collision can send a piece of equipment across a room. The radiographer needs to be especially aware of this situation with isolettes in the nursery.

After removing personnel, clearing a path for the x-ray unit, and accounting for other equipment in the room, the projection can be planned. The projection will depend on:

- The presence of other patients
- The mobility of the patient being examined
- Access for the portable unit

The x-ray beam must be directed away from any patients that cannot be removed from the room, in addition to covering them with a lead apron. Whenever possible, the x-ray beam should be aimed at an outside wall. The mobility of the patient is ascertained by checking the patient's chart, by asking the nurse in charge of the patient, and by evaluating the patient's condition. Although the mobility of portable units varies, it is generally best to place the portable unit parallel or perpendicular to the side or the end of the patient's bed.

■ ■ RADIATION PROTECTION FOR PORTABLE RADIOGRAPHY

The radiographer is responsible for the radiation protection of the patient being radiographed, the patient's roommate if it is a semiprivate room, any visitors, coworkers (including doctors and nurses), and himself or herself. In addition to removing people from the area, other methods that can be employed involve direction of the x-ray beam; length of exposure; distance from the beam; shielding; collimation; reduction of repeats; and selection of grids, screens, and technical factors.

In protecting the patient being examined, the radiographer must reduce repeat exposures and must shield, collimate, and properly select grids, screens, and technical factors. Reduction of repeat exposures can be attained by:

- Checking positioning before the exposure to ensure that it is correct
- Checking previous radiographs or files of patients for technical factors (see Recording Technics section of this chapter)
- Using a relatively high kilovolt (KV) setting technics, which have a wider exposure latitude (wider margin for technic error).

The criteria for shielding patients do not exclude those radiographed with a portable unit, but shielding is often neglected when a portable unit is used. It should not be. All patients should be shielded—especially those with chronic conditions (such as those in traction), those receiving many examinations (such as daily chest x-ray examinations), and the young (such as nursery cases). The reproductive organs must be shielded when the patient meets these three criteria:

1. The beam comes within 2 inches (5 cm) of the reproductive organs.
2. The patient has reasonable reproductive capability.
3. The shielding will not interfere with the examination.

Collimation is another area that is not performed with as much diligence with portable units as in the radiography department. Although it is often difficult to ensure proper film-beam alignment during a portable examination, the radiographer must make every attempt to guarantee that the field is limited to the film size or smaller. When the edges of the film are not visible, the radiographer must use the collimation-SID scales built into the tube. For these to be accurate, the SID must be known, and the radiographer may need to carry a tape measure, inasmuch as those that come with the portable unit are frequently broken.

Grid selection depends on the size of the part and the KV being used. Larger parts and higher KV settings generate more scatter radiation and require a grid with a higher ratio. However, high ratio grids are less flexible. The radiographer should select the lowest ratio grid practical for the size of the part and KV selected. In general, a grid is needed for parts larger than 4 inches (10 cm), except for the chest (also see the Grid Usage section of this chapter).

Intensifying screen selection is also dependent on the size of the part—smaller parts can use slower, more detailed screens; larger parts should have faster screens. The faster screens require fewer MAS, thereby reducing patient dose. They also have the added benefit of allowing a shorter exposure time, which reduces the chance of motion (which reduces repeat radiographs and prevents additional radiation dose).

Finally, technical factors can be adjusted to reduce patient dose. The KV can be increased and MAS decreased so that the density of film remains the same but the dose decreases. Increasing the KV 15 percent will allow the MAS to be decreased by one-half. However, the radiographer must consider the scale of contrast that will result (increasing the KV decreases the contrast, causing a longer scale of contrast) and the increased scatter that is generated with higher KV settings. If the increased scatter requires a higher ratio of the grid, then the entire purpose of increasing the KV (to reduce dose) will be defeated—higher ratio grids require higher MAS settings (to compensate for the scatter they absorb).

The radiographer is responsible for the radiation safety of visitors and, if the patient is not in a private room, roommates. Visitors must leave the room. If other patients in the room are ambulatory, they should leave the room also. If the other patients cannot leave the room, they must be given a lead apron. Also, whenever possible, the beam should be directed away from them.

Radiographers can never assume that other health-care workers know as much about radiography and radiation protection as radiographers themselves do. Radiographers are still responsible for the radiation protection of other workers, including nonradiologist physicians, even if the others have many years of experience. Other workers must be warned well in advance that an x-ray exposure is about to be made so that they can remove themselves from the area. If a worker cannot leave the area (as in an emergency case in which a respiratory therapist is ventilating a patient), he or she must be given a lead apron and lead gloves (if necessary) and moved away from the primary beam. In short, other workers must be given the same protection that radiographers give themselves.

Radiographers can apply the three basic methods of radiation protection to themselves: time, distance, and shielding. The time that any radiographer is exposed to radiation can be reduced by rotating all radiographers through high-radiation areas—including portable radiography. The larger the distance between the patient and the radiographer, and the radiographer and the x-ray tube, the lower the radiographer's dose will be. If the distances are doubled, the exposure will be reduced to one-fourth. Therefore, the radiographer should maximize these distances. The exposure cord (which must be at least 6 ft long) should be fully extended. If the radiographer can stand outside the patient's room and around a corner, this greatly increases the path the x-rays must follow to reach the radiographer and further reduces the dose by forcing the x-rays to bounce (and lose energy) off the floor, ceiling, or walls. The radiographer should also wear a lead apron (preferably of 0.5-mm lead equivalent) and, if necessary, lead gloves. Some radiographers do not wear a lead apron, but stand behind the portable x-ray machine for protection. This should not be done. It places the radiographer closer to the beam than is necessary, and most units have a fair amount of empty space in them, which could allow the beam to penetrate the machine easily and strike critical areas.

■ ■ POST-EXAMINATION ROOM PROCEDURES

After the portable examination is complete, it is the radiographer's job to return the room to the condition it was in when the radiographer entered it. Chairs, tables, televisions, and medical equipment must be put back in their places. Roommates and visitors must be brought back, and the patient's chart and bed must be put back in order. However, given the uncontrolled environment in which portable x-ray examinations are performed, many radiographers develop and check their work before returning the portable unit to the department. If the unit is to be left while the radiograph is being checked, it should not be left in the patient's room. If the examination is being done in the intensive care unit (ICU) or cardiac care unit (CCU), it must not be left in the room. Because radiographers are usually the only ones who know how to move the unit (and if it is self-propelled, the keys should not be left in the machine anyway), should some patient emergency arise, the huge portable unit could block vital access to the room or patient. When the portable unit is to be left while the radiograph is being checked, it should be left in the hall, out of everyone's way.

▮ ▮ THE IMPORTANCE OF CONSISTENCY

Each radiograph in a series (such as daily chest examinations or examinations to check on fracture healing) should be as consistent as possible. The radiologist should be provided with radiographs similar in density, contrast, and positioning in order to make the most accurate diagnosis possible. If the radiographs are not consistent, an important condition may be missed; and if it is not demonstrated, no one may ever know (or the condition will be discovered too late on another film). Radiographers should record their methods and the technical factors used for each portable examination. These files must then be consulted before the next examination. Also, the radiologist should not have to demand this consistency or send radiographs back for repeat exposures because a comparison cannot be made: A professional radiographer provides this level of quality and service automatically.

TECHNICS FOR PORTABLE RADIOGRAPHY

GENERAL TECHNICS

Relatively high KV technics should be used for portable radiography. This provides the radiographer with wider exposure latitude (a wider margin for error). It may also allow for a reduction in MAS, which will decrease exposure time (and reduce repeat exposures caused by motion) and decrease the patient's radiation dose. However, increasing the KV increases scatter and produces lower contrast (a longer scale of contrast). Reducing scatter requires a grid, a higher ratio grid, or use of an air-gap technic (which is described later). Each of these methods is difficult to use with portable examinations. As far as the contrast is concerned, the radiographer must be careful not to decrease it to the point that it produces an undiagnostic radiograph.

RECORDING TECHNICS

The technical factors used on every portable examination should be recorded. This record should then be consulted, along with the radiograph, before any subsequent films. The originals should be checked for the projection employed, density, contrast, and detail. If these factors are acceptable, the same ones can be used on the next films; if not, they can be corrected. This approach ensures consistency if the methods are optimal, reduces repeat exposures by using a method that has been proven (which reduces patient dose), and allows corrections and improvements to be made.

Although there are numerous variations in the methods used to record portable examination technics, there are two general ways to do it. One way is to keep a generic technic chart, much like those used in many radiography departments. The examinations are usually listed on separate pages. On each page are ranges of patient size (e.g., 10 to 14 cm, 15 to 17 cm, and 17 to 21 cm). Then the MAS, KV, screen, grid, and SID are listed for each range. Another way is a patient-specific method. This involves recording the technic used for one particular patient. The technic may be written on the radiograph or in a card file or logbook arranged alphabetically. The best method is probably a combination of the two. Radiographers can consult the generic technic chart for the preliminary examination and record the technic used on the film. Subsequent examinations can copy or improve on first radiographs, depending on their quality.

There are two key factors to this system. First, everyone must record technics, and second, everyone must use them. If some radiographers in the department use this system and others do not, it wastes time (when someone looks up a technic that is not there), increases the patient dose by increasing repeats (when mistakes are duplicated because previous radiographs were not consulted), and gives the radiologist inconsistent results. The other key factor is that all of the following information must be present to make subsequent radiographs match earlier ones:

- MAS
- KV
- SID
- Screen speed (if more than one is available)
- Grid ratio (if a grid was used)

It is also helpful if there is a description of any nonroutine positions used, which are sometimes required for patients receiving traction therapy. The description should contain the following information:

- Patient position (e.g., prone, upright, upright 45 degrees) and projection (e.g., AP, mediolateral, inferosuperior)
- Position of the part (e.g., oblique, pronated, inverted, flexed)
- Size, type, and position of the cassette, including any angle between the part and film
- CR, including the degree and direction of any angulation, and the entry point (or the exit point)

TABLE 7–1. SID CONVERSION TABLE

Original SID in inches	New SID in inches									
	36	40	44	48	52	56	60	64	68	72
36	—	1.23	1.5	1.78	2.08	2.42	2.78	3.16	3.57	4
40	0.81	—	1.21	1.44	1.69	1.96	2.25	2.56	2.89	3.24
44	0.67	0.82	—	1.19	1.39	1.62	1.86	2.11	2.39	2.68
48	0.56	0.69	0.84	—	1.17	1.36	1.56	1.77	2	2.25
52	0.48	0.59	0.71	0.85	—	1.16	1.33	1.51	1.71	1.91
56	0.41	0.51	0.61	0.73	0.86	—	1.15	1.3	1.47	1.65
60	0.36	0.44	0.53	0.64	0.75	0.87	—	1.13	1.28	1.44
64	0.31	0.39	0.47	0.56	0.66	0.75	0.88	—	1.13	1.26
68	0.28	0.34	0.42	0.5	0.58	0.68	0.78	0.88	—	1.12
72	0.25	0.31	0.37	0.44	0.52	0.6	0.69	0.79	0.89	—
76	0.22	0.27	0.33	0.4	0.46	0.54	0.62	0.71	0.8	0.89
80	0.2	0.25	0.3	0.36	0.42	0.49	0.56	0.64	0.72	0.81

For greater consistency and ease of use, the method of recording both technical factors and atypical positions should be standardized. Index cards or log sheets that have room for technics on one side and positions on the other will encourage radiographers to use them more than if they have to devise their own method or format.

▪ ▪ SID CONVERSION TABLE

Table 7–1 uses the inverse-square law to convert changes in the SID quickly. To compensate for a change in SID and maintain film density, find the original SID in column 1. Move along that row until you are in the column for the *new* SID. Multiply your original MAS by the factor in the box. For example, if your original SID is 40 inches, and the new SID is 52 inches, multiply your original MAS by 1.69.

▪ ▪ GRID USAGE

Grids are needed when scatter radiation obscures the image. Scatter lowers the contrast of the radiograph (makes the scale of contrast longer). Grids should be used when:

- The KV exceeds 80 KV
- When the part thickness is greater than 4 inches (10 cm)
- When the tissue density increases (e.g., a muscular part generates more scatter than a part filled with air)

The radiographer must consider not only when to use a grid but also which grid ratio to select. Common grid ratios are 5:1, 6:1, 8:1, 10:1, 12:1, and 16:1. As the grid ratio increases, the amount of scatter removed by the grid increases. However, higher ratio grids also remove some of the useful radiation. Therefore, as the grid ratio increases, the MAS must be increased, which also increases the radiation dose to the patient (KV can be increased instead, which will save the radiation dose to the patient, but this will increase scatter even more). A general grid conversion chart follows:

From no grid to 5:1 ratio	increase 2 times
From no grid to 6:1 ratio	increase 3 times
From no grid to 8:1 ratio	increase 4 times
From no grid to 10:1 ratio	increase 4.5 times
From no grid to 12:1 ratio	increase 5 times
From no grid to 16:1 ratio	increase 6 times

As the KV increases, scatter increases, and the ratio of the grid being used should be increased. There are some practical limits, however. An 8:1 grid usually provides acceptable clean-up of scatter up to 90 KV. Beyond 90 KV, a 10:1 or 12:1 ratio grid should be used. A 16:1 grid does not remove much more scatter than a 12:1 grid, but it requires much more MAS. The increased need for MAS may strain the output limits of a portable unit and increase the radiation dose to the patient.

The number of lead lines per inch, or per centimeter, that a grid has affects the radiographic image. When a stationary grid (i.e., nonreciprocating or non-Bucky) is used, the lead lines will be visible on the radiograph. This can be distracting to some radiologists. To reduce the visibility of the lines, the radiographer can select the grid with more lines per inch or per centimeter. Grids with more lines per inch have lead strips that are thinner and less noticeable than those with fewer lines.

The most difficult task in using a grid for portable radiography is maintaining the correct relationship between the grid and the CR. The CR may be angled along only the long axis of the grid (Fig. 7–4). The problem in portable radiography is with unintentional CR angulation across the short axis of the grid. This happens easily in the uncontrolled environment of the patient's room and will result in a loss of most, if not all, of the image. If the patient is lying supine on top of a grid cassette, a slight shift in weight to one side will tilt the grid. This will cause grid cutoff (loss of the image). The short axis of the grid will have been angled in relation to the CR. The only solution to this problem is careful positioning of the grid and CR and proper support of

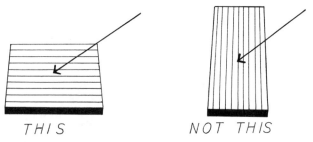

THIS   *NOT THIS*

FIG. 7–4. Permissible CR angulation when using a grid.

the grid. The radiographer must ensure that the grid is properly positioned in relation to the part and the CR. The patient must be watched to make sure that the correct position is maintained. If the grid cassette is positioned vertically, a number of commercially available cassette holders may be used, or the grid cassette may be supported with sandbags or other immobilization devices. If the patient is holding the grid cassette, clear instructions regarding its position must be given. Emphasis should be placed on the importance of *maintaining* the position. The extra minute or two that are needed to position the grid cassette carefully will reduce the patient dose and save the many minutes required to repeat the examination.

There are some radiographers who advocate turning a cassette backward as a substitute for a grid. The principle is that the back of the cassette attenuates the scatter radiation. This is not entirely accurate. The back of the cassette attenuates the beam. It will stop lower energy-scattered x-rays, but it will also stop lower energy-straight x-rays. And the results are not as predictable as are those for a grid. The result may be the need for a repeat exposure or an increase in the technical factors to offset the amount of the desirable beam that will be absorbed. Both of these factors will increase the dose to the patient. Therefore, this procedure cannot be endorsed, especially as a substitute for proper planning and preparedness.

▓ ▓ OBESE PATIENTS

The radiographer's skills can be tested on the obese patient, especially when a portable radiograph is needed. Positioning these patients properly can usually be accomplished with some extra effort. Setting the technical factors is a different story. The problems include penetration, the limited output of the portable unit, scatter, and the low contrast (longer scale of contrast) from the scatter and the patient's tissue.

Penetration of the part can usually be obtained with the settings available on modern portable equipment. The radiographer must, however, resist the urge to increase the KV too much. Although the patient may appear large, a great increase in KV to increase penetration may not be needed. Also, the higher KV will lower the contrast (lengthen the scale of contrast) more, and with obese patients, it is usually longer than desired already.

Although the current output of portable units is much higher than older ones (such as the 15-MAS type), the severely obese patient may strain the limits. To counteract this problem, the radiographer should select the highest speed-intensifying screens available. Also, the lowest possible grid ratio should be employed. However, because too much scatter radiation is a problem (from the patient size and increased KV), there are limits on how low a grid may be employed. As mentioned earlier, an 8:1 grid can usually be used with KV values of 90 or less. With an obese patient, this may be lowered to 85 (or even 80) KV because much more scatter is created in larger parts. Using a 5:1 or 6:1 grid on an obese patient, with 80 KV, may not be possible, even though a smaller increase in MAS is required for these grids. A possibility that is usually reserved for use when everything else has failed is to double-expose the film. When the beam penetrates an obese patient, the equipment is at its limit, the patient cannot be brought to the department, and the radiograph is still lacking density, the film can be exposed twice. To do this, the radiographer must estimate half the MAS needed to expose the film adequately. The x-ray tube's Anode Cooling Curve must also be checked to ensure that two exposures of this magnitude can be made in succession. If so, then the first exposure is made, it terminates, and the radiographer immediately makes a second exposure. In order for this method to be successful, the patient cannot move until the second exposure has concluded. This includes breathing. The patient is not allowed to breathe between exposures for those examinations that require suspended respiration.

There is an alternative to using a grid cassette for reducing scatter radiation, but it, too, has limitations. Instead of a grid cassette, or in addition to a grid cassette for very obese patients, the radiographer may use the air-gap method. This method is commonly used for lateral cervical spine radiographs. It reduces scatter to the film by placing the film about 10 inches (25 cm) from the part. The angle of the scattered x-rays causes many of them to miss the film (although a few are absorbed by the air). This method does result in a large amount of undesirable magnification of the part unless the SID is increased to counteract it. However, increasing the SID requires an increase in MAS (due to the inverse-square law), which further stresses the equipment.

When radiographing obese patients, the radiographer must realize that, although rare, there are some people who are so large that diagnostic radiographs cannot be obtained. When these situations arise, the radiographer should consult with a radiologist to avoid needlessly exposing the patient to radiation.

▓ ▓ SPECIFIC METHODS

▓ CHEST EXAMINATIONS

The chest examination is the most common portable radiographic procedure. The portable chest examination is frequently one anteroposterior (AP) projection, even though the routine for other patients is a posteroanterior (PA) and a lateral projection. This procedure presents six items for special consideration:

1. The patient's position
2. Positioning the patient's shoulders
3. The placement of the film
4. Medical equipment
5. Unintentionally lordotic radiographs
6. The SID

The typical position for a patient receiving a portable chest examination is seated upright in the bed. Before performing this examination, the radiographer should check the patient's chart or check with the patient's nurse to determine whether there are restrictions on placing the patient in an upright position. Some patients are restricted to lying flat, whereas others have limits as to how far upright they may be placed. For example, the patient's condition may allow a seated position of no more than 45 degrees. When this is the case, the radiographer should note on the history or on the radiograph that the patient was not fully upright. This affects air-fluid levels, depression of the diaphragm, and the position of the pulmonary vessels.

Even when the patient can sit upright in bed, the construction of most hospital beds prevents the patient's torso from being perpendicular to the floor. The radiographer may make the exposure with the patient in this position. Again, it should be noted on the history or the radiograph that the patient was, for example, 85 degrees upright. There are two other alternatives. If the conditions permit, the patient may sit on the edge of the bed for a PA. The patient can wrap his or her arms around the film (Fig. 7–5). Wrapping the arms around the film not only supports the film but also helps in rotating the shoulders forward to remove the scapulae from the lung fields. If the top of the film is not above the patient's shoulders, a pillow may be placed in the patient's lap to raise it.

The second alternative to the nearly upright AP chest position is to place a pillow, or pillows, behind the patient and under the cassette to bring the patient fully upright (Fig. 7–6). Immobilization may be required, depending

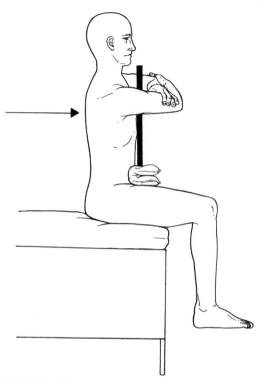

FIG. 7–5. PA projection, upright portable chest.

on the patient's ability to maintain the position. Because the film is mainly held in place by the patient's leaning against it, the film must be observed just before the exposure to ensure that neither has moved out of position.

Some radiographers neglect some of the finer positioning points when performing portable examinations. Two of these points involve the shoulders. The clavicles should be positioned below the apices, and the scapulae should be removed from the lungs no matter what position (AP or PA) is used and regardless of whether the examination is portable or performed in the department.

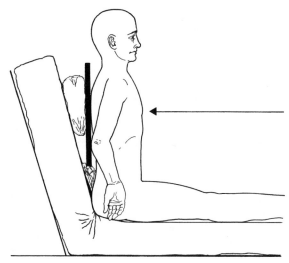

FIG. 7–6. AP projection upright portable chest.

Therefore, the shoulders should be depressed and rolled forward. Depression of the shoulders is easily accomplished. The shoulders may be rolled forward for a PA chest, as described earlier. For an AP projection, patients can place the backs of their hands on the sides of their hips. This alone is usually sufficient to remove the scapulae from the lung fields, but additional rotation is easily accomplished from this position.

Placement of the film, or cassette, is another point of interest in portable chest radiography. Many radiographers use a 14 × 17 inch (35 × 43 cm) cassette crosswise (the long axis of the film is parallel to the transverse axis of the body) for an AP portable chest examination. They use the cassette crosswise even though they would have used it lengthwise (the long axis of the film is parallel with the mid-line of the body) if they had performed the examination in the department. Although there is nothing inherently wrong with using the film crosswise, there is no real reason *to* use it crosswise, except for hypersthenic (larger than average size) patients. The hypersthenic patient's lungs are shorter than normal and wider at the base than normal. Radiographs of all other patients can be performed with the film lengthwise.

Other film placement concerns include the condition of the patient, position of the ID markers, the temperature of the cassette, and objects between the cassette and the patient. Special care must be taken when radiographing elderly patients, especially those that are malnourished. Their skin is thin and can be very brittle; a cassette being positioned against them could easily tear their skin. To avoid interference with the lung fields, it is best to place the cassette with the identification markers in the shoulders. This is true whether the film is crosswise or lengthwise, or whether the projection is PA or AP. Another concern is the temperature of the cassette. It is often colder than the patient and can be uncomfortable when it touches bare skin. It is helpful to place the cassette in a pillowcase to avoid this temperature shock to the patient. An alternative is to place the cassette behind a bed sheet. This can produce another problem: Sometimes there are objects, like heating pads, between the bed sheet and the patient. The resulting artifact causes the film to be repeated. The last film placement concern involves the action of placing the film behind the patient. Frequently, this involves the patient's leaning forward slightly and the radiographer's pushing the film down between the patient's back and the bed. If the radiographer is not careful, and the patient has monitor leads or tubing near his or her shoulders, the leads or tubing can be stretched and dislodged as the film is pushed down behind the patient. It is better to have the patient lean as far forward as possible, position the film, and then have the patient lean back against it.

Patients needing portable radiography often have various medical apparatuses attached to them. The radiographer must check for:

- Intravenous tubing
- Electrocardiogram wires (ECG leads)
- Nasogastric tubes
- Chest tubes
- Tracheostomy tubes and respirators

The radiographer must look for these items and examine them to determine whether they are pinned (or otherwise attached) to the bed sheets or pillows. The most critical of these items is the chest tube. A chest tube is inserted to drain the chest cavity for re-expansion of the lungs. The radiographer must ensure that the placement of the film does not put pressure or tension on the tubing, thus running the risk of dislodging it. Neither should tension be placed on nasogastric tubes, because it is very uncomfortable for the patient to have them reinserted. Another serious concern is dislodging IV catheters. This measure is especially important for elderly patients who have poor or collapsing veins. A tracheostomy tube should never detach, inasmuch as it is tied in place around the patient's neck. It is possible to disengage the respirator tubing from the tracheostomy tube. In fact, it is easy, because this is a loose connection that uncouples rather than stress the tracheostomy tube. The tube should be reconnected immediately if this happens, and the incident should cause no harm to the patient. Although it is embarrassing, it is not nearly as critical if an ECG lead is disconnected, because it is a monitor, not a life-support system, and is easily reconnected.

The unintentionally lordotic AP projection chest examination is another common problem in portable radiography. The greatest cause is that the CR is more horizontal than it should be (Fig. 7–7). This is a result of working in the uncontrolled environment of the patient's room, where it is difficult to place the CR perpendicular to the film. The most accurate way to place the CR perpendicular to the film has been mentioned—measure from the corners of the collimator to the corners of the film. However, some radiographers obtain good results by standing back a few feet and ensuring that the bottom of the collimator is parallel to the film.

The last major concern in portable chest radiography is the SID. The radiologist is accustomed to seeing department-produced radiographs with a 72-inch SID. The charts for calculating heart size are based on this distance. If the distance is not 72 inches (or whatever is standard for a department), this should be noted on the history sheet or on the radiograph. This approach will allow

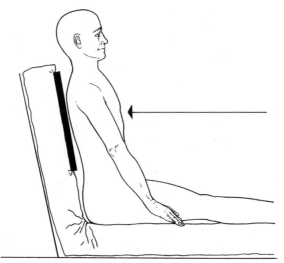

FIG. 7–7. Portable chest with its most common problem, an unintentional lordotic projection. Note that the beam is horizontal but the film is <u>not</u> vertical.

the radiologist to make any needed adjustments in the interpretation of the examination.

■ EXTREMITIES

Methods for demonstrating the extremities with a portable x-ray unit are listed in Chapter 6. The descriptions are the same as those for immobile, trauma patients. One difference, however, is the patient in traction therapy.

Patients in traction therapy usually present problems for the radiographer. The traction bars, cables, and pins can prevent normal positioning. These parts may prevent the film from being in contact with the patient. The bars or cables may prevent a normal lateral projection from being made. The overhead bars may prevent the typical 40-inch (100-cm) SID from being used. To solve these problems, the radiographer must refer to the basic principles of positioning and to the SID compensation chart.

With many patients in traction, one position will be difficult or impossible to attain. The radiographer should remember that two projections 90 degrees apart are best. Preferably an AP or PA and lateral should be taken, but if these projections are not possible because of the patient's traction, maybe two oblique projections will suffice. If that is not possible, obtain one routine projection (AP, PA, or lateral) and the next closest projection to 90 degrees from the routine position. For example, assume that the patient's femur is in traction, with metal bars along each side of the thigh. A routine AP femur should be obtained and the next closest projection to a lateral. The lateral projection may be only 75 degrees different from the PA rather than 90 degrees, but there is often no other choice.

When modifying routine positions for traction cases, the radiographer should diagram or describe successful methods so that other radiographers can duplicate them and provide consistency for the radiologist. Also, many patients in traction are able to assist the radiographer in the performance of the examination. They may be able to hold the cassette and, because the examination has been performed on them many times before, may automatically place it where it needs to go.

Because patients in traction receive a number of radiographic examinations, extra radiation-protection measures should be taken. In addition to protecting the reproductive organs, the radiographer should shield the blood-forming organs, eyes, and thyroid.

Radiographers must take extra care when working around traction therapy equipment. In some situations, blocks are placed under one or both ends of the patient's bed. These blocks can easily be knocked out from under a leg by the bumpers on the portable unit. The weights used to apply traction can also be of concern. Many of them are C-shaped, so that it is easy to add more weights by sliding them on. It is also easy to subtract weights, especially by accidentally bumping into them. When examining a patient in traction, the radiographer should note the location of weights, pulleys, cables, supporting structures, and blocks before the x-ray unit is brought into the room.

▦ ABDOMEN

The abdomen is one of the more difficult areas to radiograph with a portable unit. The difficulty is not in the unit itself or in positioning the patient; the difficulty is in positioning the cassette, with the patient on top of it, in the patient's bed. If the patient leans even slightly to one side, the grid (which is required for abdominal studies) will produce cutoff that renders the radiograph useless. It is sometimes helpful to place the patient on a backboard (such as the ones used for trauma patients), with the grid cassette on top of the board. This approach adds some stability but is not foolproof. Some portable units come with a cassette tunnel. When many exposures are needed, as with an intravenous urogram (IVU) or intravenous pyelogram (IVP), the cassette tunnel makes the job of changing films easier because it is left under the patient and the cassettes slide in and out from the side. These tunnels do not add much stability to the patient by themselves. They can, however, be used with a backboard. It is also easy and inexpensive to have one made, inasmuch as they are simply wood boxes with a radiolucent front.

▦ ▦ SPECIAL AREAS

Special areas of the hospital, such as isolation, the nursery, the ICU, and the CCU, require particular attention for radiographers performing portable examinations. In general, patients in the nursery, the ICU, the CCU, and protective isolation should be examined before general medical or surgical patients. Patients in strict, respiratory, wound (also called drainage/secretion), contact, acid-fast bacilli (AFB) (i.e., tuberculosis), total body fluid (TBF), or enteric isolation should be examined last.

If the type of isolation is not marked outside the patient's room, the radiographer must first determine the patient's type of isolation. The procedure for protective isolation is different from the procedure for the other types of isolation. For patients in protective isolation, the x-ray unit, including the wheels, should be disinfected *before* the radiographer enters the patient's room. Protective isolation is designed to protect the weakened patient from germs that healthy people are carrying. Although the portable unit will be disinfected, these patients should be among the first that are examined for the day (however, they are usually examined after patients in the ICU, CCU, and nursery). For patients in the other classes of isolation, the procedure is reversed—the unit is disinfected *after* the examination.

The protective clothing requirements for each isolation case are usually posted just outside the room. However, in general, a radiographer needs the items listed in Box 7–1 for each type of isolation.

Protective clothing must be disposed of properly, and the radiographer must wash his or her hands after the examination and before taking care of another patient (except for patients in protective isolation).

BOX 7–1
PROTECTIVE CLOTHING FOR ISOLATION

STRICT, CONTACT, AND PROTECTIVE ISOLATION
  Gown
  Gloves
  Mask
  Shoe covers

RESPIRATORY AND AFB ISOLATION
  Mask
  Gown

ENTERIC, WOUND, AND TBF ISOLATION
  Gown
  Gloves

Radiography of patients in isolation (except for protective isolation) is easier with two people. One person comes in contact with the patient, whereas the other touches only the machine and uncontaminated objects. It is best to place the cassette in a sterile pillowcase rather than have it come in contact with the patient.

When one radiographer is performing an examination on a patient in isolation, extreme care must be taken to prevent contamination of the control panel and cassette. For safety, *everything* should be decontaminated after the examination.

Nursery patients and newborns (NBs) do not have the same immune capabilities as adults. Therefore, they should be among the first patients examined for the day. Although the portable unit will be disinfected, it should not be driven through other patients' rooms and then through the nursery. The NB needing radiography will almost certainly be in an isolette, a covered bed that allows for easier control of the baby's environment. Isolettes are usually on wheels and weigh much less than a portable x-ray unit. The radiographer must be careful when maneuvering around isolettes not to send one sailing across the room. Isolettes are radiolucent, so it is easy to radiograph the baby through them. Positioning, whether the patient is upright or recumbent, requires two people. It is best to enlist a nurse to move the baby while the radiographer positions the cassette. Extra radiation-protection measures should be taken in all newborn examinations, including chest radiographs.

Patients in an ICU and CCU are usually in serious condition. They should be among the first patients of the day. The radiographer should check the patient's condition with the nurse and obtain the nurse's assistance, if necessary. Stress to the patient, including noise and patient movement, should be minimized. The portable unit should never be left in an ICU or CCU room while the radiographer develops a film. Should the patient need emergency treatment, no one will know how to move the unit out of the way. Finally, patients in an ICU and CCU who receive serial radiography examinations (e.g., daily chest radiographs) require additional radiation-protection measures.

▪ ▪ SUMMARY

Portable radiography is not much different from trauma radiography. In both cases, radiographers must adapt the equipment and positioning to the patient and the situation. The methods in Chapter 6 can be used for both portable and trauma examinations. Although the radiographer is not working in the controlled environment of the x-ray department, with study, careful planning, and careful performance, he or she can obtain results that approach, and sometimes meet, the standards for radiographs produced by fixed x-ray units.

▪ ▪ SELF-ASSESSMENT TEST

DIRECTIONS: Supply answers, in your own words, to each of the following questions:

1. What equipment, film, and so forth do you need to perform portable AP chest and lateral chest radiographs on a patient in a double-occupancy ICU room?
2. Describe two different methods for obtaining a 40-inch (100-cm) SID with a portable unit that does *not* have a measuring device attached to the tube or collimator.
3. Describe two different methods of ensuring that the CR is perpendicular to the cassette during portable radiography.
4. What three criteria will determine the direction in which you will aim the x-ray tube during portable radiography?
5. What are a radiographer's radiation-protection responsibilities toward these individuals during portable radiography?
   a. The patient
   b. The patient's roommate
   c. The patient's visitors
   d. Other health-care workers
   e. Nonradiologist physicians
6. Why should a portable radiography unit never be left unattended in the patient's room in the position to make an exposure?

7. Normally, you would use 32 MAS at 70 KV for an abdomen, with a 40-inch (100-cm) SID. However, because of the conditions in the patient's room, you must use a 56-inch (142-cm) SID. What MAS must you use to maintain the same density as on a 40-inch (100-cm) radiograph?

8. In Room 1 in your radiography department, you would use 25 MAS and 75 KV for a particular part, with an 8:1 ratio grid. You must do the same part using a portable unit that has the same output as Room 1, but the only grid cassettes you have are equipped with 5:1 ratio grids. What MAS must you use to maintain the same radiographic density as in Room 1?

9. What is the main reason why portable AP chest radiographs inadvertently resemble lordotic chest radiographs?

10. What are three things a radiographer can do to reduce the radiation dose during portable radiographic examinations?

▓ ▓ BIBLIOGRAPHY

Ballinger, PW, and Frank, ED: Merrill's Atlas of Radiographic Positions and Radiologic Procedures, ed 9. CV Mosby, St Louis, 1999.

Bontrager, K, and Anthony, B: Textbook of Radiographic Positions and Related Anatomy, ed 4. CV Mosby, St Louis, 1993.

Appendix 1

SYMPTOMS AND SIGNS OF DRUG ABUSE*

*Mixed intoxications produce complex combinations of signs and symptoms.

SYMPTOMS AND SIGNS OF DRUG ABUSE

Drug	Acute Intoxication and Overdose	Withdrawal Syndrome
CNS Stimulants Cocaine, amphetamine, dextroamphetamine, methylphenidate, phenmetrazine, phenylpropanolamine, STP[†], MDMA[‡], Bromo-DMA[§], diethylpropion, most amphetamine-like antiobesity drugs.	*Vital signs:* temperature elevated; heart rate increased; respirations shallow; BP elevated. *Mental status:* sensorium hyperacute or confused, paranoid ideation, hallucinations, delirium, impulsivity, agitation, hyperactivity, sterotypy. *Physical exam:* pupils dilated and reactive, tendon reflexes hyperactive, cardiac arrhythmias, dry mouth, sweating, tremors, convulsions, coma, stroke.	Muscular aches; abdominal pain; chills, tremors; voracious hunger; anxiety; prolonged sleep; lack of energy; profound depression, sometimes suicidal; exhaustion
Opioids Heroin, morphine, codeine, meperidine, methadone, hydromorphone, opium, pentazocine, propoxyphene, fentanyl, sufentanil	*Vital signs:* temperature decreased, respiration depressed; BP decreased, sometimes shock. *Mental status:* euphoria, stupor. *Physical exam:* pupils constricted (may be dilated	Pupils dilated; pulse rapid; gooseflesh; lacrimation, abdominal cramps; muscle jerks; flulike syndrome; vomiting; diarrhea; tremulousness; yawning; anxiety

with meperidine or extreme hypoxia), reflexes diminished to absent, pulmonary edema, constipation, convulsions with propoxyphene or meperidine, cardiac arrhythmias with propoxyphene, coma.

CNS Depressants
Barbiturates, benzodiazepines, glutethimide, meprobamate, methaqualone, ethchlorvynol, chloral hydrate, methyprylon, paraldehyde

Vital signs: respiration depressed; BP decreased; sometimes shock. *Mental status:* drowsiness or coma, confusion, delirium. *Physical exam:* pupils dilated with glutethimide or in severe poisoning, tendon reflexes depressed, ataxia, slurred speech, nystagmus, convulsions or hyperirritability with methaqualone, signs of anticholinergic poisoning with glutethimide, cardiac arrhythmias with chloral hydrate.

Tremulousness, insomnia, sweating, fever, clonic blink reflex, anxiety, cardiovascular collapse, agitation, delirium, hallucinations, disorientation, convulsions, shock

SYMPTOMS AND SIGNS OF DRUG ABUSE (continued)

Drug	Acute Intoxication and Overdose	Withdrawal Syndrome
Hallucinogens LSD,‖ psilocybin, mescaline, PCP¶	*Vital signs:* temperature elevated, heart rate increased, BP elevated. *Mental status:* euphoria, anxiety or panic, paranoia, sensorium often clear, affect inappropriate, illusions, time and visual distortions, visual hallucinations, depersonalization, with PCP hypertensive encephalopathy. *Physical exam:* pupils dilated (normal or small with PCP), tendon reflexes hyperactive. With PCP: cyclic coma or extreme hyperactivity, drooling, blank stare, mutism, amnesia, analgesia, nystagmus (sometimes vertical), gait ataxia, muscle rigidity, impulsive or violent behavior; violent, scatologic, pressured speech.	None

Cannabis Group
Marijuana, hashish, THC,** hash oil, sinsemilla

Vital signs: heart rate increased; BP decreased on standing. *Mental status:* anorexia, then increased appetite; euphoria; anxiety; sensorium often clear; dreamy, fantasy state; time-space distortions; hallucinations may be rare. *Physical exam:* pupils unchanged; conjunctiva injected; tachycardia, ataxia, and pallor in children

Nonspecific symptoms including anorexia, nausea, insomnia, restlessness, irritability, anxiety, depression

Anticholinergics
Atropine; belladonna; henbane; scopolamine; trihexyphenidyl; benztropine mesylate; procyclidine; propantheline bromide; jimson weed seed

Vital signs: temperature elevated, heart rate increased; possibly decreased BP. *Mental status:* drowsiness or coma; sensorium clouded; amnesia; disorientation; visual hallucinations; body image alterations; confusion; with propantheline restlessness, excitement. *Physical exam:* pupils dilated and fixed; decreased bowel

Gastrointestinal and musculoskeletal symptoms

SYMPTOMS AND SIGNS OF DRUG ABUSE *(continued)*		
Drug	Acute Intoxication and Overdose	Withdrawal Syndrome
Anticholinergics *(continued)*	sounds; flushed, dry skin and mucous membranes; violent behavior, convulsions; with propantheline circulatory failure, respiratory failure, paralysis, coma.	

†STP (2,5-dimethoxy-4-methylamphetamine).
‡MDMA (3,4-methylenedioxymethamphetamine).
§Bromo-DMA (4-Bromo-2,5-dimethoxyamphetamine).
‖LSD (D-lysergic acid diethylamide).
¶PCP (phencyclidine).
**THC (delta-9-tetrahydrocannabinol).
Source: The Medical Letter, vol. 29, Sept. 11, 1987, with permission.

Appendix 2

MEDICAL EMERGENCIES— WOUNDS

MEDICAL EMERGENCIES—WOUNDS						
Type	History	Pathology	Symptoms and Color	Points of Identification	Transportation	Complications
Bite (human, animal, or insect)	Bite of a reptile or rabid human or animal. Sting or bite of poisonous insect.	Tissue degeneration at site of wound. Muscular paralysis. Venom has a drastic effect on respiratory nerve centers.	Type of wound: Snake—two-fang wound. Human—shape of denture. Dog—laceration; patient shows rabid disposition. Insect—elevated wheal with pain and	Shape of wound; odor of colon bacillus about the wound in human bite; presence of stinger.	Keep patient quiet; avert apprehension; keep muscles of the area elevated and at rest.	Infection introduced by pathogenic organisms. Venom of toxic nature depresses victim. Death delay in treatment.

Brush burns or abrasions	Friction of body against rough surface.	Surface effaced with nicks and dotted with small drops of blood.	itching or burning sensation, or double red dot. Skin discolored. Surface peeled off with fine beadlike dots of blood. Skin may be permeated with foreign material.	Surface of the skin is brushed completely away, or remains very lightly attached to the area.	Use loose applications of sterile dressings held in place by loose-fitting triangle.	Infection. May retain rough, unsightly scars.
Contusions	Blow or fall.	A bruise (hematoma) or petechial area with	Skin surface is rough; the area includes a	Skin is not broken. Underlying tissues may be	Keep part well elevated. If there is additional abrasions, cover	Destruction of underlying tissue if hematoma is

MEDICAL EMERGENCIES—WOUNDS *(continued)*

Type	History	Pathology	Symptoms and Color	Points of Identification	Transportation	Complications
Contusions *(continued)*		underlying injury	large or small hematoma (depending upon the extent of injury).	slightly or markedly crushed.	with loose-fitting bandages.	not aspirated early. Infection if skin is punctured or probed.
Gun shots	Accident in care of a gun. Victim of deliberate gunfire.	Wound of single outer puncture site with deep injury consisting of twisting and tearing of tissue.	Aperture is small. Powder burns occasionally are found.	Puncture site. Deep wound shows characteristic twisting of the deeper tissues.	Keep patient very quiet; head slightly lower than body. Treat for shock. Watch temperature, pulse, respiration, and blood pressure if blood has been lost or patient is in shock.	Shock; internal hemorrhage; tetanus bacillus infection.

Lacerations	Accident wherein sharp instruments have cut and torn an area of the body.	Jagged or torn and roughened edges of tissues. May include avulsion of certain parts.	Injury has produced area of two raw or bleeding edges of the skin. Blood may be oozing or spurting from the wound.	Wound edges are jagged and irregular. Wound may contain amount of debris or dirt and usually is infected.	Edges of wound may be united with flamed strip of adhesive tape. Cover the area with loose dressings held by triangle or cravat bandage. Tetanus toxoid or antitoxin as required.	Infection and septicemia. Wound usually heals with very unsightly scar if not properly sutured.
Puncture	Accidental or intentional piercing of body with pointed object.	Tissues are pierced. Small opening through the tissues provide an excellent course or inlet for infection.	Area usually manifests no bleeding. Trauma of tissue usually evident.	Puncture site is very small. Object usually withdrawn with fair amount of ease.	Cover the area with sterile dressings and triangle or cravat bandage.	Infection of the anaerobic type (tetanus bacillus) and septicemia.
Stab	Injury by a blunt or	Size of hole in the tissue	Evidence of the	Large, very deep puncture	Keep patient very quiet with head	Internal hemorrhage

MEDICAL EMERGENCIES—WOUNDS *(continued)*

Type	History	Pathology	Symptoms and Color	Points of Identification	Transportation	Complications
Stab *(continued)*	pointed object, incurred during a fight or acquired by a fall or push.	varies with the size of the instrument. Foreign material and pathogenic bacteria of anaerobic nature are usually introduced.	instrument that was used, such as knife, ice pick, etc. Victim shows pallor, syncope, and later collapse.	site. Instrument may still be in wound. Victim may be pinned to an object by the force of the blow.	and chest slightly elevated. Treat for shock. If chest is involved, watch TPR and blood pressure.	from, or damage to, organs underlying site of wound, such as puncture and collapse of lung, abdominal visceral injury, or severance of nerve. Pulmonary hemorrhage. Infection of body by anaerobic organisms.

Source: Adapted from Thomas, CL (ed): Taber's Cyclopedic Medical Dictionary, ed 15. FA Davis, Philadelphia, 1985, pp 2119–2121, with permission.

Appendix 3

THE INTERPRETER IN FIVE LANGUAGES

LANGUAGES WITH PHONETIC PRONUNCIATIONS

English

Hello. I want to help you. I do not speak (English) but will use this book to ask you some questions. I will not be able to understand your spoken answers. Please respond by shaking your head or raising one finger to indicate "no"; nod your head or raise two fingers to indicate "yes."

Spanish

Translation

Saludos. Quiero ayudarlo. Yo no hablo español, pero voy a usar este libro para hacerle algunas preguntas. No voy a poder entender sus respuestas; por eso haga el favor de contestar, negando con la cabeza o levantando un dedo para indicar "no" y afirmando con la cabeza o levantando dos dedos para indicar "si."

Phonetic

Sah-loo'dohs. Ki-air'oh ah-joo-dar'loh. Joh noh ah'bloh es'panyohl, pair'oh voy ah oo-sar' es'tay lee'broh pahr'ah ah-sair'lay ahl-goo'nahs pray-goon'tahs. Noh voy ah poh-dair' en-ten-dair' soos res-poo-es'tahs; pore es-soh ah'gah el fah-vohr' day kohn-tes-tahr', nay-gahn'doh kohn lah kah-bay'thah oh lay-vahn-tahn'doh oon day'doh pahr'ah een-dee-kahr' noh ee ah-feer-mahn'doh kohn lah kah-bay'thah oh lay-vahn-tahn'doh dohs day'dohs pahr'a een-dee-kahr' see.

Italian

Buon giorno. La voglio aiutare. Io non parlo italiano, ma userò questo libro per farle qualche domanda. Non potrò comprendere le Sue domande. Per favore risponda con un cenno di testa. Alzi un dito per indicare "no;" muova la Sua testa su e giu o alzi due dita per indicare "si."

Translation

Phonetic

Bwon jih-or'noh. Lah vol'yoh ah-yoo-tar'ay. Ee'oh nohn par'loh ee-towl-ee-ah'noh mah oo-say'roh kwes'toh lee'broh pehr fahr'lay kwall'kay doh-mahn'dah. Non poh'throh kohm-prehn'deh-ray lay soo'ee doh-mahn'day. Pehr fah-vohr' ay ray-spohn'dah kohn oon chay'noh dee tes'tah. Ahlt'zih oon dee'toh pehr in-dee-kar'ay noh; moo-oh'vah la soo'ah tes'tah soo eh joo oh alht'zih doo'ay dee-ta pehr in-dee-kar'ay see.

French

Bonjour. Je veux bien vous aider. Je ne parle pas français mais tout en me servant de ce livre je vais vous poser des questions. Je ne comprendrai pas ce que vous dites en français. Je vous en prie, pour répondre: pour indiquer "non," secouez la tête ou levez un seul doigt; pour indiquer "oui," faites un signe de tete ou levez deux doigts.

Translation

Phonetic

Bon-zhoor'. Zheh veh bih-ehn' voo ay-day'. Zheh neh parl pah frahn-say' may too ahn meh sehr-vahn' d' seh lee'vrah zheh vay voo poh-say' day kehs-tih-on'. Zheh neh kahm-prahn'dray pah seh keh voo deet ahn frahn-say'. Zheh voo ahn pree, poor ray-pahn'drah; poor ahn-dee-kay nohn, seh-kway' lah teht oo leh-vay' on sool dwoit; por ahn-dee-kay wee', fayt on seen deh teht oo leh-vay' duh dwoit.

LANGUAGES WITH PHONETIC PRONUNCIATIONS (continued)

German

Translation

Hallo! Ich möchte Ihnen helfen. Ich spreche kein Deutsch, aber ich werde dieses Buch benützten um Sie einiges zu fragen. Ich werde Ihre Antworten nicht verstehen. Deshalb antworten Sie mir indem Sie Ihren Kopf schütteln oder heben Sie Ihren Finger um "nein" auszudrücken; nicken Sie mit dem Kopf oder heben Sie zwei Finger um "ja" auszudrücken.

Phonetic

Ha-loh! Ich möhh'tuh ee'nuhn hel'fuhn. Ich shpre'huh kīn doitsh, ah'buhr ich ver'duh dee'zuhs bookh bā-nüt'zuhn um zee ī'ni-guhs tsoo frah'guhn. Ich ver'duh ee'ruh ant'vor-tuhn nihht fer-shtay'uhn. Dās-halb' ant'vor-tuhn zee meer in-dām' zee ee'ruhn kopf shü'tln ō'der hāb'uhn zee ee'ruhn fing'uhr um nīn ows'tsoo-drük-uhn; nick'uhn zee mit dām kopf ō'der hāb'uhn zee tsvī fing'uhr um ya ows'tsoo-drük-uhn.

THE INTERPRETER IN FIVE LANGUAGES

English	Spanish	Italian	French	German
What is your name?	¿Cómo se llama?	Come si chiama Lei?	Quel est votre nom?	Wie heissen Sie?
How old are you?	¿Cuántos años tiene?	Quanti anni ha?	Quel âge avez-vous?	Wie alt sind Sie?
Do you understand me?	¿Me entiende?	Mi capisce?	Me comprenez-vous?	Verstehen Sie mich?
Answer only . . .	Conteste solamente . . .	Risponda solamente . . .	Répondez seulement . . .	Antworten Sie nur . . .
Yes No	Sí No	Si No	Oui Non	Ja Nein
Show me . . .	Enséñeme . . .	Mi faccia vedere . . .	Montrez-moi . . .	Zeigen Sie mir . . .
Which side?	¿En qué lado?	Quale lato?	Quel côté?	Auf welcher Seite?
Right	Derecha	A destra	A droit	Rechts
Left	Izquierda	A sinistra	A gauche	Links
Sit down.	Siéntese.	Si sieda.	Asseyez-vous.	Setzen Sie sich.
Stand up.	Levántese.	Si alzi.	Levez-vous.	Stehen Sie auf.
Do you feel dizzy?	¿Tiene Ud. vértigo?	Ha delle vertigini?	Avez-vous le vertige?	Ist Ihnen schwindlig?

THE INTERPRETER IN FIVE LANGUAGES (continued)

English	Spanish	Italian	French	German
Have you any difficulty in breathing?	¿Tiene dificultad al respirar?	Ha difficoltà di respirare?	C'est difficile à respirer?	Fällt Ihnen das Atemholen schwer?
Have you any pain?	¿Tiene dolor?	Ha dolori?	Avez-vous mal quelque part?	Haben Sie Schmerzen?
Where does it hurt?	¿Dónde le duele?	Dove le duele?	Où avez-vous mal?	Wo haben Sie Schmerzen?
Do you have pain here?	¿Le duele aquí?	Ha dolori qui?	Avez-vous mal par ici?	Haben Sie Schmerzen hier?

Source: Adapted from Thomas, CL (ed): Taber's Cyclopedic Medical Dictionary, ed 17. FA Davis, Philadelphia, 1993, pp 2370–2391, with permission.

Appendix 4

CASE STUDIES

▨ ▨ **CASE 1**

▨ **PATIENT CONDITION**

A male construction worker has fallen from a scaffold that was 30 feet above the ground. On entering the radiography department, you observe the following:

1. The requisition history states "fell 30 feet; 5 milligrams Demerol given IV" (10 minutes ago).
2. The patient's breathing and color appear normal.
3. No open wounds.
4. His speech is slightly slurred, and his answers to your questions are rather long and he tends to lose track of what he was saying.
5. He appears sleepy.
6. He complains of pain in both feet, both knees, both hips, and his lower back.
7. The heels of both feet are swollen and bruised.
8. The patient states that he feels that he can move his left hip, but not his right hip. He says that his right hip is much more painful than his left.
9. He states that he has had no fractures in his lower extremities and that the only surgery he has ever had was an appendectomy.
10. The accident happened 40 minutes ago.

▨ **ASSIGNMENT**

1. Write a history for this patient using medical terms.

327

2. List and describe additional observations you may want to take:
   a. Before beginning the radiographic examinations
   b. During the radiographic examinations
   c. After the radiographic examinations
3. What are the patient's most probable injuries?
4. Select the methods you will use for the examinations that have been ordered for this patient:
   a. Right and left foot
   b. Right and left calcaneus
   c. Right and left knee
   d. Right and left hip
   e. Lumbar spine
   f. Place the positions in the order you will perform them.
   g. How will you perform these examinations while minimizing the possibility of causing additional injury?

CASE 2

PATIENT CONDITION

You have been called to the emergency room to perform portable examinations on a gunshot victim. On arriving, you find the following:

1. The patient has been shot in the abdomen, left shoulder, and right chest.
2. A respiratory therapist is ventilating the patient.
3. The patient is unconscious.
4. The patient's breathing is shallow and rapid.
5. The patient's face is gray.
6. Bleeding from the gunshot wounds is currently under control.
7. The physician has found entry wounds but has not positively identified exit wounds.
8. When the patient was shot, he was thrown backward through a window, and pieces of glass are scattered across the sheets on his cart.

ASSIGNMENT

1. Write a history for this patient using medical terms.
2. The physician has told you that she wants radiographs of the chest and abdomen but has not ordered specific examinations. Select the examinations and methods you will use to demonstrate the injured areas.
3. Place the positions in the order you will perform them.
4. List the cassettes and equipment you will need to perform these examinations.
5. Describe any special problems or concerns that this case presents.

CASE 3

PATIENT CONDITION

A 4-year-old girl ran away from her mother at a shopping mall and fell down five stairs, landing on her head. She is sent to the radiography department with a requisition for skull and facial bone examinations. While talking to the mother and the girl you find:

1. The girl is not taking any prescription medicine, nor was any given in the emergency room.
2. The girl is pale.
3. The girl's breathing is 12 respirations per minute.
4. The girl appears tired, but the mother says this is not her normal nap time.
5. The girl does not readily answer you when you ask her name and age (although her mother says she knows both and is not usually shy).
6. There is a swollen and bruised area over the frontal bone.
7. There are no open wounds or bleeding.

ASSIGNMENT

1. Write a history for this patient using medical terms.

2. What are the injuries you would expect to see in this case?
3. Select the methods you will use to perform the examinations that were ordered.
4. Describe the special problems this patient presents and the methods you will use to solve them.
5. During the radiographic examination, the girl begins to vomit profusely. Describe the actions you will take when this occurs.

▨ ▨ CASE 4

▨ PATIENT CONDITION: PART 1

A female patient has been involved in a head-on A/A. She was driving 45 miles an hour when—as she describes it in a lengthy, slurring fashion—the car just went into the other lane and struck a parked car. She states that she was wearing a seat belt. She also says that she was on her way home after work and that she often has trouble sleeping, so she stopped for one drink. She also tells you that, as she got to her car to leave, she took a few pills to help her sleep. She says she took them when she left so that they would take effect just as she got home. That was 1 hour and 15 minutes before the accident, and the accident happened 30 minutes ago. She says the pills were "pheno-barbi-something."

▨ ASSIGNMENT

1. What injuries would you expect from this type of accident?

▨ PATIENT CONDITION: PART 2

On examining the patient, you find the following:

1. She is wearing a cervical collar.
2. Her right eye and nose are bruised and swollen.

3. Her nose does not lie in the MSP.
4. Her right foot is bruised, and she says she cannot feel anything below her right hip.
5. The anterior side of her right knee is greatly swollen and deeply bruised.
6. She can feel her left leg and can move the toes on her left foot.
7. She can move the fingers on both hands.
8. She cannot move her right hip or leg.

ASSIGNMENT

1. What additional observations should you make?

PATIENT CONDITION: PART 3

You check and find no popliteal or dorsalis pedis pulse on the patient's right leg. The popliteal and dorsalis pedis pulses on the left leg are 84. The patient is slightly pale; her breathing appears to be normal.

ASSIGNMENT

1. Write a history for this patient using medical terms.
2. What radiographic examinations do you think should be performed?
3. Select the methods needed for these examinations.
4. Place your selected methods in the order in which they should be performed.
5. During the performance of the radiographic examinations, the patient becomes paler, complains of feeling light-headed, and appears restless. She asks for some water, and her breathing becomes more rapid but shallower. What actions do you take? What condition is she experiencing?
6. Describe any special problems this case presents and your solution for them.

▨ ▨ CASE 5

▨ PATIENT CONDITION

A male patient is sent to the radiography department in a wheelchair with an order for right knee and right lower leg studies. His right knee is flexed about 30 degrees. He states that he was jogging, and his left leg began hurting at the lower third of his shin. Because of this problem, he began placing more stress on his right knee. After another mile, his left knee was hurting more and his right knee suddenly locked in its current position. He has not had fractures, injuries, or surgery on either leg before.

▨ ASSIGNMENT

1. What injuries do you suspect from the patient's history?
2. What additional actions will you perform before the radiographic examinations?
3. Select the methods you will use to perform right knee and left lower leg examinations.
4. Describe the special problems that this case presents and how you will solve them.

CASE STUDIES ANSWERS

1. Pt. fell 30 feet from a scaffold. Color and resp. normal. Pt. appears drowsy. Pt. complains of pain bilaterally in feet, knees, and hips (right is more painful than left); also in lower back. No previous injuries. Previous surgery: appendectomy.
2. a. Pulse rates for popliteal and dorsalis pedis on both legs. Evaluate mental status.
   b. Monitor leg pulse rates and observe for changes in mental status and for signs of shock.
   c. Pulse rates for popliteal and dorsalis pedis on both legs, respiration and color.
3. Traumatic flat feet, fractured calcaneus, impacted fractures near the knees, fractured femoral necks (especially the right), fractures of the transverse processes of the lumbar spine, compression fractures of the lumbar spine.
4. a. Horizontal beam projection (HBP) anteroposterior (AP) and lateral feet.
   b. HBP lateral calcaneus and plantodorsal projection axial *calcaneus.*
   c. AP and HBP LM knee.
   d. AP right and left hips, AP pelvis, Clements-Nakayama method for right and left hips (if the patient does *not* have injuries of the left leg, a Danelius-Miller method for the *right* may be possible).
   e. AP lumbar spine, HBP lateral, and HBP L5-S1.
   f. Lateral first, starting with the lumbar spine, then the hips, knees, etc. Then the APs.

g. By using HBPs and by moving the legs as little as possible for the APs.

CASE 2

1. Gunshot wounds to the abdomen, left shoulder, and right chest. Pt. is comatose, probably in shock. Pt. was thrown through a window, and many pieces of glass are present.
2. AP chest and AP abdomen.
3. AP chest then AP abdomen.
4. 14 × 17 inch (35 × 43 cm) cassette and 14 × 17 inch grid cassette. Markers.
5. Because we are trying to demonstrate foreign bodies and some types of glass will show up on radiographs, as much of the glass as possible should be removed. Ideally, there should be no glass between the patient and the film. The markers should be placed along the side of the films at the same level as the bullet wounds. Because a grid is being used, extra care will have to be taken to ensure that it is perpendicular to the CR.

CASE 3

1. Pt. fell down five stairs, striking her head. There is a bruised, swollen area over the frontal bone. She is drowsy and does not respond to questions; face is gray; resp. 12 per minute.
2. Possible fracture of the frontal and a concussion, possibly a subdural hematoma.
3. AP skull (pediatric patients are usually reluctant to lie face down on the x-ray table), both lateral skulls; Towne method for skull, Water's for facial bones and lateral facial bones.
4. Restraining the patient will be a problem; having the parents in the room may help. Because the patient has a good possibility of a concussion or subdural hematoma, she should never be left alone in the room and her consciousness should be continually monitored.

5. Ensure a clear airway, turn the patient's head to the side, and provide an emesis basin. Notify a physician, because the vomiting may be related to the head injury.

■ ■ CASE 4

■ PART 1

1. Anterior skull injuries if her head struck the windshield, possible cervical spine injury, too. Depressed fracture of the sternum and possible injury to the knee, femur, and hip if the legs struck the dashboard.

■ PART 2

1. Popliteal and dorsalis pedis pulses of the right leg. Evaluate for injury to the brain (e.g., vision, hearing).

■ PART 3

1. Pt. was involved in an A/A. Pt. is drowsy—this could be due to skull trauma. Pt. appears to have injured right eye, nose, right foot, and right hip. Popliteal and dorsalis pedis pulses are *absent* on the right leg; they are 84 bpm on the left leg. Breathing is normal, slight pallor. Pt. can move fingers of both hands and left leg.
2. Cervical spine, facial bones or right orbit, nasal bones, right foot, right knee, and right hip.
3. HBP lateral cervical spine. Assuming that the patient must be radiographed in the supine position, AP cervical supine and AP open-mouth cervical spine, reverse Rhese position for right orbit, reverse Waters (or modified reverse Waters—skull AP, CR angled 40 degrees cephalic), HBP lateral nasal bones, AP right hip, AP pelvis, Danelius-Miller right hip, AP and lateral right knee, and AP and lateral right foot.
4. Cervical spine; orbits; nasal bones; AP pelvis, hip, knee, foot; HBP lateral hip, knee, and foot.

5. Place the patient in a Trendelenburg position because she is probably going into shock.
6. Monitoring consciousness, not leaving the patient alone; equipment will be needed for HBPs.

▦ ▦ CASE 5

1. Stress fracture of the distal third of the left leg, cartilage damage or a loose bone fragment in the right knee.
2. None.
3. AP and lateral left lower leg, AP right knee with a curved cassette or PA partial flexion positions, and lateral knee.
4. The flexion of the right knee makes the routine AP knee less valuable and makes obliques of this knee of questionable value.

Appendix 5

ANSWERS TO SELF-ASSESSMENT TESTS

1. The radial artery is the most common location for taking a pulse. The index and middle fingers are placed on the anterior surface of the patient's wrist on the lateral side (at the distal end of the radius, near the navicular). The thumb cannot be used because it has a pulse of its own, which could be confused with the patient's. Counting for 15 seconds and multiplying by 4 to obtain the beats per minute may be acceptable. Counting for 30 seconds and doubling that rate is more accurate and desirable.

    Other locations for pulses are the carotid, femoral, temporal, dorsalis pedis, and popliteal arteries. Of these, the carotid artery is most often used. It is found on either side of the thyroid cartilage. The femoral pulse is located about 2 inches medial and 3 inches inferior to the anterior superior iliac spine (ASIS). The temporal pulse is about ½ inch anterior and ½ inch superior to the external auditory meatus (EAM). The dorsalis pedis pulse is on the dorsal surface of the foot, at the top of arch, on the medial side of the first metatarsal. The popliteal pulse is in the middle of the posterior surface of the knee.

2. Try to obtain a pulse at a point distal to the fracture. Record the rate and time. This should be done as the patient enters the department, as he or she leaves the department, or when movement of the part or patient

causes the radiographer to suspect that damage to blood vessels has occurred.

3. The typical pulse rate for adult men is 70 to 72 beats per minute, and for adult women it is 78 to 82.

4. Tachycardia describes a pulse rate higher than normal (more than 100 beats per minute); bradycardia describes a pulse rate lower than normal (less than 60 beats per minute).

5. Higher than normal pulse rates are seen in pediatric patients (often 110 to 120), patients who are standing, those who have fevers, or those who have just exerted themselves. Simply entering a hospital may raise some patients' heart rates. Being nervous, having just been in an accident, or the onset of shock may also raise the pulse rate.

6. Lower than normal pulse rates are sometimes found in tall patients, geriatric patients, resting or recumbent patients, and those in excellent physical condition.

7. The strength, weakness, or absence of the pulse should be noted in addition to its speed. A strong, rapid pulse may be caused by nervousness, whereas a weak and rapid pulse may be a symptom of shock.

8. Normal breathing varies from 12 to 20 respirations per minute, with the average being 15 or 16. Children under 5 years old normally breathe more rapidly than adults.

9. Tachypnea is rapid breathing (25 or more respirations per minute). A measure of fewer than 12 respirations per minute is considered bradypnea (slower than normal breathing). Dyspnea is difficult or labored breathing. Apnea is absence of breathing.

10. Typical adult oral temperature is 98.6° Fahrenheit (37° Celsius), with the normal range being plus or minus 1°.

11. Typical adult male blood pressure is 120/80. The range for normal systolic pressure is 100 to 140. The normal diastolic range is 60 to 90. Females, children and elderly people generally have lower normal blood pressures.

12. a. Obtain the patient's previous and current history—old fractures, surgery, how the patient was injured.

This information helps the radiographer in selecting procedures and helps the radiologist when reading the film.

b. Verify the correctness of the examinations ordered— was a left knee accidently ordered when the right knee was injured? Does the patient need a shoulder, humerus, clavicle, scapula, or A-C joints?

c. Assess the patient's condition. This pertains to the patient's ability to cooperate with the examination. Check for medical conditions that will require special care or more frequent observation and review.

d. Obtain the patient's vital signs. This is done to document the patient's entry and exit conditions, to assess the patient's condition, and to provide a baseline to refer to if the patient's condition should change.

e. Convey a caring and empathetic attitude.

13. What happened to the patient? What type of accident or trauma occurred? Where is the patient injured? Where was the impact point (or points)? Where is the pain? When was the patient injured? Has the patient ever been injured before in the same area as the current injury? Has the patient had surgery in that area before?

14. a. Mental status: Evaluate by questioning the patient and using the guide in this chapter (or on the Quick Reference Card).

b. Respiration: Evaluate by counting the respirations and by observing the patient.

c. Skin color: Evaluate by observation.

d. Presence of open wounds or bleeding: Evaluate by questioning the patient or other health personnel, and by observation.

e. Degree of sensation or the presence of pain: Evaluate by questioning the patient and by observation.

f. Musculoskeletal integrity: Evaluate by questioning the patient and by observation (both are aided by knowledge of the types of injuries that commonly occur from different kinds of trauma).

g. Patient mobility: Evaluate by questioning the patient and by observation.

15. The radiographer's legal concerns when examining a trauma patient include responsibility for the patient's well-being when in the radiographer's care, using methods that minimize the chances for additional injury to the patient, and being able to provide evidence that the radiographer's performance was equal to, or better than, that provided by any reasonable radiographer (in other words, documentation that what was done was proper). These goals can be accomplished by careful entry and exit patient evaluations, close observation as dictated by the patient's condition, use of suitable alternative methods when the routine procedures could cause additional injury, and written proof that these procedures were followed, which includes the date, the time, and the initials or signature of the radiographer.

▪ ▪ CHAPTER 2: SELF-ASSESSMENT TEST ANSWERS

1. Respiratory arrest. Call a cardiac arrest code and initiate CPR.
2. Shock. Place the patient in a Trendelenburg position, place a blanket over the patient, ensure that the patient has a patent airway, and call for a physician.
3. An artery has been severed. Apply direct pressure to the artery. If the bleeding does not stop after 5 minutes, call for assistance.
4. Difficult or labored breathing.
5. Open, clear, without obstruction.
6. Supine with the feet and legs raised (or the head and shoulders down).
7. Bleeding.
8. Insufficient circulation (which has many causes).
9. Fainting.
10. Paleness, or loss of color.
11. In respiratory arrest, the lungs and diaphragm cease to function but the heart continues (until lack of oxygen causes it to stop also). In cardiac arrest, the heart stops beating. Therefore, with respiratory arrest, the

pulse will continue for a few moments, but in cardiac arrest, there will be no pulse.

12. Hypovolemic shock is caused from a loss of blood volume, which can be from external or internal hemorrhage. Neurogenic shock involves the nervous system and can be related to mental or physical factors. Traumatic shock is a result of injury; generally, the more severe the injury, the greater the shock or the greater the chance of shock.

13. Arterial bleeding is pulsing, bright red blood. Venous bleeding involves dark red blood that does not pulse. Capillary blood oozes rather than flows.

14. Vertigo is a sensation of movement, or of the surroundings moving; dizziness is a light-headed feeling.

15. In one-person CPR, two respirations are given for every 15 chest compressions; in two-person CPR, one respiration is given for every five compressions.

■ ■ CHAPTER 3: SELF-ASSESSMENT TEST ANSWERS

1. 3
2. 2
3. 1
4. 1
5. 2
6. 4
7. 4
8. 1
9. 1
10. 2

■ ■ CHAPTER 4: SELF-ASSESSMENT TEST ANSWERS

1. Trauma injuries are those caused by external force or violence.
2. Automobile accident.
3. Fracture.

4. A bone no longer in its normal articulation; out of joint.

5. Injury from a blow or from striking an object. It usually means a blow to the head, which can cause unconsciousness and damage to the brain. It can also be used in reference to the spine or inner ear.

6. The first stage of healing that can be radiographically demonstrated (other than swelling). The stage of healing where calcium is being laid into the bone matrix.

7. A fracture in which the bone breaks through the skin.

8. A fracture in which the bone does *not* break through the skin.

9. Bone displacement; being out of alignment.

10. A fracture with two or more fracture lines, resulting in three or more fracture fragments.

11. A star-shaped fracture; a fracture with lines radiating from a central point.

12. A fracture, usually of a vertebral body, in which the bone is squashed.

13. A fracture, usually of the skull, in which the bone is pushed in.

14. A fracture resulting from abnormal strain placed on normal bone.

15. A fracture found only in the flexible bones of children in which one side breaks but the other does not.

16. Another name for a greenstick fracture; probably derived from the round protrusion on the side of the bone that is broken.

17. A fracture in which strain at a joint has pulled a piece of bone away from the segment where it attaches to a tendon.

18. A partial dislocation; usually one bone has moved inferiorly (caudally) from its normal position.

19. A transverse fracture is parallel to the transverse plane, an oblique fracture is at an angle to the long axis of the bone, and a spiral fracture's lines run up and around the shaft of a bone.

20. Compound fractures break through the skin, comminuted fractures have more than two fracture fragments, complicated fractures are those which have associated injuries to internal organs, and compres-

sion fractures involve the collapse of a vertebral body.

21. Stress and pathologic.
22. Greenstick and epiphyseal.
23. Limited or no movement of a limb; swelling at the site of the injury; pain at, or distal to, the injury; bruising at the injury site; deformity of a limb; no pulse distal to the injury; loss of feeling at, or distal to, the injury.
24. Direct fractures occur at the point of impact or trauma, indirect fractures occur some distance from the impact point.
25. Because of indirect fractures, the radiographer must be concerned with an area larger than that of the impact point. This means that the radiographer must carefully evaluate the patient, carefully move the patient, and include the entire part or area in the radiographic examination.

▦ ▦ CHAPTER 5: SELF-ASSESSMENT TEST 1 ANSWERS

1. a. The patient's head may strike the windshield, dashboard, or steering wheel. It could also pass through the windshield. Damage can occur to the brain, frontal bone, facial bones, and cervical spine. The possible injuries include epidural hematoma, subdural hematoma, skull fractures, rhinorrhea, otorrhea, facial injuries. Facial bone fracture concerns involve subcondylar fractures of the mandible and fractures of the mandibular symphysis. These fractures can allow the tongue to obstruct the throat and block the airway. Fracture of the zygoma is also a concern because it is the main support between the cranium and the maxilla. A fracture here can also involve the inferior and the lateral portions of the orbital rim. Also possible are spinal column injuries.

   b. Thoracic injuries can include the heart, great vessels, and lungs; fractured ribs; a fractured sternum; or fractured clavicles. Fractured ribs may puncture a lung, causing atelectasis, pneumothorax, hematopneumothorax, or hematothorax.

    c. Abdominal trauma from front-end collisions can be caused by the steering wheel. Some injuries may also be produced by lap-type seat belts. The spleen and liver are often involved. If the pelvis is fractured, there is always the possibility that the bladder is ruptured.

    d. The lower extremity injuries include aviator's astragalus, the patella, condylar or impacted fractures of the femur, and posterior rim fractures of the acetabulum.

2. a. Whiplash (or forced extension of the cervical spine), brain injuries.

    b. Damage to thoracic organs (heart, lungs, and great vessels), and the ribs and sternum.

    c. Possible injury to the kidneys.

    d. There are no extremity injuries that are common or typical in rear-end impact automobile accidents.

3. a. Typical head and neck injuries from side impacts involve the cervical spine, sometimes the brain. When the brain is involved, it can be a concussion or shearing and momentum injuries.

    b. Damage to the ribs, atelectasis, pneumothorax, hematopneumothorax, or hematothorax.

    c. Injury to the spleen and to the kidney on the side of the impact.

    d. If the arm was at the patient's side, the injuries could include fractures of the forearm, intercondylar fractures of the distal humerus, fractures of the midshaft and proximal humerus, and possibly fractures of the clavicle and scapula (especially from the humeral head being forced into, and fracturing, the glenoid fossa). If the window was rolled down and the arm was resting on the door, the injuries may include comminuted fractures of the elbow, impacted or intercondylar fractures of the distal humerus, impacted fractures of the humeral head, and damage to the glenoid fossa. In the lower extremity, the hip and pelvis are major concerns. The force can cause intertrochanteric fractures and impacted fractures of the femoral head, or it may force the head of the femur into the acetabulum, causing it to burst and send fragments internally. The force may also fracture the pelvis. This can result in damage to the urinary tract (especially the bladder), reproductive system, circulatory system, and lower abdominal organs, as well as fractures of the iliac wing.

4. Linear or depressed fractures of the vertex of the skull, with or without damage to the brain, and a bursting fracture of the atlas (C1). Compression fractures of the vertebral bodies and fractures of the transverse processes of the vertebrae, especially the lumbar spine. Separations of the A-C joint or shoulder joint, and fractures of the clavicle, scapula, or humerus.

5. a. Linear or depressed fractures of the skull at the impact point, with or without underlying brain damage. Contrecoup injuries may also be present. Also, shearing forces to the blood vessels could produce subdural or epidural hematomas. Damage to the cervical spine can range from strained muscles to displaced fractures. Also, shoveler's fracture is possible.

   b. Single or multiple rib fractures, atelectasis, other injuries to thoracic organs, sternum injuries, cardiac tamponade or widening of the mediastinum, and compression fractures of the thoracic spine.

   c. Injury to the spleen, the liver, the bowel, the kidneys, and the lumbar spine.

   d. The hand suffers the greatest amount of damage. Hand injuries range from insult from foreign bodies to crushing injuries to traumatic amputation. In the wrist, Colles' fracture may be seen. Also, fractures of the forearm, injuries to the elbow, and injuries to the shoulder area. Most of the work-related injuries to the lower extremities involve the feet. Traumatic flat feet, Lisfranc's dislocations, fractures of the calcaneus, and fractures or dislocations of the ankle are seen. Also, bimalleolar and trimalleolar fractures, dislocation of the ankle, damage to the knee and the femoral condyles, and possibly, Malgaigne's fracture of the pelvis.

6. a. Concussions, facial damage, nasal bone fractures, zygomatic arch and mandible fractures. Blowout fractures of the orbit; injuries to the anterior neck;

and fractures, dislocations, and whiplash injuries to the cervical spine.

b. Single rib fractures, multiple rib fractures, atelectasis, and pneumothorax are all possible. Also, compression fractures of the thoracic spine; sternoclavicular separations or separations of the sternum, clavicle, and first rib; stress fractures of the ribs.

c. Spleen, liver, kidney, bowel damage, and compression fractures of the lumbar spine.

d. Injury to the hand, dislocated fingers, and avulsion fractures of the phalanges, baseball finger (also called mallet finger or dropped finger), boxer's fracture, injuries to the thumb, Little League elbow, and dislocated shoulders. Traumatic flat feet or fractures of the calcaneus, dislocations of the talonavicular or talocalcaneal joints, stress fractures of the midshaft of the metatarsals or of the calcaneal tuberosity, ankle sprains, lower leg injuries, stress fractures at midshaft or at the distal one third of the tibia, damage to the tibial plateau, ski-boot fractures, and (of course) knee injuries.

▪ ▫ CHAPTER 5: SELF-ASSESSMENT TEST 2 ANSWERS

1. Front-end impact. Other injuries could involve the femurs, hips, sternum, ribs, cervical spine, face, and skull.
2. Colles' fracture. Other injuries could include the forearm, elbow, distal humerus, shoulder, hip, and coccyx.
3. The posterior skull should be included because injury can occur at points opposite to the impact also.
4. The force (through a shock wave) can be transmitted through the body, causing injury as it goes.

▪ ▫ CHAPTER 6: SELF-ASSESSMENT TEST ANSWERS

1. a. Anteroposterior (AP) right hip, AP pelvis, Clements-Nakayama method for right hip (this is needed because the other injuries to the legs will prevent the

left leg from being abducted), AP and lateral femurs, AP and lateral lower legs, AP, lateral and oblique right foot.

b. AP right hip, AP pelvis, Clements-Nakayama right hip, AP right femur, AP right lower leg, AP left femur, AP left lower leg, horizontal beam projection (HBP) LM right femur, HBP LM right lower leg, HBP LM left lower leg, HBP LM left femur, HBP AP right foot, oblique right foot, HBP LM right foot.

c. Sandbags, a vertical cassette holder, or similar devices will be needed for the HBPs; sponges may be needed to raise the legs for the HBPs.

d. The film will have to be supported on the Bucky for the Clements-Nakayama method and for the HBPs.

2. a. Both partial flexion elbow positions, lateral elbow.

b. Does not matter.

c. A sponge, sandbag, or other support for the forearm when performing the partial flexion position that demonstrates the distal humerus.

d. The forearm will need support for the position described in c.

3. a. A minimum cervical spine routine that includes AP, AP open-mouth, and lateral positions; upper, lower, and oblique ribs; RAO and lateral sternum.

b. An HBP lateral cervical must be taken first. If a physician interprets the radiographs and gives permission for the patient to be examined in the routine way, then the AP cervical, AP open-mouth cervical, and oblique cervical spine radiographs may be obtained. The rib and sternum radiographs may then be performed in any order. If the patient must be radiographed in the supine position she came in, then the minimum cervical spine routine is completed, possibly with substitute oblique cervical spine positions. AP rib projections would have to be made, and a substitute oblique sternum and HBP lateral sternum.

c. Weights, or some other means of applying traction to the arms for the lateral cervical spine; a grid cassette for the substitute oblique sternum and a vertical cassette holder for the HBP lateral sternum, if they are taken.

d. Same as c.

4. a. A PA, or AP, wrist (depending on the position of the arm), oblique wrist, lateral wrist, AP shoulder internal and external rotation, if possible, or AP shoulder and Y-view of the shoulder.

  b. Shoulder first, then the wrist.

  c. An upright film holder or upright Bucky. If the patient is examined in the supine position, sandbags or sponges may be needed to support the wrist or cassette or both for the wrist projection.

  d. The entire examination may be best done in the upright position. If not, the wrist positions will have to be adapted to the part.

5. a. Cervical spine: AP, AP open-mouth, and lateral. Thoracic spine: AP and lateral. Lumbar spine: minimum AP and lateral, lateral L5-S1, if possible. Skull: AP, left lateral and Towne. Facial bones: left lateral and modification of the reverse Waters (instead of rotating the head, angle the CR 40 degrees cephalic). Chest: AP and lateral. Elbow: AP and lateral, obliques if possible.

  b. HBP lateral cervical spine, AP chest, and possibly an HBP left lateral skull. These should be developed and interpreted by a physician. Assuming that the patient will be radiographed in the supine position, the remainder would be HBP lateral projection of the reverse swimmer's position (especially if the lateral cervical spine did not demonstrate all seven cervical vertebrae), facial bones, chest, thoracic spine, and lumbar spine. (It may be the procedure in some departments to have these interpreted by a physician at this point.) Then the AP skull, Towne skull, modified reverse Waters, AP cervical spine, AP open-mouth cervical spine, AP thoracic spine, AP lumbar spine, and the left elbow series.

  c. Sandbags, sponges, vertical cassette holders, grid cassettes, or similar devices will be needed for the HBPs. Weights or some other method of applying traction to the arms will be needed for the lateral cervical spine (although it may not be possible to apply traction to the injured left arm).

  d. It may be necessary for the AP projections to be made through the backboard. This will also make the HBPs difficult, because the bottom of the cassette must be lower than the patient. The elbow positions will have to be adjusted to the patient's condition and the amount of movement in the left arm.

▪ ▪ CHAPTER 7: SELF-ASSESSMENT TEST ANSWERS

1. Two 14 × 17 inch (35 × 43 cm) cassettes, vertical film holder (or similar device/equipment for the lateral chest), three lead aprons (one for you, and one for each patient), tape measure or ruler to measure source-to-image-receptor distance (SID) if there is not one on the portable unit.

2. Use a tape measure or ruler; use the collimator light (select the correct film size, at 40 inches, then move the unit until the size of the light field matches the size of the film).

3. Use your eyes to ensure that the bottom of the collimator is parallel to the cassette, or make the distance from three corners of the cassette to three corresponding corners of the collimator equal.

4. The presence of other patients, the mobility of the patient being examined, and access for the portable unit.

5. The patient: reduce repeats, collimate, shield, use correct exposure factors, use correct positioning, use lowest ratio grid that will produce a diagnostic film, use highest speed screens available, check previous portable films or files for technical factors used by others.

   The roommate: remove from the room if possible, aim central ray (CR) away if possible, shield.

   The patient's visitors: remove from the room.

   Other health-care workers: remove from room (if possible), aim CR away from them, shield, move them as far from the CR as possible.

   Nonradiologist physicians: same as for other health-care workers.

6. In case of an emergency, it would be in the way and no other personnel know how to move it, nor should they have to waste the time needed to move it.

7. 63 MAS (62.722, to be exact)

8. 12 MAS
9. Patients not being positioned fully upright (torso 90 degrees to the floor).
10. Wear a lead apron (preferably of 0.5 mm lead equivalence), stand as far away from the tube as possible—stand outside the room and if possible, around the corner.

INDEX

*THE SE   ___   OF
EATING DISORDERS*

'*The Secret Language of Eating Disorders* should be compulsory reading in every establishment dedicated to the welfare and care of the sufferers of eating disorders. It is simply the best and most enlightened book of its kind that I have read.

I wish everybody could have access to Peggy's methods of treatment and recovery. She has not only given back my daughter's life to her, but mine to me.'
Nyree Dawn Porter OBE, Actress

'We have been integrating as much of the Montreux approach as we can in our outpatient practice. The results thus far have been unbelievable! The therapy we are doing has taken on a whole different form at a completely different level that is draining but incredibly exhilarating!'
Dr Laura A. Lees, Clinical Psychologist, Lees Psychological Services, Body and Mind Center for Eating and Weight Disorders, Wisconsin

'May I congratulate you for your book which is absolutely fantastic . . . I am so enthusiastic about it and I feel it could help so many desperate parents, young girls, and doctors as well . . . thanks for your very human approach to this dreadful illness.'
Mme. Marie-Pascale Jory, Paris, France

The Secret Language of Eating Disorders

*The Revolutionary New Approach
to Understanding and Curing
Anorexia and Bulimia*

Peggy Claude-Pierre

BANTAM BOOKS

LONDON · NEW YORK · TORONTO · SYDNEY · AUCKLAND

THE SECRET LANGUAGE OF EATING DISORDERS
A BANTAM BOOK : 0 553 505254

Originally published in Great Britain by Doubleday,
a division of Transworld Publishers Ltd

PRINTING HISTORY
Doubleday edition published 1998
Bantam edition published 1998

Set in 10/12 pt Sabon by
Phoenix Typesetting, Ilkley, West Yorkshire.

Bantam Books are published by Transworld Publishers Ltd,
61–63 Uxbridge Road, London W5 5SA,
in Australia by Transworld Publishers (Australia) Pty Ltd,
15–25 Helles Avenue, Moorebank, NSW 2170,
and in New Zealand by Transworld Publishers (NZ) Ltd,
3 William Pickering Drive, Albany, Auckland.

Reproduced, printed and bound in Great Britain by
Cox & Wyman Ltd, Reading, Berks.

*With love and respect
to my darling daughters
Kirsten and Nicole,
who trusted me with their lives*

*In loving memory of Diana, Princess of Wales,
for her selfless caring and compassion
for humanity – and for having the
courage of her convictions*

We are all angels with but one wing,
And only by embracing each other can we fly.

—LUCIANO DE CRESCENZO

Acknowledgments

CERTAINLY ANY AUTHOR writes through the lens of her own life experience. I have been most fortunate to have been helped and influenced by many extraordinary individuals.

Thank you:

To my parents, who have always shown me the courtesy of respect and encouragement even when they may not have understood; for the platform of gentle wisdom.

To my husband David Harris, for his love, patience, vision, and valuable insights in the formation of this book.

To Mischa and Darius, for bringing such sunshine and joy to all who know you.

To Terry Almeida, for her brilliance and years of dedication, giving back always to the children in need.

To the three Maggies who have been in my life at one time and always: my aunt Margaret McGill, my dearest friend Maggie Kalyk, and my invaluable colleague and friend Margaret Dobson.

To my wonderfully diverse siblings who taught me much that I needed to know about human nature.

To Howie Siegel, for believing in me.

For their unfailing support, optimism, and compassion: Celine; Sarah; Irma; Karim; Noah; Alison; Diana; Sonja; Gerry; Colin; Mona; Corrina; Chahalis; Agnes; 'Erin,' John, and Paulo; John Pyper; Brenda Loney; Val Williams; Sam Travers; Bill Naughton; and the wonderful, unselfish staff of the Montreux Clinic.

In memory of special angels Ennis Cosby of New York, Christy Henrich of Missouri and Kathy D'jaime of Australia.

To some individuals of our time who exemplify humanism: Alfred Adler, Abraham Maslow, Carl Rogers, Teilhard de Chardin, Mother Teresa, Elisabeth Kübler-Ross, Jimmy and Rosalynn Carter, Bill Cosby, Pierre Elliot Trudeau, Marie Campion of Ireland, Dr. Gerald Russell of England, Dr. Keith Karran of Utah, Dr. Charles Brooks of Virginia, Dr. Craig Pratt of Ohio, Dr. Dan Smith of Illinois, Dr. Edward Feller of Rhode Island.

For an unusual level of integrity and sensitivity in journalism: Jan van den Bosch of Dutch National Television, Hans Hubner of Spiegel Television (Germany), Alan Goldberg and Lynn Sherr of *20/20* (ABC) and Oprah Winfrey.

I owe a debt of thanks to writer Susan Golant, who came to the rescue when I needed her most.

To everyone at Times Books for their unbridled enthusiasm, patience, and humor: Peter Osnos, Peter Bernstein, Carie Freimuth, Carl Raymond, Mary Beth Roche, John Rambow, Don Bender, and especially my editor extraordinaire, Elizabeth Rapoport; thank you for your insight and brilliance.

Special thanks to my agent, Beth Vesel.

Contents

Author's Note

THESE WRITINGS ARE SET FORTH without arrogance or exclusivity with the hope that someone, somewhere, may glean meaning from them and effect positive change. I have no pretense of superiority, only a passionate desire to communicate what I have learned through my personal experience in order to mitigate against the self-destruction of those in our society with eating disorders. I hope that what I have learned in working with these individuals can be used to increase our understanding of the true nature of these insidious conditions and serve as a catalyst for positive change in others as well.

I have written this book in the hope of helping victims of eating disorders everywhere. It has been my privilege to work with wonderful medical doctors, psychiatrists, and other therapists as we have struggled together to cure these devastating conditions. I wish to emphasize that I am not myself a medical doctor and I do not intend the advice I give in this book to replace the advice of a doctor. Particularly in the case of eating disorders, which have taken the lives of so many, I believe that it is absolutely essential that victims and their loved ones work closely with caring physicians and other members of the health care community who can monitor their health and progress. I hope that this book will help sufferers build a stronger, more effective partnership with their doctors as they work toward wellness.

You will note that throughout this book I refer often

to the 'victims' or 'sufferers' of eating disorders. Some people have told me, in this welcome era of patient empowerment, of their concern that these terms connote weakness and passivity. This is not my intention. As will be explained more fully later, I believe there is an essential difference between those people struggling with eating disorders and those battling physical illness such as cancer or heart disease.

The people in these last groups are often told that they have an important role in their own recovery. They may be told to refer to themselves as, for example, 'cancer survivors' to emphasize the progress they have already made toward wellness. They are encouraged to take responsibility for many aspects of their recovery, to be more assertive with their doctors, to actively seek out the support of others, to do everything they can to favor their return to complete health.

In contrast, people with eating disorders, while equally blameless for their condition, generally have enormous difficulty asking for help. They wish desperately to be able to be assertive, to demand support from others, but for reasons I will explain shortly, they do not feel themselves worthy of help, and in fact their own minds usually prevent them from requesting it.

I believe that in the initial phase of treating an acute eating disorder, it is imperative to remove all burdens and expectations from the patient. In this case, making the ill person responsible for his or her recovery can be a recipe for failure. It is their inability to ask for desperately needed and wanted help that makes these people true victims.

You will note that I frequently refer to the victim of an eating disorder as 'she.' I do this because eating disorders affect females disproportionately; of the estimated eight million people in the United States with this affliction, one million are male. I have treated more girls and women in my practice than boys and men. However, I wish to emphasize that eating disorders are no less cruel in males, and I suspect that many men and boys suffer even more because they feel they are an almost freakish minority and because the sensitive natures that predisposed them to the eating disorder in the first place make them lifelong targets for social embarrassment. I want this book to reach out to them as well and have included stories from many of the boys and men I've treated.

I have had the good fortune over the past twelve years to learn so much from the hundreds of patients I have helped reverse their anorexia and/or bulimia. Many of them have been gracious enough to allow me to include their stories, artwork, and personal communications. I wish to note that I have changed their names and identifying characteristics to respect their privacy. I have done the same for the numerous letters I received from victims, their families, and their friends.

They are my inspiration. I am devoted to them with every cell of my being.

The Secret Language
of Eating Disorders

Introduction

FOR MOST PEOPLE, eating disorders are a great mystery of our time: an enigma to the medical and psychological professionals as well as to those who have had to live with the bizarre and often tragic behavior of its victims and the sufferers themselves who cannot explain their actions. Paradoxically, much of the mystery has arisen less because we lack the knowledge or wisdom to understand what drives people to destroy themselves, but because we are all too ready to explain their behavior in some of the most authoritative and misleading clichés of our culture.

In a world so fixated on images, so prone to reward selfishness, so ready to equate success with self-promotion, it is hardly surprising that eating disorders are often construed as simple vanity taken to an extreme.

In a society so aware of the violence of everyday life, of the victimization of women and children in particular, we are easily misled to the simplistic conclusion that eating disorders are, at least partly, the result of childhood trauma (sexual and otherwise).

In an era in which the triumphs of medical science have encouraged us to use a pill for every physical or emotional disorder, we readily expect that eating disorders also will eventually yield to medical progress and medication.

In this book, I intend to examine these and other

powerful beliefs about the true nature of eating disorders.

I have spent over a decade, both personally with my daughters and in professional practice, struggling with the conundrum of eating disorders. I now believe that these conditions and the behaviors they engender can be fully understood, provided one takes the necessary steps to look beyond the obvious. Because I have been able to intervene successfully in many apparently hopeless cases, I have begun to articulate, first to myself and now increasingly to others through the work of the Montreux Counselling Centre, what I have come to call the secret language of eating disorders. I have gleaned a deep understanding of how the interplay of social situations and psychological dispositions lead people to this particular 'rational irrationality.'

This book seeks to explain the origins of eating disorders, what I have come to call Confirmed Negativity Condition (CNC). Then I will elucidate the therapeutic process I have developed that enables victims to create a new interpretation of their world so that they see that self-destruction – the unconscious impulse toward suicide that lies beneath the symptoms of eating disorders – is no longer a necessary response to their misperceived role in society.

The true dawning of my understanding of eating disorders began with my struggle to save the life of my daughter Nicole. I recall sitting on the bathroom floor, counting the one-inch black-and-white tiles to distract myself. My back was – literally and figuratively – against the wall; fear and helplessness numbed my mind. I held a pen and notebook in my hands. Although I could feel the cold from the tiles seeping through me, I was relieved because it kept me awake. I knew that if I fell asleep, my daughter's life could slip away.

For three days I had known that, according to all the statistics on anorexia, Nikki would not survive. I had read every book I could find on anorexia and had a good grasp of how mainstream medicine understood it. Many, many professionals had told me that anorexia could not be cured, that my child would have to live with it to the end of her shortened life. I had read that it most often affected intelligent, gifted people. After desperate months of searching, I finally understood that no one I had contacted or interacted with could offer a viable solution to reverse Nikki's condition. I knew that Nikki would almost certainly die.

Somehow, I realized I had to divorce myself emotionally as a parent from my daughter and develop a clear mind in order to sustain a positive and unconditional caring toward her. A parent is naturally anxious and emotional under these circumstances, but I knew that Nikki had no strength to accommodate anyone's perceived or real emotions. I knew also that I could not present a false front, because Nikki was too intelligent and would see right through it. Therefore, it was necessary to present as a whole that part of me that was objective and impenetrably calm. Given that I would have to exhibit a strong platform of unmitigated stability, I had to deny myself my humanness until she was entirely safe again.

Since I was working to complete my degree in psychology, I began a form of research paper, a diary on my observations of the peculiar behavior that had overtaken my own child. My thirteen-year-old daughter was not herself. I started to chronicle her behavior and then

5

to compare it to the girl I knew. There was little time, and I could make no mistakes. This was a chess game in which the stakes were incredibly high – those of life and death.

With the first word I wrote, sitting on those cold tiles of the bathroom floor, I stepped into a foreign land without benefit of passport or road map – only my good intentions. As I noted the disturbing aspects of my daughter's self-negating behavior, which I will explain more fully in the next chapter, I slowly came to realize that she was driven by two minds, one positive, one negative. Intuitively, I felt that for her to survive, I had to feed the positive mind and starve the negative. This is what we do now, each day, for every one of our patients at the clinic.

For five months, I stayed awake with Nikki whenever she was awake, for fear of her loneliness and the risk of suicide. I began to realize the extent of the guilt she felt whenever she ate. I understood then that the unknown enemy she perceived was more than she could contend with on her own and concluded that in order to fight it, I had to present it to Nicole as a separate entity.

I also began to see that her behavior was in some way related to her concern for me and her sister, whom we had just brought through anorexia together three months earlier. In order to save Nikki, I had to use my own vulnerabilities as a bridge. Nikki took precedence over everything in my life except her sister.

During the following months, I realized that I had a mission, not just in relation to my daughter but to the wider public.

Today, I believe with all my heart that much of what is commonly presumed about eating disorders is largely

6

mistaken or touches only on a superficial level of understanding. The toll of our confusion and misinterpretation has been high. Believing that theirs is a condition that can at best be managed as a lifelong scourge, we have allowed sufferers of eating disorders to die. We have been complicitous in victims' beliefs that they have no value as human beings. In one contemporary Western European country, the government has considered allowing anorexics to legally end their lives, believing – wrongly – that they need be terminal cases. What more damning statement of the worthlessness and devaluation of a human life could be made? We have compounded the suffering of eating disorder victims by holding them, in part or in whole, to blame for their condition.

Eating disorders remain the condition with the highest mortality rate in psychiatric practice. Between 10 and 25 percent of its victims die or are allowed to die. Those who do not die experience lives of almost unimaginable anguish.

Sadly, the suffering caused by eating disorders extends beyond its victims. All too often, families and other loved ones are tortured by the mistaken belief that they are somehow the cause of the victim's condition. They feel guilty, devastated. Families are destroyed, unnecessarily.

It is my dearest hope that once the wider public understands the true nature of eating disorders, this crushing onus of blame will be lifted from victims and their loved ones, freeing them to focus on recovery.

Because eating disorders appear to confirm powerful stereotypes and, in turn, provoke equally powerful eruptions of blame and guilt, these clichés, and the sense of failure they induce, prevent us from seeing the subtle, immensely consuming, but in the end quite straightforward social and psychological mechanisms that drive some people to behave so apparently deviantly and irrationally. As some of the great thinkers of our time have elucidated, apparently deviant behavior can make perfect sense to those involved.

Although sufferers of eating disorders have been subject to negative caricatures of selfishness and victimhood, they are in reality purveyors of the most positive virtues available to humankind. These are lives to be cherished. Sensitivity and caring are not new in man. Poets and artists through the ages have described and ached for humanity. What is disturbing is the frequency and intensity with which this caring manifests itself in eating disorders in our contemporary global reality.

I am humbled by the intense suffering of the victims of eating disorders and those who love them and awed by their uncommon courage against all odds. It has been my privilege to play a role in these victims' recovery, to see their personalities and sense of self-worth evolve. Every one of them came to us insisting that she deserved to die, that she was a useless human being, that surely someone else even sicker than she merited her spot at the clinic. As each person emerges, I continue to be astonished by her unique lovingness and pained by the thought that her life had been so readily discounted.

My role is to serve merely as a conduit to translate a secret language I have, by default, become privy to. Certainly mine is only one interpretation and reflects only those who wish it to; those who feel they cannot ask help for themselves.

This book is written with the optimistic belief that man is inherently good and would wish to respond to these victims from a sense of social responsibility. There is no blame to be attached to anyone in this message. Surely, we are all struggling to find the answers, we are all working toward the same goal: the eradication of Confirmed Negativity Condition and eating disorders.

My hope is that *The Secret Language of Eating Disorders* will build bridges among all of us united in this cause. I have the greatest respect for parents and those individuals in the helping professions who work in this field and the greatest belief in the commonality of our cause, the human conundrum.

The poet A. E. Housman said it thus:

> *If truth in hearts that perish*
> *Could move the powers on high,*
> *I think the love I bear you*
> *Should make you not to die.*

PART I

The
Negative
Mind

I

The Beginning of Montreux

My journey as a therapist for eating disorders seems, in retrospect, both planned and spontaneous. I knew from a young age that I would become a psychologist. The well-being of the world's children has always been my primary focus.

As a young woman, I was fortunate enough to have two incredible daughters. When they reached early adolescence, I resumed work toward an advanced degree in psychology at the university. I ended an incompatible marriage and moved to a new town to accelerate my studies, leaving behind a comfortable home for a small apartment. I had planned to have Kirsten, then fifteen, and Nicole, thirteen, join me, but Kirsten initially stayed behind to live with my parents and finish her school semester.

KIRSTEN

It was during those intervening months that Kirsten developed anorexia. One evening, my mother alerted me to the problem of my daughter's diminishing weight. Kirsten was studying until two or three in the morning, which was not unusual since she had always been a hard-working student. But my mother had noticed that Kirsten had large dark pools under her eyes, and she had lost a tremendous amount of weight in a short period of time. Hearing this, I asked Kirsten to join me.

When she walked off the plane, I was shocked to see that my daughter, who was five foot nine, now weighed less than a hundred pounds. She must have lost over twenty-five pounds while we had been apart. Going back to school was out of the question; she needed help – now. I told her, 'Honey, you know you are staying with me.'

She just looked back at me and said simply, 'Yes, Mom, I know.'

Under the surface, I was in a state of panic. I immediately took Kirsten to a doctor to check her electrolyte balance. He was the first in a procession of professionals. They all told me the same thing: Kirsten had anorexia and there was no cure for it. At best, an anorexic lived with it – that was called maintenance.

'How serious is it?' I asked. I knew the mortality rate was high. The doctor shook his head to indicate that Kirsten's prognosis was bleak.

I started reading everything I could about anorexia. I wanted to discover how I had failed this child. 'What did I do wrong to make her hate herself so much?' I asked over and over again. Until I understood that, I would not know what the right help was. Everything I read told me that bad parenting, childhood trauma, sexual abuse, and a string of other 'issues' were the cause.

Had our temporary separation caused Kirsten's illness? I felt remorse and extreme guilt. Naturally, as a single parent I assumed total blame for my daughter's illness, and the ensuing parade of psychiatrists did nothing to change my mind.

However, I balked at the psychiatrists' conclusion that Kirsten was being manipulative and selfish, that she was losing weight on purpose to get my attention. I had known this child all her life; I could not accept that she could change so radically from the kind, giving person I had always known her to be. Kirsten had always been unusually sensitive to and aware of other people's needs, in fact she was diligent about attending to them.

I asked my daughter to explain what she was thinking and feeling so I could understand how to help her. She told me that there seemed to be some other louder thought pattern in her head that made no logical sense. Yet Kirsten had always been a very logical child. It became obvious that she did not understand what was happening to her and was powerless to stop it. She said she felt she was going crazy. The medical doctors told me that she could not go on much longer in this manner.

I soon became aware that Kirsten felt terrible guilt about anything connected with food. Whenever I tried to persuade her to eat, she either refused, or tears would roll down her cheeks while she struggled to force the food down to please me. I remember taking her to a restaurant for a muffin. She ate it, but as we were leaving, I could tell she was feeling immense guilt about it. As we drove away I asked her, 'Kirsten, I'm good enough for a muffin. What makes you think you're not good enough for a muffin?'

We stopped at a traffic light. She said, 'Mom, see that light over there? You see that it's green. Logically, I know it's green, but my head tells me it's red, and I'm not allowed to go. That's the best analogy I can make for you about something that makes no sense to me. That's why I'm doing something so illogical.'

She gave me similar clues about how her head operated. Later I realized that Kirsten's traffic-light analogy first made me understand that two minds were warring inside Kirsten's head. She was a determined person, and

I kept trying to persuade her to fight against whatever force was barring her from eating in peace.

The first two months were the most frightening. Occasionally at night, while Kirsten was sleeping, I would go quietly into her bedroom to check on her. Under her blankets, she was skeletal. I would slowly replace the blankets so she would not know I had been there, and she would not be concerned about my worry for her. It was hard to believe that she could survive; she was down to about eighty-four pounds. Fear almost paralyzed me.

She told me sadly one night, 'Mom, you've never lied to me in your life, so I'm going to listen to you, even though the pressure is more than I can bear sometimes. Everything in me tells me not to trust anybody or anything at this point, but I've always trusted you. I'll continue to trust you, whatever it takes.' To this day, I know that's what brought her through, and I stand in awe of her incredible courage against the unbelievable negativity of her mind.

In retrospect, I realize that her decision to trust me unconditionally was the turning point. She kept going to the doctors because I asked her to. Over the next six months, I worked with her every day. She even came to my university classes with me; I was loath to let her out of my sight. Intuitively I knew she should not be alone; otherwise this negativity, whatever it was, would gain strength in her mind when she was by herself.

After every meal, she would talk to me about the illogical thought patterns she could not get out of her head. She was direct about how she felt. Sometimes, she would look at some minuscule bit of food on her plate and tell me, 'Mom, this hurts so much. I shouldn't be eating it. I should be eating a quarter of it. That's all I deserve.' She felt almost subhuman, less than the rest of us. She never knew why she was less deserving, but she just knew she was.

In the first three or four months of her illness, Kirsten was suicidal and frightened, as if eating had some great negative consequence. I talked to her constantly. She was gentle, never abusive. Together we tried to work it out. For every illogical word or act, I responded gently with a logical discussion of the reality of the situation.

She cut off her hair and dyed it purple. At the time I did not pay much attention because I saw it as a natural consequence of being an adolescent. She dressed in layers as though she were trying to arm herself to fight the world; her natural gentleness began seeping away. It was as if she were on a search for self as she kept trying on different modes of appearance. She would wear outside what she seemed to lack inside for strength. (I would later learn that this is characteristic of many people with eating disorders.)

Since we had just moved to a new city, initially she no longer had any friends. I noticed that this normally outgoing girl did not even try to make new ones.

She became extremely agitated. She had to move all the time. If she needed to stay in one spot, she would walk in place; she could not sit in a chair without jiggling around excessively. She exercised all the time. I did not think that was such a problem, so I was not as on top of it as I might have been. Later I would know better.

Several times Kirsten made statements that told me she perceived herself to be the adult in the situation, capable of making decisions that seemed rational to her but were anything but. At other times, she would say, 'Mom, just let me go, just let me die. This is too hard; I can't fight it.' I never heard, 'Mom, help me.' She never asked for help; I gave it to her, but she did not feel she was allowed to expect it.

She would never say that she was worried about me, but she was always trying to make life easier for me.

Then Kirsten started losing the ability to make any decisions, any choices at all; it was as if she had lost faith in her ability to choose. She second-guessed every possible decision or choice. When I asked about her preferences, she would respond, 'Mom, what do you think?' 'What will serve other people better?' She could not make the simplest choices about the most basic issues: what to wear, what restaurant to go to, what to eat. She was unable to create any of her own structure at all.

It was such an unrelenting nightmare. Not only was I terrified that my daughter was losing her life, but I was convinced I was the cause of her torment. Everywhere I went, I felt and accepted the stigma. The public knew that someone had to be blamed – the parent, the child, or both. I was overcome by the numbness of hopelessness. How could my child be dying in front of me? I knew I had to do something, but I did not know where to begin. The information I was getting made no sense. So little of it seemed to apply to Kirsten. Certainly, I would not accept that my daughter's anorexia was incurable. On occasion I glimpsed an idea that felt right, but essentially I felt terribly, terribly alone, left to stumble along an unfamiliar road in a strange country, whose signs were in a language I could not understand.

I found myself of two minds. On one hand, I was petrified that someone could live with such agony – I was witnessing an emotional state that was unspeakably cruel on a continuous basis. On the other hand, I was irritated that I had allowed myself to see doctors as gods; I had expected physicians to have an answer for everything. Of course doctors are not wholly responsible for this deity complex; we put them on the pedestals ourselves. But how could I accept it when they told me my daughter was going to die, that she could never be cured? How could anybody give up on a psychological illness?

The doctors' explanations of Kirsten's illness were based on happenstance and theory, not on strict experience. I had so many questions: Why does an eating disorder affect one child and not another in the same circumstance? I had read that most siblings of anorexics did not get the illness themselves. Did sexual abuse cause it? I knew that Kirsten had not been abused. Family trauma was another commonly cited cause, but I knew that my daughter viewed my divorce as a positive event, not a traumatic one. I started searching for venues that would prove these issues to be the cause because I wanted desperately to find an answer that could reverse the consequences.

Never was I convinced that anorexia was primarily about weight. When Kirsten was sick, she expressed fears about getting fat, but it was not her main focus. She was much too composed to complain about her looks. She would tell me, 'I need to be thinner. I don't know the reason why,' and then she would start to cry.

Given the public view that anorexia attacked adolescent girls, a group famously obsessed with looking right and fitting in, I assumed – wrongly – that Kirsten's illness was in part bound up with concerns about body image. I now know that anorexia does not depend on gender, age, or looks.

I considered taking Kirsten to an eating disorders clinic. Every one that I investigated had a program based on behavior modification. The theory was that if you changed a person's actions, you would change the person. At these clinics, the therapists taught the patients that there were consequences to their behavior. They were given specific goals, such as finishing a particular dish, and told that if they did not achieve the goal, there would be a consequence or punishment. They would be prohibited from seeing their parents, using the swimming pool, or engaging in some other enjoyable activity.

I felt intuitively that I had to separate Kirsten's actions from their consequences. My daughter was experiencing such intense punishment internally already that for me to inflict more would be counterproductive to her recovery. Logically, behavior modification did not seem reasonable, at least for this child.

For six months, I talked Kirsten through every meal and prepared all of them myself. At each meal, I would distract her with funny stories to take the onus off the fact that she was eating.

Kirsten's little sister, Nicole, was an enormous help; she did everything to please her sister. She spent every spare moment sitting with Kirsten, talking and joking with her, giving her things, trying to make a difference. Nicole became a completely selfless person during her sister's illness and stood by her with every possible fiber of her being. I would later realize that she was being inadvertently set up for her own fall.

We combated Kirsten's illness with unconditional love and support. I refused to react to any rare bad behavior except with soothing statements like 'I know you didn't mean to do that.' I would never get angry under any circumstances. Intuitively I felt that something in Kirsten was testing me to find out how willing I was to be there for her. Kirsten was trying to let me know that she deserved nothing, but she was so gracious that the signals were not always apparent. It was a successful day if I just kept her alive.

I was becoming more and more physically exhausted. I felt it was unsafe for me to sleep. What if something happened to Kirsten when my back was turned? I had tried to engage yet another specialist for insight, but he had neither the time nor the inclination. He was probably exhausted and disillusioned himself from the dearth of answers. 'You're just one of many. I have no time,' he told me, and I was devastated.

I felt that I was operating on base instinct. If I could only find the cause, then I would know how to reverse Kirsten's anorexia. I used to comfort myself with this thought, but in my more selfish moments, I longed for some respite. I lived in a void of uncertainty and desperation. The most lonely thought is that there must be an answer, but my daughter might die because I could not find it in time. I fought for my own sanity during this time as much as I did for Kirsten's.

Ultimately, it was Kirsten's incredibly logical, lawyer-like mind that helped bring her through. Anorexia knows no logic, and part of Kirsten's mind would insist repeatedly that she was not allowed to eat, or that she could subsist on some ridiculously small amount of food. I would argue her through it for hours, and she generously let me.

'Honey,' I would attempt to reason with her, 'what would you expect me to eat for a day?' I had to explain the logic of the situation every time. 'Write down for me what you eat; would you be happy if I ate only that much?'

Later I realized that asking her to write out her daily menu may have been a mistake; I know now that in creating a written table of contents, the negative part of her mind could use it to reprimand her for her indulgence. (At some point in therapy, however, this can be a positive, even worthwhile interim structure.)

Slowly she became stronger. The dread drained from me as the days marched on and she became more confident. Eventually I realized she would make it, at least this time. But almost every book I had read warned me of the high rate of relapse, so I felt I could not really relax. My aim was not only to save her life, but to find out how to prevent a recurrence. What, then, was the trigger?

I began to suspect that relapse occurred when this negative mindset was somehow ignited; the trigger was something other than the anorexia itself. It seemed improbable that anorexia was a direct result of a single issue or even accumulated issues; perhaps it was the straw that broke the camel's back. Now I know: It is not the ten issues that finally become too much, but rather one's attitude toward and perception of the issues that brings on the manifestation of the condition. A person's negative mindset becomes increasingly pessimistic and subjective so that it searches out any issue to turn into another negative to feed itself. On its hunt for confirmation, it perverts any issue wherever it can because it is so hungry for negativity.

During that year, I continued to attend classes to become a psychologist and kept taking Kirsten with me. My field of interest was children. I was engaged in a major research project that involved twenty-six countries, studying how to prevent recidivism in juvenile delinquents released from prison. Two nations, Japan and Sweden, invited me to study with them for a year each. I was finding that kindness, not punishment, worked miracles. Later I would see this as a metaphor for my own work with victims of eating disorders.

It was another six months after Kirsten's weight had stabilized and the doctors declared her out of the woods that I could begin to feel safe about her. I know she suffered more than she ever told me. She has always had immense courage. Kirsten told me later that it took her almost another year after she had regained her weight to feel she had an assured self with internal guidelines that she could live with comfortably. Even though she was over the manifestation of her condition, she had needed that year to gain strength, to become as whole as every person ought to be.

NICOLE

Within three months of Kirsten's recovery, I started recognizing the signs of an eating disorder in her little sister. Kirsten's illness had fortunately fine-tuned my antennae. Nicole began making excuses to avoid meals, subtly at first, then more noticeably. She would tell me she had eaten elsewhere and that she was just so full she couldn't eat, or that she had had a huge lunch and wasn't hungry for dinner. She began taking extended walks, sometimes disappearing for half a day; I would later discover she had been walking the whole time to burn off calories.

Even though her illness presented itself in a different way – she was evasive where Kirsten had been mostly straightforward – I began having an unhealthy fear about her. I was unable to sleep because I knew intuitively that, although I tried to deny it, Nicole too was in the grips of an eating disorder. The signs became too many, too often, to deny it any longer. I would see Nicole opening a can of tuna and pretending to make a sandwich. Later I would find the whole thing thrown out upside down in the garbage, so I would not readily notice that the can was still full.

Once I made the decision to face my inconceivable reality, I experienced again the dread I had just released myself from – dread that permeated me to the core. I was unsure if I had the physical energy to pull another daughter back from the precipice. I had been so exhausted for so long. Would I have the strength? Could I outlast this illness once more? I was frightened that I would be unable to, but certainly Nicole deserved the same efforts I had made for her sister.

Nikki's illness was a nightmare that I could never have anticipated. At the worst, I was ready for a rematch of what I had gone through with Kirsten. I now know that the severity of an eating disorder depends on the sufferer's personality. As it turned out, Nicole's condition was many times worse than Kirsten's had been. Without the work I had done with Kirsten, I would have gone into Nicole's case completely unprepared. I thank Kirsten for teaching me. I was still, however, woefully unready.

From the beginning, Nicole was intensely suicidal and she went into a downward spiral very quickly. She was in a deep depression, which I now realize is partially caused by the lack of nutrition inherent in anorexia.

From the beginning, I knew I had to be with Nicole twenty-four hours a day or she would not survive. I tried to continue with school as I had with Kirsten, but Nikki refused to come along. She did not want people to see her; she was a failure, an imposter, inadequate in every way, a fool. It was a desperate situation. I had no means to invite anybody to help me deal with Nikki's illness, no money, no confidence that anyone else would take it seriously enough to protect Nicole. I knew of no clinic that would watch my child like I would. Without constant supervision, I knew she would find an occasion to harm herself.

She hated me. She hated everybody. She lashed out while simultaneously refusing all aid. 'Don't you dare help me. I don't deserve it,' she yelled. Once when I was rocking her with my arms loosely around her, she cried out, 'Don't ever come near me. Go away.'

'You don't have to love me,' I replied. 'You don't need to worry about that. I will always love you.'

She broke down and began to cry on my shoulder. 'I don't know why I said that. I don't think it. I don't mean it. I don't know why I'm doing this. I love you so much, and I would never want to hurt you.'

Shortly after that, I realized that for the both of us to survive the ordeal, I had to leave my emotional self out of the picture. I knew better than to take Nicole's remarks personally. Every night I sat up trying to devise a way to separate my emotional mother self from my daughter in order to create the objectivity I knew I needed for her survival. I decided to create concrete steps for myself to follow to keep me balanced in order to buffer Nikki's condition.

I went to town and bought myself a thick notebook of lined paper and told myself that I was doing an immense research project. My diary would record Nikki's every move, behavior, bite of food, and emotion as well as my reactions. Having a well-defined task with a beginning, middle, and end gave me some hope in a bleak situation. My rational self needed this, because my emotional self could find no end to Nicole's illness; therefore I did not know where I would find the strength to fight it. My rational self had to choke back the sobs and panic that surged through me.

At night I crouched on the bathroom floor; the cold floor tiles and the stark lighting would keep me awake. I pored over a list of everything the textbooks said about the causes and characteristics of eating disorders and compared them to what I was seeing with Nicole. Nothing in her behavior computed with the theories. I played with the 'begging for attention' hypothesis for a while. The public conception was that manipulative people used self-starvation as a 'cry for attention.' In this sense, a cry for help was construed as futile, but why would it be? I was certainly attentive to Nikki, yet her self-deprivation continued. Anorexia was no ordinary distress signal.

Theory 2 postulated that Nicole was selfish. That certainly did not make any sense; Nikki was the least selfish person I knew. She had just helped save her sister's life, and she was just a child.

Theory 3 supposed that Nicole was another example of 'the best little girl in the world,' a perfectionist running herself into the ground to please me because, supposedly, that was my expectation. But how could the Perfect Little Girl suddenly turn into her antithesis, as far from obliging as she could be? I had never implicitly or explicitly demanded perfection from her. Our relationship had always been warm and loving.

I took Nikki to psychiatrists and psychologists, but they would only frighten her, telling her that she was failing fast. Before long, she was given every possible psychiatric label. Finally, the threat of their involvement would make her try to eat more than usual, but even so, she soon weighed much less than her sister had at her worst.

Every night, I continued to write in my diary, to argue the experts' theories on paper. I still assumed that anorexia primarily affected teenage girls, so I compared my own feelings at that age with what Nikki was experiencing. Like her, I remember feeling undeserving, convinced that everyone else was better; I was unworthy of being in their company. I had not wanted to inflict myself on them. Though I had not become anorexic, I could see that same mindset intensify itself in my daughter. I had had inklings of this inclination in Kirsten when she was sick.

I was becoming more convinced that there was an underlying condition that predisposed people to eating disorders, not a life issue, but an interpretation of life caused by an inherent mindset. Could this explain why many people who live apparently worse lives come through relatively unscathed? I began waiting for the moments Nikki would sleep so I could work on my theories. I started adding and subtracting. This endeavor distracted my mind from the pain and apparent futility of trying to cure Nikki's anorexia and gave me purpose.

Two months into Nikki's illness, I began to find notes from her all over the apartment in every container. Most were written in the third person: 'Nicole is a fat pig.' 'Nicole is no good.' 'Nicole doesn't deserve to live.' 'Nicole deserves to die.' 'Nicole needs to be tormented.' Why was she not writing in the first person, I wondered, why not, 'I am a fat pig?' No sooner would I throw the notes away in horror than the jars would fill up with them again.

My own health began to suffer. I slept only an hour and a half a night. What worse torture than lack of sleep? One night I purposely disrobed in front of a mirror and looked at my reflection. At that moment, I vowed to myself that I would make sure this body would die before I would let my darling child die. It was a pledge not to commit suicide or give up for even a moment. I was truly drained, but as long as there was a breath in me, there would be in her.

I made myself the platform for Nicole's survival. Anything else I may have needed – including finishing my doctorate, which I wanted to do so desperately – I had to put aside. There was no choice. I never blamed Nikki. I never felt the need. I was not angry with her for a second. I knew my daughters had not brought this on themselves; they were as confused about their condition as I was.

Psychiatrists, however, seemed intent on fixing blame. One diagnosed Nicole as schizophrenic after a seven-minute interview. Others prescribed every kind of medication, seven or eight drugs at the same time, none of which she took – she refused them all, and I would not force her for fear of undermining her faith in me. Although I felt medication was not the answer for my child, I did not have the faintest idea what was.

Nikki's behavior became progressively more bizarre. She would throw a plate at my head after she had eaten something off it or break a window because she was so upset at eating. She trembled in fear, crouched in corners of the room. It was as if there was a presence beyond the two of us that was so negatively powerful. Nicole kept saying, 'Mom, you can't fight it. It's stronger than us both.' That would send shock waves of alarm through me, but I knew intuitively it was imperative that I remain composed to her, that I present only strength and serenity. I don't know where it came from.

Nikki's body somehow sensed she needed potassium, so I drove her, sometimes for hours, hunting for the 'right' banana. We would stop at six or ten or thirteen stores. I thought the right banana would be medium sized, yellow, with few marks. I was terribly wrong. To Nikki, the 'right' banana was unfit for human consumption: blackened, hidden under others, destined to be thrown in the garbage, with only an inch of edible fruit. She could convince herself that she was not really eating if she allowed herself to consume such a lowly castoff. It was frustrating, frightening, and exhausting.

One morning at 4:00 a.m., I was writing in my journal, sitting on the cold bathroom floor, when I heard Nikki creep into the kitchen. When I followed her, she had disappeared. Then I heard a sound. I found her under the table, eating dog food out of a dog dish. We had no dog.

I did not know where the dish or the dog food had come from. She was on all fours, weeping, as she crouched down to eat. I went over to her and held her and begged, 'Don't do this, darling. You don't need to do this. We will figure this out.'

She just sobbed in my arms and held on. 'I don't know why I do this. I'm so bad.'

'Honey, why are you so bad?' I asked.

'You don't understand. I just am.'

'What have you ever done that's so bad? You've been such a good girl all your life – a wonderful child.'

'I don't know the answer,' she replied, 'but I know it's in my head all the time.'

I brought her back to bed and stayed with her. I knew I had to negate every possible bad thing her head told her. I also had to assume she was hearing negative thoughts constantly. She was obviously unable to reach out for help, even though she wanted it. Something was holding her back. Certainly she did not want to die.

At first I would wait until Nikki said something, and then I would answer her with logic. Soon I began to make comforting statements even when she said nothing. I would give her positive reinforcement, assuming that what was going on in her head was silent to me but terribly loud and powerful to her. She started letting me into her game of fooling the negative voice. She eventually realized that I was strong enough to work with her against it. Her negative thoughts became an 'it,' because in separating 'it' from her, I could fight it: United, 'it' could stand. Divided from her, 'it' might fall.

I presented analogies to better explain the situation of her mind to her. I pictured 'it' as a wolf stalking a flock of sheep. The wolf determines which sheep is the weakest and tries to separate that sheep from the fold. I used distraction or any other means to outsmart the wolf. I had to prove to Nikki that I could do it, that she could lean on me, that I would never give in, even as her mind bombarded her with cruelty.

One windy and blustery November day, Nikki slipped out of the house in a thin coat, telling me I was not allowed to come with her. I followed her without her knowing it, as I often would afterwards, the wind wiping away the sound of my steps. Nikki was concentrating on her forced march to burn off calories.

She hesitated when she saw a frail lady waiting to cross a major intersection. Even in her misery she tried to be kind. She tentatively approached the woman. Because the wind was so loud, the woman did not hear her coming. I knew Nikki had wanted to help the woman cross the street. She reached down to hold the woman's elbow. The woman turned and began to hit her with her purse. Nikki fell back in shock. She pushed herself even further that day because the woman had not let her help her. She must have done something wrong. On two other occasions she collapsed on the street. I carried her home, never knowing if she would still be breathing when we got there. In my head, I begged for her life: 'Please, someone, anyone. Just let her live. Take me instead. She is just an innocent child.'

I tried yet another specialist. I sent her up to his office. After twenty minutes, Nikki came running down to the car where I was waiting. Sobbing, she got in, slammed the door, and said, 'Let's leave here, Mom.'

'What's wrong, honey?' I asked.

'He wants to talk to you. He told me you were to blame for everything. He never even met you!'

In less than twenty minutes this doctor had decided he knew my child's life. 'Nikki, let's go up and see what he has to say,' I said gently.

'Are you sure you're strong enough?' she asked. Sick as she was, Nikki was trying to protect me! Why? Had I shown her vulnerability?

The doctor was as cold as his white lab coat. Nikki asked him, 'How is my mother to blame? Tell her please, because it makes no sense to me.'

I was so choked up by her pain that I could barely control myself. I asked the doctor, 'Would you like to know what I think of my daughter? Would you like to know about us?'

'Not particularly,' he responded. 'Your daughter is sick because you haven't been able to handle your life.'

'I am handling my life just fine, thank you,' I said. 'I need help handling hers.'

'Nicole will live a subquality life,' he continued. 'You'll have to manage her condition, and she might die.'

I told him that I had always been strong, that I was committed to curing her. I began to sound defensive, I'm sure, and he said 'I'm not interested in dealing with you. I will deal with your daughter and I will not confide in you anything that goes on between me and her.'

That was too much for Nikki. She raised her voice to him, 'My mother has never done anything wrong that I know of. She's not to blame for this condition. You're insensitive! And you don't know me at all! It's fine that my mother knows anything you and I talk about. I am bad. Are there any secrets to be ashamed of?'

I said, 'Honey, let's go. He just thinks differently than we do.' I saw no sense staying with someone who was negative from the start. Who would be her structure if she were separated from me? In any case, Nikki refused to go back to see him.

After a while, Nikki's negative thought pattern, though cunning, became predictable, and I could fool it relatively easily. And so I began to trick what I had come to see as 'the mind below the actual mind.' I realized Nikki could not allow herself to eat if she had a plate of food in front of her, so I would take her out to dinner and order for myself. Everybody must have thought I was crazy, but I was conscious only of the task in front of me. I would cut chicken, her favorite, into small pieces and put them on a side plate under my left elbow so nobody else could see. I was not admitting to her negative mind that food was in front of her. It was 'mine,' and she did not have to take responsibility for it. I would look the other way as she slipped tiny pieces into her mouth. If I covered everything with a napkin so only one piece was visible at a time, she would take it. Slowly, ever so slowly, I was feeding her.

I looked for other strategies. I started saying, 'Darling, while you were out for a walk [she would never admit that I had followed her; we both pretended I had stayed home], somebody called [nobody had, really]. Some friends want to come over for tea. Would you mind coming with me to buy ingredients for a cake?' I am sure

32

she became the best baker in six counties. Everybody started sending her cookbooks. (I later learned that anorexics 'eat' vicariously; they pore over cookbooks all the time, watch cooking shows, and cook food for other people without consuming any food themselves.)

I would never actually make the tea – no one came – but my ruse gave Nikki a reason to bake. When the batter was ready, she would allow herself to eat a little of it (which wasn't, technically speaking, 'cake'), and fool the negative that way. Later, I would ask her if she would cut the cake so when 'people came,' we would have lady-like finger slices. That was a way for her to eat some of the crumbs – those were not 'cake' either – without her negative thoughts making her responsible for allowing herself the favor of eating.

At about the same time, I also realized I had to weigh Nikki backward and never divulge her weight, although she would demand to know. Nikki was less able to respond to logic than Kirsten had been. I could not reveal her weight because no number would be good enough; she would always have to be less than whatever she currently weighed. When she was sixty-eight pounds, I tried to reason with her. 'You know that you're in an impossible physical position. You can't last like this. You thought you were low enough at eighty. Now you're sixty-eight. Logically, you know better.'

'I don't know anything,' she replied angrily.

'If you have to be lower than eighty, are you satisfied at sixty-eight?' The negative condition was caught red-handed. 'If you weighed only twenty pounds, would your negative condition be satisfied?'

She started to cry. 'No. Only if I'm dead.'

That night in my journal, I wrote that I knew this was a track to death. I began to question the famous myth

33

that being model thin was the anorexic's ultimate goal. We were not dealing with a fashion statement here.

So much repetition. So much reiteration. So much counteracting the negativity inside Nikki. So much reinforcing that small kernel of hope I knew was there. In some moments, Nikki was desperate to respond. I could often see the pleading in her eyes. Through the small bits of food, she would have occasional bits of joy. The day she 'graduated' from 1 percent to whole yogurt, she was laughing and crying at the same time. Everything was a baby step, because there were only baby steps. It takes incredible patience in a society that has no patience. I wrote in my research journal, 'The turtle wins the race. . . . It takes time, but you'll only get there with patience.'

One day when I was near the breaking point, I left Nikki with a dear friend for a half hour, just to do something 'normal' for myself. It seemed a long time since I had interacted properly with society. I took my newspaper and went out to a restaurant. It was three in the afternoon. I imagined the place would be reasonably empty. In fact, a few people were having coffee there.

One of them, a woman whom I knew only slightly, came over to me and asked, 'Could I talk to you for a moment? I want to ask you something.' I told her I did not have much time. She pulled down my newspaper/shield and asked, 'Don't you feel like a total loser, having two out of two daughters anorexic and you a counselor?' I cannot remember my response, but I do recall feeling the world did not understand us. I spent a few more nights pondering how I might have failed my daughters. Poor mothering genes?

But then I began using the notion of guilt for my

research. If I felt guilty and I could not find a clear reason for it, then how could I wonder at my daughters' guilt? Both were equally unreasonable. My children could not tell me why they felt guilty; they just 'knew' they were because somehow they were bad. That week I let go of guilt. I found it useless except as a motivator, and I was already quite motivated!

My journal became my best friend. It was my only sanity. It cherished my fear and pain yet nurtured my logic. Without its comfort, I would not have survived. It heard me and forgave me everything. In it I set out a long-term plan for how we would get through the next six to eight months. They were the roughest of my life.

One particularly exhausting day, after Nikki had been yelling obscenities at me, she demanded plaintively, 'Mom, what do you see that I don't see?'

God, I thought, she is giving me an ultimatum. 'Nikki,' I replied, 'give me your happiest moment ever.'

She remembered it easily. It was walking on the board-walk in Montreux in Switzerland. 'The sunlight was shining through the leaves in the trees and the board-walk was all mottled. I felt such a complete peace and understanding with myself and everything.' Nicole felt honestly that if happiness were related to peacefulness, that was her best moment.

This gave me insight: Nikki was striving for peace and contentedness. She wished she could bring that moment and that feeling back. I held that thought. I presented a dream to her that I was certain, if I could get her better, I would make a reality. I was desperate, so what might have seemed extreme did not seem so then. I told her that, as I had told Kirsten, I was going to get her better. There was no alternative to that. I was uncertain how, but I was beginning to get a good sense of it. Then, after she got better, I would develop a practice that would get other children better. I told her that I would get my doctorate in psychology so people would believe us. I told her we would call the practice Montreux.

Nikki was wonderfully excited about that and held on to my dream; it distracted her. I used it as a continuing theme in her care, by presenting concrete hope. It would give her something to live for. I told her that eventually we would be in a position to open a clinic. When we knew we could do it, we would open clinics all over the world so children and parents would no longer be blamed. Everyone would finally understand. I told her it would take me ten years to convince the world, and that somehow things would fall into place. People would need and want to learn so children wouldn't die.

That became Nikki's structure. I continued to feed her with several small meals at home or in a restaurant, where she was both too embarrassed to overreact and distracted enough to eat. I knew she was not allowed to say she was hungry ever, so I would say I was hungry. We ate six times a day. Slowly, slowly, I brought her back to health. During this time I sought other help as well, because I was terrified that I would be unable to pull her through despite my efforts. But these experts were either negative, apologetic, or benign at best, which at least was inoffensive, but unfortunately offered no insight or relief.

It took me a year and a half to turn Nikki around. After ten months, I knew she was going to recover. So that she would not feel like an outcast and to prepare her for reentry in society, I started a group at my home for any child or teenager who felt dysfunctional. I wanted Nikki to realize this was a common plight of the human condition; she had not been singled out for negativity. One of my patients was a recovering heroin addict, several others were anorexic or bulimic.

Doctors who had heard of my experience with my daughters began to refer patients to me. I received calls asking if I would consider talking to this mother or that child. Within two years, much to my dismay, I had a line-up of patients I could not contend with. More than anything, I wanted to get my doctorate before I buried myself in my practice. But each life placed in front of me was someone for whom I felt such compassion and understanding – I could never allow myself preference over any one of them.

MONTREUX TODAY

Montreux Counselling Centre began as an outpatient practice in 1988 as more and more referrals followed reports of my success with my own daughters. I did not put my name or number in the phone book because I did not want to invite more patients at this point. At some level I felt terribly burdened, because I had not had a gasp of air between treating my two daughters and the rest of the world's patients, and it was essential to me that I finish my degree.

I stuck to my plan and was halfway through when desperate parents placed a young anorexic child in front of me. The parents had exhausted every other viable option. Nothing was working, and their daughter was very ill. I had to make a conscious choice, once again, between my education ambitions and the life of a child. Naturally, the child was the only option. It was well worth it – what an angel this incredible child is.

As I confronted cases of increasing need, I began taking other patients into my home (and the homes of others) in order to create a more consistent atmosphere for them. Some of my early patients, and later my own daughters, became my co-workers in implementing these 'localized environments of unconditional support' for dying patients. This experience helped me devise the medically monitored, one-on-one, twenty-four-hour-a-day individualized care plan from which we work with acutely ill patients today.

The Montreux Clinic opened in 1993 in order to meet the requirements of those individuals in extreme need who, generally, had been through many other programs and who were frequently labeled 'treatment resistant.' The clinic offers outpatient services as well.

Now, four years into our residential operation, we have been particularly encouraged by the emerging eagerness of professional colleagues to embrace more positive treatment modalities. We have been fortunate to work closely with excellent treatment teams in acute care hospitals where patients must often be stabilized before they are able to travel to us.

Health care insurers are realizing the highly cost-effective nature of our work and a number of companies have funded treatment for patients in our program. (Though the treatment terms called for are longer than those of programs that concentrate merely on feeding, the per diem rate is 25 to 50 percent less than the cost of treatment at acute care hospitals; moreover, when patients recover completely, they have no need for further treatment.)

We have successfully treated hundreds of people with eating disorders. I have counseled patients as old as sixty-four and as young as three.* Our clinic offers a practical application of the theory elucidated in this book.

In several ways Montreux can also be seen as a social laboratory for positive change. If victims of what we call Confirmed Negativity Condition are indeed an altruistic segment of our society, then the gifts that they have to give the world are readily evident in the Montreux community. Their altruism is reflected in the wish of many recovered patients to become careworkers themselves. (We encourage recovered patients to investigate other avenues for several years in order to explore their own needs before working with patients themselves; currently approximately an eighth of our careworkers and counselors are former sufferers.)

For incoming patients, the possibility of spending time with fully recovered former patients helps create a bridge of hope, which is most helpful in plotting a course for the new patients' recovery. Our other careworkers come from a cross section of the professional spectrum. They are chosen for training based on their ability to provide unconditional support to those in need rather than achievement in any particular discipline; we search for qualities of kindness, compassion, vision, and patience that go beyond the expected 'norm.' Most feel that the work itself, performed in an atmosphere of positive encouragement, provides immense rewards in terms of self-development and the motivation to surpass self-expectation.

We find Montreux an incredibly inspiring environment, a testament to the capacity of the human spirit.

* It should be noted that while the vast majority of the patients who come to us for treatment do achieve complete recovery – they have completed the program – there have been a few who have left the program, of their own volition, prior to the point at which we felt it was appropriate for them to do so.

Confirmed Negativity Condition

Every day I receive letters from Julie, a young woman with severe anorexia. They are heartrending missives, and her words tear at my soul.

'*I am a bad person,*' she writes. 'I hate myself when I eat. I don't want to live because I'm too ashamed. I want to be small. . . . I want to be little, please let me be little again. I'm too afraid to live, I'm too embarrassed to be seen. I want to hurt myself. I'm no good. I'm a terrible, evil person. . . .

'It helps so to be punished; it feels so kind, like the only gift I have to offer. I don't deserve to live and I want to show you I know that. I need you to see it on my face so you can receive some assurance, some inkling of my regret, some idea that I am sorry. There is no way to tell you, no way to express my sadness, no means to make obvious the guilt in my heart, the knowledge of my evil, the compassion you deserve, the pain I have earned. Let me hurt myself, let me do good. . . .'

Another day, another note: 'I wish my mind would turn off and rest. I am junk and honestly, I deserve to die. . . . I feel like a hideous scar that ought to be removed, but still remains as a reminder of the damage that caused its appearance initially.'

And then another note: 'I can't stand myself anymore. I pray to God to help me punish myself with more pain. . . . All I hear when I do take care of myself is,

"You're disgusting. How can you let yourself be content. How dare you keep living, especially so well."'

And still another. 'I deserve only punishment, and abhor myself. . . . I am completely horrified and ashamed, repulsed and sorrowful every second I live, every moment I am.'

What makes Julie, a seemingly normal teenager before the onset of this disorder, suffer such self-abnegation, such utter self-hatred? What makes her want to starve herself into oblivion? What makes her write in the secret language of despair?

It is my experiences with my daughters, patients, and thousands of letters and writings like Julie's that have helped me discover the etiology (the underlying causes) of eating disorders. I have coined the term Confirmed Negativity Condition (CNC) to define the complex thought processes that plague the minds of those with eating disorders and others. An eating disorder is to Confirmed Negativity Condition as a rash is to measles or swollen glands are to mumps; it is a symptom of an underlying problem.

The predisposition for Confirmed Negativity Condition begins early in life, but a CNC 'carrier' does not necessarily have to develop an eating disorder. (On the other hand, as I see it, an eating disorder victim must have CNC.) Other possible self-negating manifestations of CNC may include depression, agoraphobia, panic attacks, obsessive-compulsive disorder, or somatic disorders (including any other way such victims may internalize their pain). An individual can have several of these manifestations simultaneously *with or without an eating disorder being one of them*. (Often they coexist with eating disorders and occasionally, when a patient is letting go of anorexia, she will attempt to replace it with another manifestation of CNC such as agoraphobia.) Eating disorders are of particular concern, however, given their debilitating effects and high mortality rate.

I have come to believe that CNC precedes the eating disorder and is at the root of these devastating illnesses. The eating disorder is the symptom; CNC is the affliction we must cure.

A CIVIL WAR IN THE MIND

As horrifying as Julie's situation is, it is far from rare. Indeed, I have found that virtually all people suffering from severe eating disorders experience similar secret thoughts about their unworthiness. They feel like insects trapped in a spider's web. Extricating themselves becomes increasingly impossible as CNC slowly draws out their lives.

Victims clearly are caught in an internal struggle which is often expressed as a dialogue between their being and their 'head.' One young woman wrote to me, 'I'm lost, and I mean lost. It's like someone has put me on a desert island with no survival supplies. I'm the only one on the island, me and my head. Great, I'm stuck with my #1 enemy.'

And another described how she was letting her 'head' take over her life, slowly but surely.

I know it's probably just in my head, but to me it feels like I am drowning. My head feels like a war zone and it just won't stop. Day after day I seem to be losing control over my life and it terrifies me. Even when friends come over, I just lay like a zombie on the couch, not talking or joining in with what they are doing, just listening to them and my head.

Most of the time lately, I feel too tired to fight it so I just listen. When it gets too much I end up breaking down in tears but I try to hide it.

Another wrote of how her head terrorized her. 'It doesn't matter how fast you run to escape it, you'll never run fast enough. . . . It has no features, no feelings; it is flat and lifeless yet it hates you and seeks your ruin more efficiently than anything else could. When you die, it's gone too. It just dissolves into thin air. Its only reason for existence is to wreck you.'

This civil war in the mind – what I think of as a dual mindset – was made quite plain in another woman's writings. She actually gave voice to what I call the Negative Mind – the force that takes over the lives of people with anorexia and bulimia. 'You're not going to get better,' this inner voice said to her, 'instead you'll get worse. . . . You wish someone would come along and save the day. No one would want to see you better. They'll hate you regardless. You're fat. Everyone else is tricking you. You can only listen to me and do what I tell you.'

People with eating disorders are at war with themselves. They are of two minds. The Negative Mind is totally powerful when the symptoms of the eating disorder are present. What may have begun as doubting thoughts, indecisiveness, or mild self-criticism intensifies to form an autonomous voice. It is tyrannical, hypercritical, destructive, and despair-confirming. It tells its victim:

Everyone HATES you.
You only cause trouble.
There's nothing you can do right.

You are demanding, selfish, greedy, and mean.

Things will never work out for you.

You make the world miserable.

A person like you doesn't deserve any pleasure, and eating is pleasurable.

If you try to get rid of me, I will only go and hurt someone else; and if I did that, you know you couldn't live with yourself, so I'm here to stay!!

You're fat and gross and ugly.

Your father will die in a plane crash if you eat.

You should burn in hell.

You don't deserve to live.

You should not eat because to eat is to live.

You are a burden to society.

You should die.

Not all sufferers hear the voice as clearly as others. One woman wrote to me, 'I constantly hear distant "whispers" in the back of my mind. I cannot make them out or understand them. My thoughts run in circles, do somersaults, and sometimes just "disappear." At the end of the day, I am tired from talking so much – yet I have not uttered a spoken word to anyone in many days. Just myself. My head. My body.'

The wish that someone would 'come along and save the day' is evidence of what I call the Actual Mind. The Actual Mind is a positive force, which as the essential individual is desperate to live. It is the mind of the victim before she developed CNC and is the mind she will return to once the CNC is gone. The Actual Mind is who the patient would have been had CNC been averted and her emotional development not been arrested. The Actual Mind consists of normal reactions to everyday events.

It might be helpful to think of CNC as a parasite that attempts to consume the Actual Mind, its host. Such a parasite can seem to obliterate the true gentle nature of its host or, at least, temporarily cloud it and thus confuse it, so that the naturally caring victim behaves like her antithesis, striking out at everybody in an attempt to alienate loved ones. It will feed off the host and superficially change her behavior until its presence is diagnosed and effectively treated. The Negative Mind is the tool of CNC. It is the enforcer, preying on the host, whose potential lies hidden under the facade of her often inexplicable behavior.

As CNC develops more strength, the victim will try to bargain with the Negative Mind for small favors:

'I promise not to eat supper tonight if you allow me to have this grape now.'
'I'll run for three hours if you let me have this bowl of strawberries.'
'Please don't kill my sister. I promise not to be nice to the doctor.'

The compromise is always heavily in favor of the Negative Mind.

Often the victim of an eating disorder, caught in the crossfire between the Negative and Actual Minds, will suffer for years without dying. It is difficult to imagine the miserable quality of life as an eternal hostage, being relegated to begging for mercy, for every tidbit, as a supplicant on the street. As Milton put it so succinctly in *Paradise Lost*:

The mind is its own place, and in itself
Can make a heaven of hell, a hell of heaven.

46

With this bargaining, the Actual Mind relinquishes its place progressively to the Negative Mind and diminishes over time. As my correspondent Julie had said, 'Day after day I seem to be losing control over my life and it terrifies me. . . . Most of the time lately, I feel too tired to fight it so I just listen.' As the CNC becomes more entrenched, the Negative Mind controls what little is left of the victim's identity. She is permitted nothing in her own interest.

Understand, however, that even though the Negative Mind is extremely domineering, at no point is the victim entirely without her Actual Mind. She is merely without most of its power. A small part of it manifests even when the Negative Mind is in control. In the acute stage of an eating disorder, the Negative Mind may be so powerful that the Actual Mind almost disappears. But the fact that the victim is still alive indicates its presence and, in fact, suggests the starting point for recovery. (See Chapters 5 and 6.)

When under the control of the Negative Mind, the Actual Mind is terrorized and paralyzed. It seems incapable of stopping itself from falling more deeply into an abyss of nonbeing. One of the dictates of the Negative Mind is to prohibit the Actual Mind from reaching out for help. The victim is undeserving of succor.

However, also bear in mind that the parasitic Negative Mind is able to host itself only in someone who is essentially altruistic and does not want to be a burden to family or society by reaching out for aid. It would be unusual for such a person to ask for help in the first place, even before CNC develops into an eating disorder.

When a person is held in thrall to an eating disorder, her Actual Mind is at the mercy of her Negative Mind. Still, the Actual Mind is the true potential mind of the patient. From my experience, it will exist again after the victim has reinterpreted herself and has learned to balance her perspective about her role in society.

THE SUBJECTIVE WORLD OF THE ANOREXIC

To be subjective about a remark or an event is to personalize it. To be subjective means to translate everything through the prism of one's personal reality. In the case of the individual who develops an eating disorder, to be subjective means to pass every event through the distorting lens of the Negative Mind and to turn the event against oneself. Indeed, CNC is the culmination of negative subjectivity turned against oneself. This hypercritical subjectivity will cause the victim to interpret every comment made to her as a negative reflection on her, or it will make the victim assume blame for every event, no matter how objectively unrelated to her.

Consider, for example, the parents who may ask their anorexic son to help them babysit. 'We have to go to the store now. Will you look after Tommy for an hour?'

The anorexic may think, 'Oh God, they want to talk about something behind my back. They're just pretending that it's about looking after Tommy.' Victims of CNC assume that they are excluded from everything because they feel unworthy. Therefore, they naturally assume that everyone else will be talking against them.

Imagine, further, the situation in which a mother complains of a headache. The child with an eating disorder will blame herself for her mother's pain and wonder what she had done to cause it. Or if someone said to an anorexic woman, 'That dress really suits you,' her subjectivity might prompt her to reply or think to herself, 'Oh no! The one I wore yesterday was horrible.' Suddenly there is no right thing to say.

On the other hand, to be objective means to interpret an event or statement realistically without assuming responsibility or a negative interpretation.

An individual who is able to take an objective perspective might respond to his parents' request for babysitting with: 'How nice. Mom and Dad can have an hour together, and I'll have fun with Tommy. I haven't played with him for a while,' or perhaps more typically adolescent, 'Why do they always stick me with the babysitting? I'm entitled to a life too!' The headache would be met with the response, 'I'm sorry you don't feel well. The aspirin is on my dresser,' and the compliment about the dress with, 'Thanks. It's brand-new. I love it too.'

Because of the anorexic's persistently negative subjective reality, it becomes difficult for family members and society in general to find the correct language with which to talk to her. With each statement, no matter how seemingly benign, the victim gleans yet more material to confirm her negative beliefs about herself.

She becomes progressively less capable of any rational perspective or even of making choices. She will defer to others and become increasingly anxious, afraid that any decision she makes will be the wrong one. As my daughter Kirsten wrote ten years after her recovery, 'I remember being suspicious and intimidated at every turn; I was hesitant and almost incapable of relating to anyone or anything.'

I sometimes think of victims of eating disorders as willow wands who bend whichever way the wind blows. One recovered patient wrote:

> I changed my personality to become what I thought each person wanted me to be. I didn't think enough of my own identity to share it with others and I constantly tried to adapt myself to their needs. I imagined that everyone expected perfection from me, and I strove to become the perfect daughter, friend, student.

I have heard many people describe eating disorders as a consequence of low self-esteem. As I discuss in the next chapter, I believe the problem goes far deeper. In fact, I find that individuals with eating disorders have *no* sense of self or identity except for the fulfillment of their extremely subjective perception of other's expectations. A middle-aged anorexic told me on the phone recently, 'I am weary and frightened to open the door each morning. I never know who I am or what I'm going to have to face, and I'm exhausted from trying.' She later wrote to me, 'I am 40 years old but I feel like I am 4. Daily I vacillate ceaselessly between wanting to live and wanting to die because I do not know how to live.'

This woman has been arrested emotionally and developmentally. Psychologically, she is still a child with an unformed sense of self.

Many individuals with eating disorders will try to make themselves 'perfect' solely in order to please others. Only in emotional maturity do we develop the necessary objectivity to realize that it is indeed impossible to make oneself or life perfect. Describing his relationship difficulties with friends and loved ones, Jeremy wrote in his journal:

> I try to anticipate and meet their every need before they can even so much as suggest there might be one. I daren't be anything less than a perfect friend or they will leave me, I fear. . . . Generally it is easiest to be alone because then there is no one to interrupt my quest for perfection. But in this quest I drive others away who are sensing my loneliness and want to mend it. I force my high standards on them. I expect their homes and things to be perfect. If they are not, I will clean house for them while they are trying to just sit down with me, share a cup of tea and a visit.

Because the Negative Mind inflicts constant chaos, the victim of an eating disorder tries to grasp any sense of structure for herself. Unfortunately, she often fails miserably because she has no balanced perspective with which to work. Society often mistakenly interprets this wish to create order as the victim's attempt to control those around her. Society does not recognize that she struggles to exist in the world because she has no personal identity beyond her failure to create the perfect world for others.

ANOREXIA, BULIMIA, AND OVEREATING

Anorexia and bulimia come from the same mindset: CNC. They are merely different manifestations of the Negative Mind. Often anorexia leads to bulimia. The body can be so starved of nutrition that it develops what we term a 'bodymind,' which overrides the anorexic's impulse to starve herself and goes into high gear to search for food.

The bulimic bodymind veers from one extreme – starvation – to the other – bingeing – generally depending on how desperate it is to save itself. Parents of bulimics often report that the victim goes into a trancelike state during a binge. As the sufferer may later relate, she devours amazingly enormous quantities of food at one sitting or 'feeding frenzy.' Loved ones may watch in unmitigated horror as the victim 'protects her territory.' Often the family is relegated to another part of the house and the door to the kitchen is closed tightly. Parents have reported chaining refrigerators and freezers against the eventuality of such unbridled eating. The victim may then also purge by inducing vomiting and may overuse laxatives to finish the job.

There are many variations on this theme. One father wrote to me about his daughter: 'Her bulimia was so bad when she couldn't get enough food that she would try to kill herself. I got an extra job to make ends meet but we couldn't meet Monica's needs. She would pawn anything that she could find to buy food, even her guitar which she loved so much. She would even take the lunches that I had packed for myself.'

Another woman suffering from bulimia and anorexia wrote, 'Presently I go weeks without eating, weeks bingeing, weeks bingeing and purging, weeks bingeing and using laxatives, etc. etc. There just seems to be no end. . . .'

Another way of purging can be overexercise, not allowing food to be accepted into the body without retribution. Intermittently, the victim becomes physically and emotionally exhausted with the effort and moves back to the starving mode.

Bulimia leaves its victims with a feeling of incredible self-loathing. Patients frequently describe themselves as 'disgusting pigs.' When an anorexic's Actual Mind becomes conscious of her body weight as it turns to extreme gauntness, she is often equally repulsed.

Chronic overeating can represent another manifestation of CNC. However, there is a vast difference between being overweight and having an eating disorder. There is a distinction between the person who is overweight but not distraught because of it, and the person for whom overeating is a manifestation of self-hatred and a lack of self. The diagnosis depends on an outside assessment and the individual's own view of herself.

A person who is miserable about overeating, who cannot do anything positive about it, and who eats out of a sense of self-loathing may well have CNC.

THE PREDISPOSITION FOR CNC

What are the origins of the Negative Mind? How does someone become hostage to a mental construct of his or her own design? I believe that it all begins with a predisposition for CNC. Those predisposed to CNC are acutely sensitive to the needs of everyone and even everything else in their environment. Whether it be in the microcosm of the nuclear family or the macrocosm of our contemporary global reality, the potential victims of CNC have somehow come to deem themselves shepherds of the flock of humanity. These children are caring of their families and the universe. They are humanists of the first degree. As concerned environmentalists, the ozone layer, poverty, sickness, and the plight of the whales all immediately capture their attention.

How does it come about that a child should take the woes of the world on her fragile shoulders? That she should wish – in fact, see it as her inalienable duty – to parent her parents or save the world? I believe that, as infants, a number of us come into this world with the predisposition to CNC; it is therefore an inborn temperament. However, not every person with the predisposition develops CNC, just as not every person with a genetically endowed predisposition for a certain cancer, for example, develops the disease.

Often the immoderate sense of responsibility that is the hallmark of a predisposition to CNC becomes apparent at an early age. Many parents, in retrospect, recall how their caring child was always inordinately worried or concerned about others, even at an age when most children believe they are the center of the universe. Parents have told me:

'I knew there was something different about her ever since she could talk. She was always so helpful. She never caused any trouble and seemed to understand everybody's needs. She stood aside. She watched, observed rather than involving herself in fun.'

'She used to do vacuuming for me when she was three and four. I never asked her to; she just tried to help out where she could.'

'I got migraines all the time. He had to help with the younger child. He just did.'

'He put his small jacket on a care worker when their flight was canceled and he and everyone had to sleep on the floor of the airport. He was only three years old at the time.'

'She sat by the baby's bed all night watching her breathe because the doctor said the baby was a bit congested. She was about six years of age when that happened. I couldn't make her go to bed.'

'She always seemed to be more mature than she needed to be. The other children always came first. I worried about it at the time but it was a great help all the same. She never complained and never seemed to suffer. She looked after us all.'

A mother recounted that her eight-year-old would not join her playmates until all the housework was done. She did not want her parents doing it all themselves. One child tried to make her house earthquake proof. Another fastidiously checked all the locks and pulled out all the plugs at night so that her parents would be safe. A six-year-old took it upon herself to toddler-proof the house. My daughter Kirsten wrote, 'I remember as a child checking all the windows, doors, the stove and the toaster when my family was in bed at night to ensure that everything was secured and turned off.'

Some therapists might describe such behaviors as symptoms of obsessive-compulsive disorder, but I do not perceive them that way; in my experience these behaviors disappear once the underlying confirmed negativity is treated.

After Nora recovered from her eating disorder, she described in an Assessment Testimonial, one of the gauges of progress we use at the clinic, how she had taken on the world's troubles from early childhood onward: 'From a young age, I worried about everything. Were my parents happy with me? Did my brothers ever feel lonely? Did my sister hate herself as I did? I felt responsible for them and attributed any of their worries or unhappy comments, no matter how remote, to something I had or had not done. I worried about things I couldn't change – terrorism, poverty, sickness, unhappiness.'

It seems as if this child's mind stands aside, watching and waiting, studying life's circumstance from another place. The child with the CNC predisposition is often described as 'the best child' or the 'most responsible one.'

HOW THE CNC PREDISPOSITION BECOMES CONFIRMED

CNC is the culmination of negative assumptions about oneself in the caring for and the sense of responsibility for the world. Whether CNC develops depends substantially on the environment.

It is natural for children to become concerned about life around them. But these wise souls take it past the obvious point, fretting endlessly about the ozone layer, recycling every last scrap in the house, and so on. Children with CNC predispositions are fertile ground for misinterpretation of society's motives. But given an intelligent mind – and it is a given that most anorexics and bulimics are extremely intelligent – why is it they are unable to put society's or their family's needs into perspective? The reasons for this are familial as well as societal.

The Microcosm of the Family

Parenting in the natural order is about instruction and guidance of a child's potential. Boundaries for safety and structure shape and program a child's attitude. The normal development of children goes through obvious stages of need. Healthy development depends on a generally supportive and structured family environment. Ideally, as a child moves forward from one phase of growth, she has learned whatever the previous phase could teach her. This will serve as a platform from which growth naturally springs.

However, children who develop without the proper guidance of an adult and the structure of a supportive family become increasingly bewildered. This occurs if a child grows without restrictions of structure, or without confidence in the platform from which she should draw strength.

Permit me to share an example from my own family to illustrate. Recently, my daughter Nicole spent several nights alone with her two-year-old son, Darius, while her husband was away on business. Shortly after his father left, Darius turned to Nikki and said, 'Don't worry, Mommy. I take care of you now.'

Had Nikki responded, 'Oh, isn't that sweet. You're the man of the house,' she might have inadvertently re-inforced her child's sense that he was somehow responsible for her welfare. If Darius were predisposed to CNC, this could unconsciously confirm an erroneous assumption about his role in the family – that he needs to parent his parents.

But instead, Nicole wisely replied with a hug, 'I'm the mommy here, sweetheart. I'll take care of you! You don't have to worry about anything.' With her response, Nicole was creating a sense of structure and safety for her son. She was helping him to put his role in the family into the proper perspective – that he is still, after all, a dependent child, and that it is not his job to take care of his mother.

Parents who are afraid to set such limits for their CNC-predisposed children, for instance, who constantly ask for their children's opinion without stating what is acceptable or what is not (for fear of offending the child), who welcome their children's misguided attempts at parenting them, or who assume their children have the wherewithal to develop their own identities without their guidance, may unwittingly feed into the development of CNC by denying their youngsters the boundaries from which to develop a self-identity. This is not meant to blame parents but rather to illustrate how easily a precociously mature child can insinuate herself into a position of responsibility within the family structure. I know with my own children, I was more willing to let them assume more responsibility than perhaps I should have.

I am reminded of a tale attributed to Buddha. He was said to have given one of his talks to a group of disciples while holding a bird in his palm. The students were fascinated by the Buddha's ability to prevent the bird from flying away and were unable to duplicate his feat. Finally, they could restrain their curiosity no longer and blurted their question to the great master. 'Why does the bird not fly away?'

The Buddha replied, 'It is quite simple, my friends. Each time I sense that the bird will take flight, I simply drop my hand a bit, and the bird has nothing to push off from.'

I wish to emphasize here that it is normal and appropriate for parents of children who do not have a predisposition for CNC to encourage their offspring's independence, ability to reason for themselves, and desire to set some of their own boundaries. Ordinary children generally respond well to this, but children with the CNC predisposition will begin to feel overwhelmed. The parents' task is to be aware of their child's innate temperament and respond accordingly, and to distinguish between developing individuality and encouraging too much independence (see Chapter 6).

If a child is unsure of the messages she is receiving from anxious parents, she, like Buddha's bird, has no platform from which to push, and consequently has difficulty creating a sense of self. This can arrest her emotional development by interfering with the growth of her identity, thus eventually leading her toward subjectivity and self-abnegation.

Indeed, as time goes by, a CNC sufferer becomes so given to the well-being and caring of the world that she spends little time developing her internal identity. This eventually leads her toward subjectivity and self-abnegation. Her external identity becomes anything necessary to satisfy what she perceives the world needs it to be. So her self-concept is based on an unhealthy, vicarious respect for others. She mentally sacrifices her need to develop her own identity for the sake of healing the world, and finally, anxiously, anticipating possible problems to prevent.

The Macrocosm of Society

I believe that today we are living in an apprehensive, unparented society. Parents are themselves anxious. The rules and roles that seemed so clear fifty years ago, even thirty years ago, no longer exist. We are always worried about something. Indeed, some of our contemporary cities remind one of a disturbed antbed: We are panicky, agitated, and traveling in all directions at once, daily confirming a hurried, stressed lifestyle.

Although we seem more electronically connected through cellular phones, faxes, and pagers, we are fooling ourselves, for we are connected only to the harried pace of society. We are actually more disconnected from the parts of ourselves that are conducive to emotional health – our caringness and concern for others. Rather than seeing life as being about survival, we are seeing it as an avoidance of the inevitable. We are too apt to castigate ourselves for our emotional problems; instead, we need to understand and accept that being human is about faltering and learning.

We seem to have become so anxiety-conditioned that we need to live as a sedated society – we seem incapable of living life without a crutch in the form of medication, be it analgesics or antidepressants. Our increasing numbness and sedation cause us to become more apathetic rather than more caring. Life is more anxiety-provoking, so we practice avoidance. But in so doing, do we teach our young, inadvertently, that there is a pill for everything emotional and physical? Do we indicate that pain, imperfection, and humanness are unacceptable elements of the human condition?

Our extended families have shrunk to near oblivion. When truncated families face serious problems such as illness, unemployment, divorce, or substance abuse, and the CNC-predisposed child has few trusted adults to turn to for advice and guidance, she may erroneously believe that the healing of her family is solely her responsibility. The more adults – family and friends – actively participating in a child's growth years, the more the child is able to grasp an objective reality, and the more the child seems to allow herself to be a child.

What do the media teach us? Violence in the media desensitizes us to others' suffering – we become helpless bystanders and we practice bystander apathy.

What do the media teach our children? Ubiquitous images glorify negativity and sensationalism while they discourage hope and instill fear. The media present a near-constant diet of pessimism, competition, contradiction, sedation, hopelessness, and doom. Given that bad news is more available and interesting, and a good news story is a rarity at most, it appears that young minds in our society, as they hurry along to keep up with the latest, are terribly vulnerable to absorbing the negative messages surrounding them.

Sensitive children with a CNC disposition are doused with pessimism and negativity that is passed through society like a contagious yawn, and they learn from society too well.

When a society's values become external, it devalues the essence of humanness. In so many ways, what the suggestible and ultimately vulnerable child will learn is mostly projected through television, tabloid sensationalism, and other entertainment and information media. These venues are available at a very early age – an age well before a child has the capacity to put what she is absorbing into proper perspective. One of the youngest patients I've counseled used to sit on his mother's lap and watch the evening news. She had no way of knowing that he took every bit of negative news deeply to heart and came to believe that it was his duty to right the world's wrongs.

Children need structure in order to survive. For their well-being it is imperative to encourage congruency with their environment, optimism, and hope despite the different perspectives in the world. If children conclude from watching the media and observing their surroundings that life is chaos, that the contradictions of doom and a no-pain existence can reside within the realm of perfectionism, this can tip them from a predisposition into full-blown CNC.

As these children struggle to create a perfect world, they become more agile at perfecting their own selves vicariously. Here lie additional tools for the development of CNC. They strive for scholastic, physical, and artistic excellence. They are the perfect students, athletes, artists, or musicians.

CNC-predisposed children excel in most venues society has provided to showcase important external values, such as school, sports, gymnastics, dance, music, and so on. In their minds, they are attempting to adhere to what they perceive as society's dictates – to please others before themselves. They do not strive to be the best because of their inherent sense of superiority and duty; they do it to try to prove their worth to others because they lack an internal sense of self.

Both of Connie's parents were lawyers, and she believed she needed to become a lawyer too. She suffered a complete collapse while in her third year of studies, not because she was incapable of the work, but because she felt she could never live up to her idea of her parents' expectations for her.

In fact, Connie's parents are wonderful people who did well in their own careers but had no wish for their daughter other than her well-being. Connie assumed that to make them happy, she had to follow in their footsteps. Subsequent to treatment, she enrolled in design school and is now an accomplished and recognized designer. I have found over and over in working with patients that the drive to create perfection for others replaces the natural maturation of self. Only when patients recover and nurture this sense can they begin to explore their own passions and loves – to discover what pleases them alone.

After working for many years with families of children with eating disorders, you realize that these children are more privy and prone to the contradictions society presents them: On one hand, it seems to them that they are obliged to attain perfection, while on the other, there is increasing unmitigated pain in the world and poverty, sickness, and death. The media make both poles abundantly accessible and unavoidable. The very language of our society depicts doom and hopelessness while subtly demanding the impossible – perfection. The child with a caring disposition, hoping to avert disaster either in her nuclear family or in society in general, runs faster and faster to appease others and prevent some potential catastrophe, because she believes she can – and must.

Sadly, the victim has no idea that all the world does not share her perspective of peace and goodwill. She has not had enough time to understand the differences between people, to perceive that humans operate within the limitations of their understanding and abilities, that offense comes more often from ignorance and unawareness than it does from intent, that just because society presents the notion that perfection is attainable, she is not solely responsible for achieving it. CNC victims learn society too well without having the maturity to moderate their understanding of it.

At the same time, however, it is important to note that many people can and do identify with the beginning stages of CNC – the desire to serve the world, the impulse to put the pleasure of others first – and have spent their lives helping others. Yet they have somehow learned to live in the world without developing an eating disorder or other self-negating condition. These individuals' lives somehow correct themselves before the Negative Condition becomes confirmed and therefore detrimental to their survival. They allow themselves the favor of being well and are able to achieve some balance in their efforts to help the world.

Ultimately, the failure of perfectionism for the CNC victim engenders a supreme sense of worthlessness that leads to the manifestation of an eating disorder. This worthlessness is expressed in the anorexic as an attempt at being the smallest and sickest and in the bulimic with ever more extreme binge/purge episodes. Both manifestations deny the victim any sense of normalcy; both are thoroughly degrading. The subtle reality of this mindset is that *sufferers need to be the best at being the least deserving*. Ultimately, they need to know: Are they the best *at dying*?

HOW CNC MANIFESTS AS AN EATING DISORDER

Imagine someone who always places herself (or what little self exists) second, who vigilantly tries to appease others before anything else. She learns to subordinate her needs and desires by learning society's values and what she must do to live up to these values.

It is an extreme risk to lend one's identity completely to other people's needs. The victim lives through anyone's need vicariously. When the need no longer exists in the chosen person, she seeks out other people in need upon which to focus her attention, caringness, and overconcern, or she manufactures need where none exists.

When one's identity is so consumed with ministering to a certain need (real or perceived) over a long period of time, it becomes even more difficult to disassociate from it. Margie developed anorexia at age sixty-four when her husband died. She had spent years attending to his severe medical condition and she had to relearn living in order to survive. With months of intervention, she successfully reinterpreted herself to live objectively, with compassion and kindness yet retaining her newfound identity. It became apparent through counseling that throughout her life, Margie had looked after her siblings, then her mother, and most recently her husband. She had identified herself only through other people's need rather than her own individual potential.

Another patient was one of five siblings. Her mother was a highly emotional person who continually lamented her plight in life and was prone to tearful outbursts. Although Carla was different from her mother, she was unaware that human nature describes itself in many ways. She became determined to create a happiness for her mother that seemed unattainable for her and, sadly, failed miserably.

Carla's mother was just being who she was. But nothing in Carla's learning to that point made her understand that people operate from different dispositions and that it is acceptable to respond otherwise to life.

It is, of course, impossible for any one individual to achieve such a magnificent objective as to completely rid the world of its ills or one's family of its woes. Caring, empathy, and compassion are wonderful attributes in any person. However, even the most altruistic person must include herself in the well-being she wishes and works toward for others. When these virtues exceed themselves to the point of self-sacrifice, the individual finds herself lost.

When a child with CNC discovers that she cannot 'save the world,' that perfection is impossible, she is devastated. She feels betrayed if parents have cancer, or heart attacks, or become bankrupt, or if relationships are less than perfect. She feels horrified that she cannot rescue the whales or the tropical rain forests. Failure begets failure. She judges herself unworthy and weak because she is incapable of solving these overwhelming problems – problems that continue to challenge the best adult minds. These disappointments and traumas, although they do not 'cause' the eating disorder (since the cause is the underlying misinterpretation of her role fundamental to CNC), can nevertheless trigger its onset.

The child's initial perception, that she can effect change, is coupled with the growing knowledge that she is, in fact, all too powerless to do so. The contradiction inherent in these two disparate forces leads her to believe that either she or the world is living a lie. She becomes increasingly subjective – everyone and everything around her reinforces her unworthiness, her defeat, her impotence – and she fails to advance in the natural growth toward objectivity. She falls into CNC.

As the confirmed negativity becomes progressively worse, subjectivity comes to dominate 20, 30, 50, 60 percent of her thoughts. Without early intervention, when subjectivity overbalances objectivity, when it constantly seeks ways to feed itself and becomes increasingly successful in doing so, the eating disorder manifests and quickly grows dangerous.

The CNC sufferer becomes incapable of handling responsibility for the pain in the microcosm of her own family and in mitigating what she sees as the pain of the world. Yet despite her incapacity, she still feels she must somehow be responsible. She therefore unconsciously decides to resign. She becomes despairing of survival in her perception of what society requires. She does not want to come to this conclusion but sees no recourse. At this point in her demise, she feels it is her just deserts. As the victim heads toward self-destruction, her Negative Mind grows in importance and magnitude.

Understanding the motivating forces behind the eating disorder behavior helps to translate it. It can be broken down to a relatively simple formula:

Eating means having food.
Food means having life.
I should not have life because I do not deserve it.
I do not deserve life because I have failed humanity.
Therefore I do not deserve food.

As a victim moves from CNC to a manifestation of eating disorder, her mind will increasingly deteriorate her sense of worth. She indicates her lack of faith in her identity by severely cutting back on food. She has lost confidence in herself and her decision-making ability since she has lost faith in her own validity in the world. She becomes isolated from friends because she believes she is less than they are and does not want to impose her ignorance and boring personality on them.

Victims love their parents so much that they feel guilty eating in front of them. They do not see themselves as worthy. They find it extremely difficult to allow themselves any pleasure since they have surely not protected their parents from all ills. To admit openly that they are allowing themselves to partake of life seems selfish. In the victim's mind, she has profoundly disappointed her parents.

Here is how Nora describes her slide into CNC and then anorexia: 'I finally just wanted to fade away completely, to remove myself from a world that appeared to be sad and cold. The restriction of food was

67

simply a way to make myself even more unobtrusive. It was a continuation of the punishment I would impose on myself for not being able to save everyone. . . . Inside my head there was a constant harsh voice, encouraging me in this downward spiral, telling me that I was nothing, that I was unworthy, that I was not doing as much as I could to contribute to everyone's happiness.'

THE PARADOX OF BLAME

When we talk about eating disorders, the concept of 'blame' seems to raise its head distressingly often. For want of a clearer answer, parents blame themselves or are blamed for being inadequate in some measure. The sufferers, already incorrigible in their own heads, are blamed for being callous enough to hurt their parents and siblings; their noncompliance during treatment is construed as intentional and volitional. But to suggest that any one person, or society as a whole, is to blame for eating disorders is an oversimplification.

Eating disorders develop unconsciously; victims are as confused as those around them when the contradictory symptoms emerge. Moreover, who is to blame if a person is born into the world highly sensitive?

To borrow an analogy from physiology, it has been determined that in any cross section of individuals, the number of taste buds in a square centimeter of tongue can range from twelve to two hundred. Some people are simply more sensitive to taste than others. Such ranges also hold true in a cross section of personalities. Some people are more emotionally sensitive than others. However, the heightened sensitivity of a CNC-predisposed individual is always directed toward the needs of others. She possesses a selfless sensitivity. Is this blameworthy? We wouldn't blame someone whose predisposition to diabetes or cancer caused her to develop the illness; why would we blame those who develop eating disorders?

Society may inadvertently contribute to the production of eating disorders, but until its members have been enlightened, can they be held responsible?

The victim is living a nightmare, internally and externally. Her beloved parents, who in her mind need support in the first place, and whose love and support she so badly needs, are in the uncomfortable throes of added chaos and distress because of her behavior. She has unintentionally made their lives a worse hell. As Julie wrote to me in some of her voluminous letters:

'I hurt people and regret the reality of what I am doing to everyone. I think of my mother and cry at the horror of creating so much misery just being alive.'

'In a weak moment I confessed these feelings to my mother and have now successfully ruined her life as well.'

'I cringe when I think of what I have done to my mother.'

One of the most tragic facts of eating disorders is that its victims become receptacles for society's inadvertent abuse. They are accused of noncompliance when they have failed a hospital program. Rarely do we hear that a system has not worked for them; rather, we are told that they have not worked for the system. I have received hundreds of letters that reiterate this point. The following is just a sampling:

'Please help us. Our daughter Hannah has failed her fourth program. Her weight dropped down to 68 pounds.'

'Celine wants to get better but she has been unable to find the solution to cure herself. She has tried and failed basically every program out there. It will come down to 1) her dying or 2) your program/miracle to cure her.'

'The doctor told Marci that she was a waste of his time, that she doesn't have a life. She has disappointed the doctor because she hasn't been able to "fix" herself, and since Marci doesn't really have a life, why should anyone try to save her?'

'I have been rejected by several hospital programs because they say my depression is so severe that they are not trained for that level. One hospital said that I am going to die from this if I keep on losing weight and then rejected me.'

'My life has been one big failure. I hate myself, and have attempted suicide three times. I plan to finish the job next fall.'

'I have not been successful with any other treatment programs I have tried, but that is completely my fault. . . . My family has pleaded with me to recover, but I constantly fail to put aside my own wishes and do the necessary things to stabilize my condition.'

'I really hate myself for getting trapped in this disease. There must have been something I could have done to prevent it. It's all of my fault that my family is hurting. I destroyed the trust that my parents had in me before.'

'I am in my thirties and have been hospitalized several times in an eating disorder unit which did not help me overcome my problem. I am not blaming them and I take full responsibility for my failure. . . . At the time of my last hospitalization, the psychiatrist said he would no longer treat me because I had let him down.

He told me that I was a failure and that I would be a chronic anorexic. Everything he told me is true. I am a failure and don't deserve to live.'

It would appear on the surface that these victims wish their deaths. It seems never to occur to us that perhaps that assumption doesn't make rational sense, that anyone wishing death for psychological reasons certainly must be misguided; that it is probable that, as many of my patients have said, they don't know how to live rather than that they don't want to.

What the general public most likely does not understand is that the victim may attempt suicide because she thinks there is no way she can live with the internal mental horror, the unrelenting pressure of the Negative Mind. If society continues to lay the onus of blame on the eating disorder victim, if therapists and others in the helping professions tell victims that they're failures, *if we turn on our own*, how can the Actual Mind not admit defeat?

Sometimes, in frustration and desperation or for the perceived protection of the victim's siblings, parents, often at the suggestion of therapists, throw the eating disorder victim out of her home – a Tough Love approach. With less protection and ability now to fend for herself, she somehow must, as must her siblings accept that their sister must be punished because she did not adhere to society's rules. She becomes doubly stigmatized.

One mother of an anorexic child wrote, 'She finally quit going to school and just gave up. And I am ashamed to admit it, but so did I. I basically threw her out of the house because of her negative influence on our other children. I love Alicia with all my heart, but

I couldn't sacrifice the other children for her.'

The concept of 'blame' disallows that imperfection is a part of the human condition. Rather than creating acceptance and support for unity and understanding for everyone's benefit, blame sets up corruption and division of family and eventually of societal structure.

When anyone blames an ill child or her anxious parents, they are operating out of the mindset of 'authority for authority's sake.' The danger is that if a therapist blames an eating disorder victim or labels her a failure out of frustration or a sense of helplessness, the family and patient may still swallow those statements whole and without question. The attitude that eating disorders are 'incurable' becomes a self-fulfilling prophecy for the victim.

Unfortunately, it seems many traditional methods of treatment worldwide put the onus of blame and responsibility on a mind that is incapable, in its acute manifestation, of taking it. The translation to the sufferer is 'I cannot overcome this. I am worthless and a failure.' As this attitude is often repeated through many more years of treatment, the Negative Mind is only more re-inforced and armed with additional ammunition. Indeed, the Negative Mind will absorb the information and use it subjectively against the Actual Mind. 'I have been rejected and I have failed – more proof that I am worthless and a burden to my family and society.'

Sufferers live in a surreal daze of misery and confusion, sometimes hoping each day will be the last. The devastation to all involved is beyond belief and in its loneliness, inhuman.

The onus of responsibility is being put on our weakest, our most sensitive. As naturally caring children, these individuals take responsibility upon themselves anyway.

When they become ill, it is heaped upon them. Does it not occur to us that blame rarely corrects any situation, but makes people feel even more subservient? Is it not likely that not only might this be wrong but that it is highly counterproductive and will just aggravate the problem?

Often what appears to be the obvious answer in the treatment of the eating disorder conundrum – attacking the external behavior of the victim – is actually its antithesis. In the case of eating disorders, seeing is not believing. In the case of eating disorders, people are not their behavior. Anorexia or bulimia is the most visible symptom of a more complicated, complex, and convoluted mindset derived from a misinterpretation of its victim's role in life.

Victims of eating disorders have always felt they must not trouble the world. They are only interested in healing society, not in hindering it. Given that excelling proves almost effortless, how can they now accept the alarming fact that they are suddenly incapable of mastering their own territory – their emotional mind? How can these individuals, who see themselves as subservient to the human race, ask for help or admit defeat in the fight for life? When they fault themselves for their plight, how can they turn to society for help?

Eating disorders offer many expressions. They are all self-negating. They are the epitome of alienation from self and society. Internally, the actual potential person dies a million deaths in shame and contrition for something she apparently has no control over. When placed necessarily in an atmosphere of unconditional forgiveness, the patient is able to begin to allow herself, though slowly and with difficulty, the right to be human – with all its accompanying foibles.

Society has inadvertently created the perfect puzzle – a person so distorted in self-image, so much in the grasp of the Negative Mind, so undeserving of help, that she must suffer psychological purgatory until we – the outsiders – understand her secret language and deliver her from her plight.

Yet, despite the horrifying aspects of CNC, it is amazing to watch the courage of victims of eating disorders. That some are still alive after battling sometimes from twenty to thirty years should be a lesson to humankind. What residue of hope encourages these individuals to get up every day and try again? Their survival would seem, by normal standards, to defy all odds!

3

Myths and Misconceptions

'More are killed by word of mouth than by the sword.'
—LEONARDO DA VINCI

'I have always been told I am a controlling perfectionist.'
'I can't be cured. I'm too bad. I'm going to have to deal with this the rest of my life. I just have to live with it.'

'It's those pictures of supermodels in the magazines that put Jamie on this incessant diet.'

'They told me my daughter is going to be released on Sunday. She's only sixteen. Her insurance has run out. They told me to prepare for her death. There is nothing more they can do.'

'I don't deserve to get well. I feel so dirty, hopeless, no-good, fat, scared, a failure, insecure. I really don't deserve to live.'

'I am disgusted with myself for being the cause of all this.'

'My daughter is 5 feet 8 inches and sixty pounds. There's not much left of her. She won't comply with anyone. She's only been out of hospitals for two four-month periods in the last three years. She has ruined the family.'

'My husband and I aren't speaking. We don't really have a relationship anymore. My kids hate me for ignoring them because my own problems were more important than they were. I've tried; can you help? It's been almost a dozen years. Our home is a war zone and my therapist refuses to see me anymore because I lost too much weight and didn't stick to the bargains we made.'

'They say I am selfish; that all I care about is how I look.'

'My doctor told me I don't want to grow up.'

'I am the worst case they have ever seen and I'm incurable.'

'She refuses to deal with her underlying issues no matter how many psychiatrists she sees.'

'I used to be the perfect child with everything going for me, but I have lost it all!'

'I'm not worth saving, but I might prove an interesting experiment.'

'I don't want my daughter to die. They say we are a dysfunctional family, but my wife and I are still together. We don't fight and we love our daughter very much. They say they can do no more for my daughter. She is only nineteen. It is not the natural order of things that she should die first. Surely something can be done.'

All of these statements are based on myths and misconceptions about anorexia and bulimia. Unfortunately, many of these myths still hold sway today and are often the basis upon which we regard and treat patients with eating disorders.

In this chapter, I hope to offer an alternative to these myths and set in their place what I have perceived is the true nature of eating disorders – CNC and the Negative Mind.

A widely held theory expounds that anorexia is in part caused by a culture that values appearance over substance and prizes women only when they are thin. Much has been said about the cult of thinness, the rise of the supermodel as a public icon, and the belief that victims of eating disorders lose weight to emulate a supposed physical ideal.

Eating disorders are eight times more common in women than in men. Surely one of the external values society offers as a venue of perfection is the female body. Women grow up being complimented more on their looks than on any other quality. We are told that most women are perpetually dieting. Yet we must be careful about assessing blame for eating disorders to this aspect of contemporary society without considering the broader context.

The deification of thinness is dangerous, but where eating disorders are concerned, it can be misleading. Indeed, this is a much more complicated issue than appears at first glance, and if a connection exists between the cult of thinness and anorexia, it is far deeper than mere vanity.

There is a difference between becoming thin for the sake of fitting into society's expectations and becoming thinner and thinner and thinner for the sake of dying. Taken to their extreme, eating disorders are, after all, a slow form of suicide.

If models in their beauteous, supposed perfection are an example to the vulnerable, why do those suffering eating disorders progress so far beyond thinness to emaciation and, ultimately, death? Why are boys and men affected? Why will one model become anorexic and another not? Why do elderly women become anorexics crippled with arthritis? Why do small children?

The distorted perception starts early – I have counseled patients as young as three years old – and I now believe that the 'failure to thrive' cited in infants can be in some instances an early manifestation of the Negative Mind. The seeds of anorexia may have been planted at a much earlier age than the one at which individuals become body-conscious.

Society's emphasis on looks clouds the more important issue that children are dying because they are trying to achieve impossible standards of perfection. As we have seen in the previous chapter, this focus on perfection is not so much for personal gratification as it is a misguided attempt to improve the world.

Rather than thinking of the supermodel syndrome as a cause of eating disorders, it is best to think of it as a possible trigger. Modeling is an area in which perfection seems attainable, one of the many venues for perfection (such as sports, academics, dance, and so on) that eating disorder victims will fit themselves into. Most teenage girls try to lose a few pounds for the sake of attracting boys in high school. Many women are constantly on a diet, unhappy with their bodies. But a girl with an eating disorder will use the ideal of the model as a way to hone her sense of perfection; boys are not on her mind. A woman with an eating disorder doesn't want to be a size 6; she wants to be a size 0. The difference is knowing how much of what society presents to take seriously.

I do believe that media and advertising images that glorify perfection and beauty contribute to many women's sense of unhappiness about their imperfectly human bodies. I would applaud a movement to curtail the supermodel syndrome. But I am not convinced that the rate of eating disorders would fall as a result; I believe that people with CNC would find another venue of perfection to emulate.

Moreover, anorexics frequently suffer from gross distortion of their body image. They will often claim they are overweight in the face of all physical evidence to the contrary. One young woman planning a third suicide attempt wrote to me that, at five foot four, she weighed 93 pounds. 'I feel fat all the time,' she said, 'but before I kill myself, I must be thin. I cannot let some undertaker see my ugly fat body.'

The DSM-IV, the latest diagnostic manual of psychiatric conditions, states, 'Individuals with this disorder intensely fear gaining weight or becoming fat. This intense fear of becoming fat is usually not alleviated by the weight loss. In fact, concern about weight gain often increases even as actual weight continues to decrease.'

I believe that the Negative Mind will not allow its victims to see themselves as they are because weight is synonymous with life. Given that victims are on an unconscious track to total self-negation (death), if they perceive themselves as fat, this will allow the Negative Mind to demand that they lose even more weight.

Anorexics will lie about whether they have eaten because the Negative Mind, which insists without reason or logic on their demise, instructs them to. They wear concealing clothes to protect the Negative Mind, to forestall confrontation with the people around them. In the few cases in which anorexics flaunt their gauntness, they are pointing out that they are more unworthy than others. They vie to be the best at dying.

Anorexia is about self-loathing and self-hatred for falling short of perfection. Nora wrote several years after her recovery, 'I didn't look at models and dream of looking like them. I didn't think that I was becoming beautiful. I thought I was the ugliest, most selfish, and horrible person.'

'Anorexia is more prevalent in females than in males because females are told that appearance is important while males are praised for other qualities.'

I do agree that women are bombarded with images of unattainable female beauty. Women's magazines are filled with articles and advertisements touting diets, weight loss, exercise machines, and so on. Beautiful women are featured in television ads that sell everything from beer to automobiles to detergent.

Though the images of 'perfect' women still vastly outnumber those extolling male perfection, I do in fact see a rise in the number of images of men, although they are perhaps more obscured. *Men's Health* and *GQ* as opposed to *Glamour* and *Vogue* – the magazine titles may not always be as direct.

Once again, however, I think we are looking at a trigger, not a direct cause. Eating disorders are not gender-based any more than CNC is gender-based.

Historically, women have been honed to be the care-givers of home and therefore of society's needs. For years, they have been the quiet support person, the one to whom the expressions 'The power behind the throne' and 'Behind every great man is a great woman' applied. So naturally, it would follow that there would be a higher incidence of eating disorder manifestation among females.

Today, society is evolving. Men can act more sensitively. We are finally a more humanistic culture rather than a culture of warriors.

And eating disorders among men are on the rise – at least one million men number among the eight million people afflicted with them in the United States. I attribute this to the ever-increasing anxiety and attitudes toward perceived stress in society (the macrocosm) and the changing rules within the nuclear family (the microcosm), coupled with the victim's sensitive, caring nature.

Perhaps men are not faced with the anxiety of society's contradictions as often because their stereotypical role is to do rather than to mediate and placate. But given the changing roles in society, men see themselves more often in the position of giving care. One young man who came into my care after years of hospitalization that culminated in institutionalization in a mental facility because of the severity of his suicidality had begun his slide toward CNC and anorexia as a young boy. His mother had suffered stomach problems so intense that she had to run to the hospital for treatment. Jonathan took it upon himself to keep his two younger siblings quiet while his mother recovered from her frequent ailments. She had not asked him to do this, but in his own mind, he saw it as his role.

Each case of anorexia is different. But anorexics all hear the same language and display the same inherent kindness. After their recovery, their Actual Minds will regain control, and these former victims will be objectively, not subjectively, kind.

'Anorexia is caused by physical, emotional, or sexual abuse.'

Abuse falls into the category of 'Underlying Issues.' These issues are real, and they need to be addressed. In this discussion, I applaud the work being done with people who have such issues. At the same time, however, I question whether these issues are directly related to anorexia. As one victim wrote to me, 'I don't know how to change. Any program I've been in was a stop-gap measure – a one- or three-month hospital stay where I'd put on weight that I'd immediately drop as soon as I was released. (Sure, I worked through many important issues – but never unraveled the behavior.)'

I keep reading that eating disorders are skyrocketing because sexual abuse is coming out of the closet. I have had patients come to me and say, 'I don't remember being sexually abused, but since I have anorexia, I guess I must have been.'

I know of one father who was accused of sexually abusing his daughter because she was anorexic. There was no evidence for believing he had molested his little girl. Even though no one in the family could see how this abuse was possible, the mother divorced him because of the groundless charge. Both child and father denied any abuse took place, and I believe them – it took me two years to put the family back together.

I do not deny that sexual abuse occurs in situations in which child and parent vigorously deny it, nor do I want to minimize the devastating trauma that can occur after sexual abuse. However, most of my patients have not been abused, and I want to set aside the common misconception that every eating disorder is the product of abuse – physical, sexual, or otherwise.

On the other hand, I have worked with several anorexics who have been sexually abused. They felt that they deserved what happened to them, they did not feel traumatized by it, and were primarily relieved that it had not occurred to someone else. Typically, they welcomed what must seem to the rest of us like cruel punishment (the work of the ever-perverse Negative Mind), and still they cared for others first – even their abusers. In truth, they lacked an accurate perception of their reality and responsibility.

Consequently, I believe it may not be the trauma of the abuse per se, but the individual's perception of reality that will cause anorexia. We can change reality only to a certain point (by addressing the trauma and distress that act as triggers), but we can try to change people's attitudes toward and perceptions of reality. In other words, we can objectify abuse, that is, try to help the abused victim understand that she did not deserve or cause the abuse, in order to preserve the sanity of the victim. Perhaps anger toward ignorance only compounds the problem and prolongs the suffering of the victim. Compassion and understanding for the limitations of human awareness would seem more likely to heal the victim than criticizing her for not condemning her abuse or her abuser.

'Anorexia is caused by distant, uncaring, demanding, or otherwise dysfunctional parents.'

There is a widespread perception that anorexia is more common in families in which rigid, exacting, uncompromising parents impose their own personalities on compliant little children. The 'best little girl in the world' stereotype conveys that nothing the child does is good enough for insatiable, demanding parents, so the child keeps trying harder and harder to please them.

This is blatantly untrue for the vast majority of my cases. In fact, I was alarmed to discover how wrong the stereotype is. It would have made it easier to find that parents were uncaring or demanding or dysfunctional, because then the answer to the eating disorder conundrum would have been much simpler.

Parents are primarily responsible for defining the world in which their children find themselves, but the emergence of an eating disorder is not in itself a response to a specific social structure within the family. Rather, I find that motivation for achievement is far more self-imposed.

I have observed that these children are determined to create the best possible scenario for the ones they love, without having been asked or pushed. Generally, the intense striving to achieve and the insatiable need for validation come from within them, not from external sources such as parents.

One girl wrote in her journal, 'I was running track before school, doing homework instead of eating lunch, doing more running after school, studying until one o'clock or two o'clock in the morning and sleeping four or five hours a night, maximum. . . . I contemplated driving my car around a corner and not turning because I had gotten a 97 percent on a project that was worth only a fraction of my final grade. I made one stupid mistake on a departmental exam and it haunted me for months! Nothing was ever good enough. And when I did achieve "perfection," it meant nothing to me.'

Another wrote, 'I cannot recognize or appreciate any of my own accomplishments. Others are always better.

Even when I achieve excellence it isn't good enough. I recently got 98 percent on my calculus final and was upset with myself for not doing better. My goals are far too high. I lose sight of what is realistic or even excellent, and strive for what is impossible. I never reach it, so I am always a failure in my estimation and that makes me unhappy.'

Moreover, young people with eating disorders work at parenting their parents; they insist on caring for the adults. As I explained in Chapter 2, parents are generally struck by the maturity of these children from a very early age and tend to lean on them because they can.

Most of the parents whom I see are incredible – extremely loving and caring. They are also incredibly human – they have flaws and faults like the rest of us. Parents are people – they are human and imperfect. Every family in the world has circumstances that play the scale of that humanness. Motivation and the effort to make things work are all that are available to any of us. Failure requires tolerance and understanding without one being labeled a misfit.

The stress of parents' divorce in particular is blamed for children's eating disorders. However, most of my patients' parents are not divorced, and most of the families I see are not dysfunctional. However, if parents have the slightest squabble, the child with CNC regards it as a crisis of the most major proportions and will try to intervene. This later gets misconstrued by many therapists as evidence of a 'dysfunctional family,' when in fact it is a reflection of the hypersensitive perspective of the child with CNC.

As I've mentioned, if anything, family traumas such as illness, divorce, or other life crises may act as triggers that help shift someone with preexisting CNC into a full-blown eating disorder. If a child is already feeling negative and subjective about what is going on in her life, she is more vulnerable and susceptible to taking these emergencies personally and feeling helpless about them. The more pervasive the pessimistic thought patterns – that is, if they dominate 60 percent of her thoughts rather than 20 percent – the more effective the trigger will be in setting off the eating disorder.

Certainly there are extremes – true dysfunctional families, and that dysfunction can act as a trigger for eating disorders. It is essential that such families come to terms with the dysfunction and seek appropriate therapy to address it. Although I believe that an individual whose CNC has been reversed will not respond to the same trigger – divorce, depression, or other trauma – by relapsing into an eating disorder, the trigger is nonetheless a potent source of stress. For the health of the whole family, it must be dealt with. I'll discuss this further in Chapter 7.

However, not every family that raises its voice once in a while is dysfunctional. Conversely, an eating disorder will be highly distressing to any family system. A cohesive and healthy family unit can be pushed to self-destruction by the very threats and misguided suspicions we have talked about.

I have found that many parents of eating disorder victims, like most parents, are possibly overanxious, but that anxiety is shaped and even inadvertently encouraged by society. Parents may rush to the doctor for every little thing; they may use a pill for every perceived problem. Is this about the child or about the 'anxiety of prevention'? Certainly, parents generally come from a place of good intentions.

Because of this, I feel it is imperative to let go of blame.

Often parents live with guilt for feeling that they have somehow contributed to and are responsible for the way their children behave. Parents are moved to shame because they have been labeled – rightly or wrongly – dysfunctional and feel they are the objects of a witch-hunt. This serves to create more agitation, stress, and negativity within an already tormented family.

These parents spend untold hours denouncing themselves for their human inadequacies while simultaneously living in the war zone of their sick children's lives. They try to carry on their jobs and lives while entertaining a nightmare within the walls of their homes, a nightmare that they are too often told is their fault and inadvertently their doing. Their most important focus, their child, is at risk of dying. Parents stand helpless in the apparent hopelessness of their situation.

In the long run, placing the blame on parents – even if they are 'guilty' of creating triggers for eating disorders – can be detrimental and dangerous to their child. It may prevent them from being available to her when they are most essential as her basic support system. Their energies will be diverted to searching for their error in 'causing' their child's condition and possible death. Their guilt will rob them of the strength to stand firm to reverse the Negative Mind, and so they may give in to what they assume are their child's needs when they are actually giving in to the condition's demands.

'Anorexia is the consequence of perfectionistic people failing in their desire to be perfect.'

Perfectionism for an individual with an eating disorder is about appeasing society and placating its expectations.

One child wrote in her journal, 'I don't feel confident with myself as a person, so I feel I have to try to conform to society's pressure to meet the expectations it places on people's acceptance based on their appearance.'

Why does a child need to be perfect? Perhaps she does because we, as a society, have told her that she *can* be, and because she feels she therefore *must* be. But there is a great difference between seeking to perfect oneself for self-satisfaction or the accolades of family or society – behavior that we would probably label as 'normal' – and the victim's attempt at perfection in order to make society, as a whole, a better place for all. A tall order, indeed!

***

'Anorexia is caused by low self-esteem.'

***

When Nicole was still ill, an old friend told her that she was conceited because she was always looking in the mirror. 'Doesn't she understand? It isn't about that, Mom,' she said tearfully. 'I was looking to find myself. I was hunting for me.'

It makes little sense to talk of self-esteem in the same breath as anorexia. As I have explained in the previous chapter, anorexia is a condition based on the lack of a fully defined self. To recover from anorexia, the victim must first develop a self before she can address her self-esteem.

I become concerned when I hear about people struggling to build an acutely ill patient's self-esteem, because that person has no clear sense of self to which to attribute the esteem. This makes the victim feel more worthless, and the parent and loved one more guilty.

Esteem will naturally begin to develop after the self has begun to emerge.

> *'Anorexia is the result of trauma from the pain of parents' divorce, adolescence, or other life crises.'*

In the case of my own divorce, it is natural to wonder whether tensions in the household before the breakup or the stress of the breakup itself were what tipped my daughters toward anorexia. Kirsten, Nicole, and I have discussed this at great length and do not believe these issues were the trigger for their eating disorders. My former husband and I did not have a turbulent relationship; it just gradually became apparent to us that we wanted different things out of the marriage. We did not have an acrimonious split-up; it was a long time coming and the girls knew and were in agreement with it. (It was our friends and neighbors who were surprised.) I've been asked if undercurrents of tension rather than overt drama might have pushed my daughters over the edge. If so, why were they well all during the years when my husband and I were living on parallel tracks yet under the same roof, and only became ill when I moved out on my own? Surely one's parents splitting up – even if my daughters acknowledged that it made everyone happier – must be traumatic; how could a family's dissolution not be a negative? Yet Kirsten and Nikki tell me they didn't see it that way. In retrospect, it is clear to us that the trigger for their illness was not my divorce but their anxiety and hypersensitive reaction to my struggles as a single parent trying to earn a degree and raise two children on her own. In typical CNC fashion, they were worrying not about themselves, but about my well-being. My struggles became their burden, although I wasn't aware of it at the time.

Of course, every divorce is unique because every marriage and family is unique, and I do believe there are children who feel traumatized by their parents' breakup. However, it has been my experience that in these cases, it is not the particulars of the divorce itself, but the manner in which the CNC-disposed child takes the blame and burdens upon herself that triggers the eating disorder. This can happen even in the most civil divorces. A divorce represents a failed marriage, and the person with CNC will inevitably see herself as responsible for the failure – or as a failure for not being able to prevent it.

It is true that the majority of eating disorders begin during adolescence. What is unique about adolescence today? Teenagers live in a more anxious society. The person with an eating disorder takes on the role of caregiver and nurturer. She has to decide many things about her future at a much earlier age. Society's message is anxiety and fear and despair.

Parents are busy trying to accommodate their child's individuality. Given the psychological onus that society places on evaluating the self, parents are perhaps less inclined to make a defined stance on what direction to push their child. Thus the child feels she is sinking in quicksand at the very time she needs direction. She cannot find a platform from which to spring.

I believe that generally today's parents turn the responsibility for decisions – 'What would you like, dear?' – over to children too early. Fewer rules, less structure, less black and white. Perhaps parents are loath to appear directive of their child's potential because in contemporary society people are generally less sure of their environment and therefore their role in it. Maybe it is out of a misled 'respect' for the child with CNC, given that we are so afraid of harming her integrity as an individual, that we do not create enough structure for her when she needs it early in life.

'Anorexia is a disease
of the "economically advantaged."'

Eating disorders have often been said to be the province of middle or upper socioeconomic classes. That may generally be true, but it is also understandable. Today there is less physical stress in living in middle- and upper-class households, but in my observation more emotional stress and more anxiety that sensitive children are bound to absorb. Perhaps parents in these circumstances are more rushed and anxious in maintaining their lifestyles. This may result in more perceived stress, which children in turn translate as anxiety.

Perhaps a child's internal interpretation of her parents' achievements creates in her the expectation that she must live up to their 'standards,' even though this does not come from parental edicts. She has constructed these 'standards' herself. The middle- and upper-income child may shoulder more responsibility, not because her parents ask her to, but because she takes it upon herself to fulfill what she perceives as their high aspirations.

I believe that middle- or upper-income children have more choices than their lower-income counterparts. Their parents' lives are not as clearly cut-and-dried as other people's may be, and for sensitive children, the proliferation of choices and expectations, real or perceived, may be overwhelming. Lower-income children seem to intuit their limitations – or have them forced upon them – and harbor fewer illusions about their reality. For such a child, the platform to build her identity may not be complicated with the confusion of the parents' search for meaning and society's pressure of expectation. The existence of boundaries, whether desirable or not, at least provides a form of stability.

Perhaps, too, children in lower socioeconomic circumstances enjoy the benefits of a larger extended family. Grandparents, uncles, and aunts may share the chore of nurturing, and as I mentioned earlier, the more adults participate in a child's growth, the more likely the child will grasp objective reality.

Nevertheless, in my practice, I see eating disorders in all socioeconomic groups. I think it continues to be more prevalent in the upper and middle classes, but I know there is no clear 'class' line anymore.

'Anorexia is a psychosomatic disorder caused by a child's refusal to grow up into an adult.'

A common misinterpretation is that anorexics are struggling to remain childlike. As purported victims of the Peter Pan syndrome, they are thought to fear and loathe adulthood. But our case histories show again and again that the fear of growing up may be a consequence of the eating disorder, but it is not a cause.

Before manifesting the condition, these young people had extraordinary capability for self-direction and social responsibility. Depending on their age, they excelled in every area. Far from reneging on adult responsibility, they shouldered too much of it to adhere to society's extended values. They appeared compliant for fear of offending others. Their primary focus was always for the well-being of others rather than themselves.

But by being the 'caregiver' and 'parent' in their own minds, CNC victims have already tried to grow up before their time. They have taken on mature responsibilities long before they acquired the adult objectivity or reasoning to recognize their own limitations, and naturally they were not up to the task.

The world is large and daunting. CNC-predisposed children have tried to make it all right for everyone and they have failed miserably in their own eyes. It is not that they do not want to grow up, it is that they do not know how. They have had responsibility and failed at it. One young girl wrote to me, as so many others do, 'I don't want to die, but I don't know how to want to live.'

Saying that a child 'refuses to grow up' implies that she is reneging on her obligation. The fact is, she is an altruistic soul, the true caregiver who believes she has already tried to grow up and failed. Her perceived monumental failure overwhelms her with the realization that she has been unable to make the world a better place for everyone else.

In Günter Grass's classic novel *The Tin Drum*, the protagonist, Oskar, gets smaller and smaller and smaller inside himself because he has no sense of self. Just like the anorexic, he gains his sense of self vicariously by being a guardian angel to an adult. When the angel fails, he does not blame the adult for ignoring his instruction; he blames himself as the poor guidance counselor.

Children are also said to become anorexic because they do not want to become sexual beings. Sexuality implies not just maturity but pleasure. Just as the punishing Negative Mind will not allow its victims food, so will it deny them any other form of pleasure as well.

Sexual maturity is also synonymous with graduating to being normal. In their minds, anorexics believe they do not deserve that privilege because they have already 'tried' adulthood and failed. Avoiding sexual maturity (or any act of normalcy) is a way of relieving themselves of the guilt they experience for failing to help the world. It is not fear of sex per se, but rather fear of further failure at responsibility and the guilt that new failures would engender. Menstruation, an indication of physiological normalcy, is not a welcome rite of passage for these victims.

The individual in the acute grip of an eating disorder is therefore asexual. I have received many letters from women who have managed to marry and even have children while wrestling with an eating disorder. They are maintaining their condition and their relapses suggest that while they have subdued the inner turmoil temporarily, they are not truly inhabiting their sexual selves.

'Anorexia is an unconscious attention-getting device, a cry for help.'

Anorexics are highly embarrassed at being noticed. They typically wear baggy clothing to disguise their weight loss.

There is, however, a contradiction here. Victims of CNC yearn for someone to understand them, but their Negative Mind will not allow them to ask for help, and they do not feel they deserve it anyway. If weight loss is the unconscious cry for attention, why don't victims stop losing weight once parents and other loved ones try to intervene, often with valiant efforts? It is because their unconscious motive is to die, not to get attention. If there were a way to die of anorexia without losing weight – a visible sign – they would do it.

My patients tell me, 'I have to die in a way that won't hurt people.' It's not that they want to die; it's that they feel they can no longer exist because they are failures in their own minds.

'People with eating disorders are selfish.
They just need to get on with their lives
and stop ruining everyone else's!'

As I hope I've made abundantly clear, eating disorder victims are the antithesis of selfish. Indeed, they are selfless to the highest degree. Unfortunately, the Negative Mind constantly accuses them of self-indulgence when they want merely to exist in the world, so any allegation of selfishness from external sources such as family or medical professionals simply reinforces and strengthens the Negative Mind's hand.

The mother of three children in England contacted me about her fifteen-year-old daughter who was dying of anorexia. Gabrielle had had the illness for a year and a half, and during that time had been hospitalized eight times. 'The doctors told her she was a spoiled brat,' this distraught mother complained to me. 'They said, "All Gabby needs is a good kick in the bottom." '

This response to an eating disorder reminds me of how people used to regard depression. We once believed that depressed people could just 'snap out of it' if they tried hard enough. And somehow we still are of the opinion that if victims of eating disorders cared enough (about their parents' or other loved ones' anguish?), they could will themselves to get better. Nothing could be further from the truth. Indeed, the problems began because these 'old souls' cared too much and they need help to find a way out of the miasma that traps them.

'Anorexia is a tool for control.'

The misconception is that by denying themselves food in the face of the vigorous encouragement to eat, anorexics are trying to control their world against others. Rather than control others, I believe victims are trying to control the remaining bit of their Actual Mind against the Negative Mind. They are losing power because the Negative Mind bullies the Actual Mind into submission.

If we ignore the existence or misunderstand the role of the Negative Mind, it can only follow that we will misconstrue whom the child is trying to control. The Actual Mind always takes the rap for the Negative Mind, since the latter is so carefully hidden from our view. Consequently, the child will understandably be mislabeled as controlling.

As the Negative Mind gains in strength, it creates internal chaos.

'On the outside, I still look like I am in control and so together, but on the inside I have nothing.'

'I have been in turmoil. I'm so completely without direction.'

'I feel myself completely shattered and I'm so afraid.'

'Emotions control my food. The life that I can't control, controls my food.'

'There is always that fear of criticism, ridicule, being scolded, losing a job, losing a friend, or failing. I'm always afraid when asked to do a job, or left with the decision of what to make for dinner that I'll do it wrong and thus be rejected.'

Controlling behaviors can be seen as a child's attempt to create a structure for herself. Indeed, at the clinic I give a mug and plate with an individual design to each patient who comes to us. This seems like a small gesture, but it's an important one. The unique mug and plate are hers alone – part of the interim structure she so desperately needs. Until that point, she is searching for any level of structure in her habits, food, and being.

The anorexic's habit of preparing food for others while refusing to eat it herself is commonly misinterpreted as a need to control her environment. Again, understanding the motivation behind the actions is useful.

This behavior demonstrates the Negative Mind's domination of the Actual Mind. Victims stand near food; they spend time focusing on it because they are desperate to be allowed it. They consciously deny themselves but subconsciously desire food because they are physiologically starving. So as they eat vicariously by preparing food for others, they also demonstrate their own unworthiness to be normal human beings. In fact, many children will adulterate their food with hot sauce, vinegar, or even chlorine cleanser to make it unfit for human consumption and only worthy of them, the unworthy.

According to DSM-IV, in the anorexic, 'weight loss is viewed as an impressive achievement and a sign of extraordinary self-discipline, whereas weight gain is perceived as an unacceptable failure of self-control.'

For normal dieters, weight loss may be considered a bona fide achievement, but for those with eating disorders, weight loss is the antithesis of achievement, despite what the victims consciously believe. Weight loss is an unconscious acceptance of failure, an acknowledgment or resignation that the anorexic is giving up the right to live. The only 'impressive achievement' is that she has proven to herself that she is indeed unworthy of life. She is controlling herself to death.

The stereotype is that these children want to control everything, but in fact they want to serve everyone and ensure the well-being of the planet. They see themselves as 'trouble-shooters' and are ever on the alert for problems to solve.

It is contradictory to be both pliable, as a common stereotype goes, and also controlling, as another common stereotype goes. It is contradictory to be both a good caregiver and listener – which implies an adult sensibility – AND someone who does not want to take responsibility for her controlling actions.

'Anorexics are to blame for their situation.
They're doing it to get back at others.'

Given that the dynamics of an eating disorder occur at an unconscious level and are as perplexing and complicating for its victims as they are for their families, the view that anorexics are intentionally guilty of hurting their beloved parents just adds to the nightmare of their existence.

When unwitting practitioners blame parents for their children's anorexia by insisting that anorexia results from favoritism, abuse, or some other symptom of family dysfunction, they often create animosity among parents toward their children, and the victims end up the losers. After such finger-pointing, parents often ask victims, 'Why have you done this to us? How could you continue to be so cruel?'

The victim will cope more easily if a therapist tries to teach her with compassion and intelligence that everyone is imperfect. And so it is healthier for all involved to translate 'blame' into 'limitations.' The individual stops hunting for wrongdoers.

The very word 'victim' implies helplessness at the

hands of another. In this case, the victimization is neither by the inadvertent ignorance and unawareness of society nor of any given individual. Eating disorders are an exceedingly negative response to a misinterpretation of one's role in the world. The victimization occurs in the negative construct the patient has unwittingly built against herself. She becomes helpless against the onslaught of the Negative Mind within her.

'Sufferers need to hold on to their condition as a crutch.'

I have often heard it described that victims of eating disorders are in some perverse way clinging to the crutch of their illness. It is more accurate to say that they are dominated and enslaved by it. They want to let go of it, but they have nothing to replace it with. As Carrie wrote in her journal, 'One reason I've held on to anorexia for so long is probably because every time I feel a bit stronger or happier, I worry and immediately retreat. It's because I feel guilty for feeling good. . . .'

Ultimately, victims are terrified to relinquish the condition because they know no other way of being. For example, Sharon wrote to me, 'I basically have resolved to accept my life as an eating disorder. It's the only thing I've ever been able to capture and call my own and the only thing no one has ever been able to take away from me.'

Therefore to give up the condition is to cease to exist – even worse than death. Anorexia becomes a negative structure – 'Who am I if not my illness?' – and an all-pervasive way of being.

'The longer you have anorexia,
the harder it is to cure.'

On occasion, this may be true because the condition has been confirmed repeatedly, possibly due to so many futile hospitalizations. With each failed program, the Negative Mind reconfirms itself and becomes more pernicious. Similarly, the longer the Actual Mind has learned to exist marginally and the longer it feels the negative comfort of that existence, the more difficult an eating disorder is to cure.

However, I have also found that it is just as difficult to cure anorexia in people who have had it for a short time as it is to cure those who have been ill for years. Once the Negative Mind has enough control to manifest an eating disorder, healing appears to depend more on the basic personality of the individual than on the duration of the eating disorder manifestation.

'Anorexia can't be cured; it can only be
managed. You'll live with it and die from it.'

Eating disorders are a silent epidemic. Anorexics have no constituency. They cannot rise up en masse to say, 'We need help.' You do not see them banding together to form research societies and associations, although others have formed these organizations on their behalf. Nevertheless, these conditions are completely reversible, though the cure requires a total re-nurturing of the afflicted individual.

However, to 'manage anorexia' is merely to maintain the condition's status. To maintain it is to invite recidivism. In order to correct the eating disorder symptom, the CNC must be addressed and reversed. This reversal requires patience, complete understanding, and as much time as each individual needs.

How can we integrate this concept into society as it exists today? How, given the vast tragedy we see before us, can we not?

4

The Acute Patient: Held Hostage
by the 'Forever' Intruder

Confirmed Negativity Condition is not cyclical; it progresses along an intensifying continuum. However, in its early stages, it can be reversed with relatively less difficulty than when it becomes more deeply entrenched. An individual whose thoughts are dominated by subjectivity and negativity 25 percent of the time, for instance, is capable of springing back to normal thinking if she encounters a positive intervention, even if that intervention is fortuitous. If this occurs again and again, she can regain a normal course in life.

At fourteen, Danielle was well on her way toward anorexia. Measuring five foot eight, she weighed one hundred pounds, and had remained in that condition for a year. But in high school, she encountered a group of new friends who were so supportive of her and so accepting that they seemed to erase the negativity that was plaguing her. 'I truly believed they were my family when I wasn't anchored by family,' she told me as she described her brush with eating disorders so many years ago.

Outpatient psychotherapeutic intervention can also be helpful during the early stages, as long as those at home are able to participate in a loving situation. (See Chapters 7 and 8.)

When accidental interventions do not occur, or if loved ones have not recognized the signs of the encroaching CNC and did not involve professional caregivers, the Negative Mind becomes more pronounced and reinforced. It fills its victim's mind with anxiety, and thoughts of unworthiness, self-deprecation, and doom. Subjectivity begins to reign, particularly if set off by triggers, which feel the negativity. Inwardly, life turns dark as the victim slides toward the confusion of emotional childhood and then the helplessness of infancy, while outwardly she frets about food and weight and exercise. She appears indecisive and withdrawing. Eventually she stops eating. Soon the condition worsens to the point of acuteness.

THE PHYSIOLOGY OF
THE ACUTE PATIENT

One might think that someone with an acute eating disorder will always resemble a famine victim – skeletal body, ribs, pelvis, and spine nearly protruding through translucent skin; abdomen bloated; eyes sunken; hair sparse; spirit broken.

While this may describe many acute patients, it certainly does not portray all of them. Bulimic patients and even some anorexics may pass for low 'normal' in weight and therefore not be so easily recognized as having a problem (see Chapter 7 for more warning signs). Nevertheless, they may be as seriously ill as those patients who weigh forty-seven pounds and appear at the brink of death.

'I was hospitalized with atrial fibrillation and severe electrolyte imbalance plus internal bleeding,' wrote one woman. 'My daughter is severely osteoporotic and she hasn't even gone into puberty yet,' wrote another. These are only a few of the physiological effects of acute eating disorders.

Indeed, an acute patient may experience the breakdown of body organs. She is at high risk for heart attack from electrolyte imbalance, for instance. And though low potassium levels are not always necessarily a marker, frequently they can indicate that a patient is in danger of dying.

Other physical indicators of acute eating disorders can include:

- bradycardia (low heart rate) and irregular heartbeat
- edema (tissue swelling from water retention) due to electrolyte imbalances
- potential kidney failure
- potential liver failure
- osteoporosis
- extreme fluctuations in blood pressure
- in bulimic patients, esophageal scarring and dental decay from excessive vomiting
- intestinal rupture from excessive use of laxatives
- insomnia

In its desperation for nutrition, the body begins to cannibalize itself. First the protective fat cushions around the heart and kidneys disappear, resulting in more potential for damage. Then, the protein structure of the muscles and internal organs is mobilized for nutrition (just as the calcium is taken from the bones). The body eventually deteriorates and wastes away.

Edema gives the victim the false impression that she is

gaining weight. Upon noticing the swelling, a victim often becomes frightened that she is gaining weight and further restricts her intake of food, thereby exacerbating the bloating and starvation in a vicious cycle.

Skin becomes dry and raw because the body lacks necessary oils. Feet can become bloodied from hours of intense exercise. Hair thins, breaks, and falls out. Nails split. In extreme cases, a soft downy growth of hair called lanugo appears all over the skin, including the face, in the body's desperate attempt to maintain warmth in the absence of protective layers of fat.

One of the first physiological markers of illness in adolescent and adult females is amenorrhea. The body stops menstruation as a way to conserve vital resources such as iron and protein. When menstruation returns, this is a valuable indication of the body's healing.

In the acute stage of anorexia, victims cannot concentrate; their eyes dart furtively, and they are usually incapable of any sustained eye contact. They are afraid of being 'read' and recognized. Nevertheless, the intellect is the last to go. Victims will often accomplish extraordinary academic feats while on the verge of physical collapse.

Parents and professionals should take care not to use this information to threaten or scare their children or patients. Telling someone she 'looks like a concentration camp victim' or that he 'could drop dead if he doesn't stop' is counterproductive. The victim already feels like a 'walking freak' and further blame-inducing language will only exacerbate her already overwhelming sense of guilt or unworthiness.

Any of these signs and symptoms require professional medical evaluation and treatment. It is essential to realize that physical appearance is not a valid indicator of the severity of an eating disorder. If you suspect a loved one has an eating disorder, make sure that person sees a medical doctor immediately.

THE PSYCHOLOGY OF
THE ACUTE PATIENT

How can anyone allow herself to fall into such a dreadful medical condition? It has been my experience that the origin of this physiological deterioration is the CNC victim succumbing to the Negative Mind. Edna, one of my correspondents, described the power of the Negative Mind in a poem she sent me:

My Mind Is a Cannibal
My mind is a cannibal,
reveling in vicious pleasure,
watching my body devour itself.
The always truthful looking-glass
has agreed to a bribe, offered by the inner-eye,
and distortion assures me that my skeleton-like state
is ravishing . . . that I am the envy of all.
Pernicious pain makes a sculpture out of me,
a ghastly creation,
which no audience would ever pay to see,
except for me.
Almost consciously,
I permit coercion to comfort me
with an insidiously vile routine . . .
leaving my emotions famished.
My bones have dried like winter's twigs.
My concave curves have draped themselves loosely in
    skin.

Like a star burning bright on the threshold of death,
I collapse into myself.
All day is night, and night . . . eternal blackness.
I die. I swallow death.
I consume it with my voracious appetite.
It eats me. It digests every part of me
(or at least all that is left).
I must be happy with death.
It loves me . . . passionately. It sings to me. Lullabies.
I will sleep soundly, safely in the moist darkness of its
   stomach. . . .

The Negative Mind is an intruder whom the acute
eating disorder patient feels she has inadvertently invited
upon herself. As one patient wrote to me, 'I don't think
there was an exact date. It felt like anorexia had sneaked
up behind me and inserted itself slowly inside me without
me really noticing it.'

It is as if she is being held hostage with a gun to her
head. Though (and perhaps because) the threats are
internal, they inspire more fear than if they existed in the
'real' world. Thus, society is generally unable to recognize and identify the enemy in the same way that the
victim does.

Science fiction has no edge over what the Negative
Mind has created to frighten its acute victim to death.
Its hold on her psyche becomes all-enveloping and all-
involving. When family or friends in all innocence
attempt to extend help, the Negative Mind necessarily
instructs the weaker Actual Mind to reject it since the
sufferer does not deserve it. To her, the mind game is very
real and terrifying. Often what seems to the victim to be
a real voice mocks, leers, threatens, and instructs her to
self-destruct.

One of my patients, Mariah, recorded the civil war inside her head as she battled anorexia and bulimia. She neither censored the voice nor could explain her actions, but felt absolutely compelled to obey the Negative Mind:

6:00 a.m. Get up you fuckhead, get up. You'll be late if you don't and you know you're not leaving till it's done [exercising].

6:45 a.m. Fifteen more minutes. Come on you fat pig. You're **tired???** You can't be, I won't let you. If you don't go the full hour you're not eating anything today.

8:00 a.m. Get off the bus now, you have time to walk the extra five blocks and not be late. You'll burn off the milk you had in your coffee this morning.

12:00 p.m. ['Mariah, do you want to have lunch with us?'] Fuck, now what? Think bitch **think!** Just say no ('I can't, I've already said no too many times'). Go, then, but you better get rid of everything you eat.

12:30 p.m. ('Tuna sandwich, please.') Tuna! Tuna!!! **You fucking fat bitch.** Don't you know they use tons of real mayo? You can't bring up every last bit of sauce. I keep saying only solid foods. No sauce. No combination of foods or shit like that. That way you know exactly what to look for when you throw up.

Laxatives! You have to get them before you go back to work. Three big boxes. ('I have to go out tonight and they'll be working by then.') Listen, bitch, you fucked up by asking for tuna. Besides, no one cares if you show up or not.

4:00 p.m. The laxatives won't be working for another hour or so, the shit is probably stored quite nicely on your ass already. You'll have to stay a half hour extra at the gym.

6:00 p.m. ('Oh shit. I'm coming home late again – she'll kill me – damn, she's going to be furious.') You deserve it though, you selfish bitch – going to the gym behind her back.

7:30 p.m. You promised yesterday was going to be the last time. You fucking bitch – you are shit and you always will be shit. They're all right about you. How can you live with yourself? You're dishonest and selfish. You never do anything right and you are a **fat! fat! fat!!!!** useless poor excuse for a human being Bitch. I hate you bitch I **hate** you. Look at yourself in the mirror and tell me I'm lying. You can't because you see what I do. You lost only 2 pounds today and it's not good enough!

Now hurry up and get rid of it. I don't care if you have to stick your whole fucking arm down your throat – you're going to get rid of it. I don't give a shit if you're bleeding. Your whole insides can come up and **you still won't stop.**

The Negative Mind speaks to its victim in a vile, degrading way while the victim herself is generally possessed of a great dignity and would not express herself in such a manner.

By the time people have become acutely ill, the Negative Mind is so real that most can actually conjure up a physical description of 'it.' My daughter Kirsten described 'it' as a 'beast' in one of her poems:

Glancing Toward Defeat
External beauty defies itself with the markings of the
    beast,
Smiles like the quick drop of sharpened knives
Scathing saws glistening upon other sorrows

Tearing apart lips
Wrenching out eyes
– leave them in bits

Internal beauty mistakeningly
Collapses when shadowed by the beast
An onlooker watching through mirrors,
The slow death of the dying
– their final feast

A marching hand in hand,
Beating tears
– label them 'pathetic'
I know, I know
let them go quietly, one slip gains a remark
to encourage further crying, if only it didn't
hurt while crying inside.

Another way the victim can reveal the torment in her
mind is through pictorial representations. We encourage
the patients at the clinic to make paintings of their
tormentors. Often many have done so even before
coming into care.

The artwork is a nonverbal way of soliciting the
alliance of the outside world in the victim's struggle.
One eight-year-old, for instance, would slip her drawings into her father's briefcase as a way to communicate
her anguish to him. Although horrified by them, unfortunately he did not know what to make of them.

Though there are many variations on the theme, the
acute patient's artwork often shows the sufferer's lack of
power. Victims are being controlled by a dark, 'evil'
demon or monster who is intent on torturing its victim
internally, slowly.

Often these artworks show red, fanning flames of what one would suppose is a 'Hell,' and some shadowy form in black. Though I treat my patients with therapy based on a humanistic psychological premise, I am scarcely surprised that some parents might think that their children are 'possessed.' They are not. This mindset and its resultant behavior become more understandable in the context of recovery. Other depictions show the eating disorder sufferer:

- in cages or jails surrounded by words of negativity such as 'loser,' 'failure,' 'fat pig,' 'guilt,' 'responsible.'
- swimming in an ocean with no hope of shore; treading water to an inevitable end.
- down a deep well with sides of slippery moss that renders scaling it impossible, yet the victim can see the light at the top.
- standing against a brick wall that covers the page with no means of climbing it. (The victim appears minuscule.)
- as a child standing on a scale with the world held on his or her shoulders.

One of my daughter Nicole's drawings, created before I was able to recognize its meaning, was of twins. One held her eyes to the future and had a red rose of life's blood at her feet (where it was elusively available) and a cross on her neck representing hope. The other looked slightly downward and dejected; she was thinner than her counterpart and held the black rose of hopelessness and despair. (This illustration appears in the inset.)

Three-year-old Zev always refers to the Negative Mind as 'the man under his hair.' That was his usual answer to his mother and me when we asked him why he would not eat. 'The man won't let me. He will be angry,' he would explain.

'Darling, you are safe now,' I would assure him. 'The man under your hair can't hurt you anymore. I'm holding you very tightly.'

'Yes, Peggy, you are holding me, but he is still hurting me.'

'How can he hurt you, darling? See, you are in my arms.'

'Peggy, he is angry that you are holding me, so he is playing drums loudly in my head so I can't hear the nice things you are saying to me.'

When anorexia is in its acute stage, the Negative Mind allows the victim no pleasure. When I first met Zev, he was forbidden by it from accepting or opening presents. Everyone else deserved them, but not him. He would put his hands behind his back if anyone would extend something in his direction. His eyes became very dark, intense, and fearful.

If he agreed to eat anything, it could not be called 'food' and it could not make him grow because he was not permitted to grow. Growing would mean extension of life.

Once when asked what he wanted to be when he grew up, this three-year-old answered very quietly and thoughtfully, 'I am not going to grow up. I am going to be dead before these pants are too short.' Incredulous, we assured him he would grow when he was supposed to. He started to cry and said, 'No, I'm not. The man told me I wouldn't be allowed to, and I'm scared of the man. He is always mean to me.'

This child never played with other children. He always stood aside and observed. His development, however, was extraordinary. He would memorize pages of the telephone book for amusement. He loved sports and could act out an entire baseball game, playing each position in turn as the ball went around the 'field.' He had spent a year and a half undergoing medical testing (before we had been contacted) which failed to turn up any organic reason to explain his refusal to eat.

In the acute phase of an eating disorder, victims have no road map for direction. They feel as if they are in a complex maze running against time, as surely they are. Sometimes their mental pain is so intense and so powerful that they will wound themselves to distract themselves from it.

Some sufferers mutilate themselves, scraping, scratching, or cutting their skin. This is an attempt to escape from the relentless hounding of the negative; the physical pain of the mutilation temporarily blots out the internal voices.

When Mariah was acute, she would scald herself in the shower because her Negative Mind told her she was not allowed to temper the hot water with cold. She was told to harm herself constantly and in the early stage of recovery, when she had around-the-clock care, she held on to people all through the night with the TV and radio on in order to tune out the Negative Mind urging her toward destruction.

Another victim wrote in her journal, 'I cut my arms and punched my legs up too. I don't regret doing it. I deserved every bit of it. I am a bad person and deserve to die.'

Victims have said that on occasion, their wounds are mistaken for suicide attempts. Though on many occasions victims found it difficult to conceive of living under the merciless regime of the Negative Mind and might have attempted suicide, at other times marking or cutting was an added form of self-punishment.

The reign of terror effected by the Negative Mind creates a conspiracy of silence in the victim which in fact unites all victims of CNC. One sufferer wrote and asked me, 'How is it that you know the secret that we are not allowed to tell?'

Eating disorder victims are desperate for help and at the same time afraid and guilty for asking for it. Carissa wrote to me, 'Please let me come to you, even if I sleep in a doorway. I won't take up much room. I'm afraid HE will make me kill myself if you don't let me come soon. I know you understand.'

Others have written, 'I feel overcome by guilt for having received your attention,' and 'How can you choose me? I am so unworthy. Should not some more deserving soul have my bed?' Even in their misery and minuscule hope for a life worth living, they are more caring of another in the same plight.

BIZARRE BEHAVIOR

As the victim becomes more entrenched in her condition, she becomes increasingly oblivious to the effect of her behavior on society. Bizarre behavior serves to isolate her both in its commanding focus of the Negative Mind and its power to alienate family and friends.

Victims experience agitated sleep both because of their physical imbalances and their constant need to forage for food, whether or not they actually eat it. For six months, my daughter Nikki slept no more than an hour and a half each night. The intense drive to find and then deny food will send the person back and forth from the refrigerator endlessly at the expense of rest.

Patients have hurled verbal abuse at me. They tell me repeatedly how much they hate me. They have spit food in my face, flung dishes at me, hit me, refused to get out of bed, and rebuffed interactions with others.

In public, it is not unusual for my patients to try to embarrass those around them. They may scream at the top of their lungs, sit down in puddles, or smear cold cream on their faces before going out in public. Patients often dress in bizarre ways, trying identities on for size. Boys might dress up in women's clothing.

In private, I have witnessed and parents have often-times reported to me exceedingly disturbing behavior: patients smearing themselves with excrement, eating garbage out of garbage cans, eating their own vomit. One patient consumed pounds of raw sausage. Another, a bulimic, wrote to me that she eats and then vomits two hundred pounds of food a day. The self-mutilation mentioned earlier is perhaps the most distressing to others.

It is important to understand that this antisocial behavior is intended to prove to the victims and others that they are worthy of alienation. They seek rejection at all costs in order to reconfirm their own sense of worth-lessness. Simultaneously, they are terribly frightened by this Negative Mind they do not understand, and embarrassed and ashamed by the negative behavior they can neither explain nor discontinue.

TRANCES

About 25 percent of people with eating disorders will go into trances when in the acute stage. A trance indicates that the victim is in the most extreme psychological state of the illness. The Negative Mind virtually overwhelms the Actual Mind. The victim has tuned out external reality and assumes a dissociative state – she is temporarily oblivious to reality.

The warning signs of an impending trance can include:

- the voice of the patient diminishing to a whisper.
- fear entering the voice or showing evidence of 'flat affect' with no modulation.
- the body beginning to immobilize. The victim may curl up in bed in a fetal position out of fear, or freeze seated in a chair.
- the person making no eye contact and being obviously preoccupied with what is happening in her mind.
- the person not answering directly and/or being slow to answer.

Trances are a consequence of the Negative Mind shutting out any possible optimism or positivity from the Actual Mind or from the external voice of loved ones. When in a trance, the anorexic person is almost completely focused on and at the mercy of the Negative Mind.

A person in a trance stares straight ahead, not even blinking or moving her eyelashes; she is open-eyed but unseeing. The bridge of the nose often becomes pinched and slightly protruded, perhaps indicating overwhelming concentration. The teeth may become clenched, and breathing turns short and rapid. It appears that the victim is listening intently to something internal; she is hearing the negative voices in her head which can take the form of loud commands against her.

Most often, at the clinic, patients go into trances during the first three months of treatment when the Negative Mind feels trapped, cornered with no back door. He (for most of my patients call it a 'he') can no longer order an external manifestation such as making the victim overexercise or vomit. He therefore doubles his efforts internally. The Negative Mind at this stage will make statements such as:

'Don't listen to them; they're lying to you.'
'They're trying to make you fat.'
'You're a selfish, ugly pig who is taking up a clinic bed that somebody else deserves more.'
'You're not sick.'
'I'm going to make you pay by making your family suffer. Your father is going to die in a plane crash because you told them you needed help.'
'Your mother is going to have a heart attack because you told them you liked that sandwich.'
'Nobody loves you. Who could?'

The patient might also hear loud clanging, music, pounding drumbeats, anything to drown out the positivity coming from the caregiver.

The victim in a trance is terrified. At this stage, she thinks that anorexia is stronger than her caregivers because that is what the Negative Mind repeatedly tells her. (For more on trances, see Chapter 5.)

TRICKS

In the person with an acute eating disorder, the Negative Mind is skilled at maintaining its status. The Negative

Mind tries to make the victim's behavior seem reasonable to cloak its real intention and convince the external world that the victim is behaving as any normal person would.

At our clinic, acute patients present our caregivers with a great variety of 'tricks.' A patient may say, for instance:

> 'I can't eat this kind of bread because it bothers my gums.'
> 'I'm diabetic, so I can't have sugar.'
> 'I'm lactose-intolerant, so I can't have milk.'
> 'I'm hypoglycemic, so I can't have fat.'

Some patients might claim to be vegetarian or vegan, hiding behind humanitarianism. Yet often these individuals tuck into steaks and hamburgers once they get better.

Patients feign a love for plain food because they are afraid that salt will make them retain fluid or that spices will have calories in them. Others deliberately overcook their food not only to make it less enjoyable but also to boil the nutrition right out of it. Some hide food in dishes, clothing, paper towels or napkins, or coat the sides of the bowl with it so it will appear to have been eaten. Others dilute juice with water.

Even when the scales are taken away, many sufferers will find ways of charting their progress toward nothingness, using measuring tapes, shoelaces, belts, or clothing. If mirrors are removed so that the victim cannot be obsessive about her appearance, she might use windows, the blank television screen, or the oven door to study her reflection.

Weigh-ins at the doctor's office can also pose

challenges. Some victims drink great quantities of water or refuse to go to the bathroom before weighing sessions. Others might weigh down their clothes with coins or rocks, or wear many layers of heavy clothing to foil the scale.

Some acutely ill victims pretend to be constipated in order to trick the physician into prescribing laxatives.

I have also seen patients go to great lengths to burn off extra calories. They may fidget endlessly. Some victims invent an incessant stream of errands that require constant motion. Others stand for long periods of time because they suppose this will burn more calories than sitting. An acute patient may refuse to wear an overcoat in winter, believing she will burn off more calories trying to stay warm. Others exercise while showering or bathing. One patient said she needed privacy; in reality, she was exercising inside her closet.

Some patients will tell me, 'I can't sleep with the light on.' They want to exercise under the sheets undetected. Or they will say on a warm summer's day, 'Turn off the fans, I'm too cold.' They believe that they can sweat the calories away.

Offers to do housework, once a sign of the person's caringness and willingness to help, can now be construed as an effort to burn off calories.

After having fallen victim to one of these ruses, we might abashedly declare, 'Hey, I just got snowed.' Nevertheless, we cannot accuse the victim of lying or manipulating us when perpetrating these self-defeating behaviors. Beyond lying to herself, she is dancing to the tune of the Negative Mind.

SMALL WRITING

People in the throes of an eating disorder might leave other clues, awaiting translation by those aware enough to detect them. Some, but not all, sufferers will change their style of handwriting; as CNC is confirmed and the eating disorder progresses, their words become smaller and smaller, almost as though they were trying to disappear altogether.

Every day at the clinic we receive dozens of letters crammed with handwriting so tiny it can require a magnifying glass to decipher. These letters might even include an apology along the lines of, 'Please forgive the size of my writing; I didn't want it to take up space.' What more eloquent statement of a sufferer's sense of non-self, of subservience to others?

As patients at our clinic work through the first two stages of therapy and move into the third (see Chapter 6), their identity, their evolving sense of self, begins to manifest even in the size of their writing, which expands and opens. This coincides with their availability to others, their openness and clarity of thought. As they grow in allowing themselves into the real world, their writing quite noticeably changes from dots of illegibility to normal-size words. They are beginning to free themselves of the warped perspective that has hounded them into subhumanism.

If we can appreciate the handwriting as an analogy of smallness – infancy – it will help us understand why the victim feels unable to cope with any responsibility, even, ultimately, the caring for herself.

The risk of suicide is twofold in the acute patient. On the one hand, the Negative Mind may have given the victim constant instructions to hurt and destroy herself because of her unworthiness. Julie wrote in her letters to me, for instance, 'It makes me want to cut myself all the more, every disgraceful, despicable, hideous second I live, every unforgivable, shameful, evil time I eat.' And later, 'No pure, kind mind can comprehend one as evil as I. And so, is it not my responsibility, my most important obligation, the only thing I have to offer, to so rightly die, to finally spare you?' The strength of the Actual Mind will determine how well a victim can fight off these directives.

Usually when a patient comes to the acute stage she is also exhausted with the efforts of holding at bay the Negative Mind. Think of a deer separated from the herd, chased by a pack of wolves. Eventually he loses hope of a way out and gives up. Risk of suicide is high with acute patients because they are so weary of fighting.

As one young woman wrote to me, 'I'm 24 years old and have had an eating disorder for 8 years. I've been in and out of the hospital for this a dozen times. . . . It's not that I don't want to get better, I do. It's just that I have tried so many things and it just seems hopeless. . . . Suicide is looking better and better every day. I'm not sure what else to do.'

And another one wrote, 'Lately I've decided not to fight it anymore. I've dropped 13 pounds in as many days. . . . I'm writing my will and am readying my personal affairs. I just can't fight it anymore. This isn't a cry for help because it's too late for me.'

We can also look at the condition itself as an unconscious form of slow suicide. An eating disorder is a relinquishing of the right to live cloaked by the Negative Mind in an irrational logic.

SOCIAL WITHDRAWAL

Social interaction depends on communicating on many levels. Some victims seem to communicate quite well, but in reality, they have become wonderful actors. They pretend that they are happy and present a front of normalcy when they are hiding 'terrible secrets' inside. 'I play-act my entire day until I am home and can lapse back into the behavior that I've known for so long as me,' one woman wrote to me.

'I have been able to keep my behavior hidden from my family, which, in the end, only makes the situation that much more agonizing,' another one wrote. 'My guilt is intolerable. . . . I do my best to appear well. I have become too good an actress, but I know it cannot last.'

For the most part, acute patients can no longer hide the intensity of their preoccupation with food or their lack of self-image. Most often, they isolate themselves from anyone who does not understand their predicament including friends, family members, and society in general. 'For the longest time, I didn't care if anyone knew about my problem,' one woman wrote. 'In fact, I was even able to help a few people because of my openness and knowledge about it. But recently, I've lapsed back into hiding.'

Patients with eating disorders know they cannot be normal, and as their condition progresses, they become more lonely and separated from their support systems. One young woman wrote, 'I feel as though I am not a very pleasant person to be around. I am ashamed of who

I am and what I have become! Ugly, fat, selfish, guilty, and an unfriendly personality. *Unlovable.* An overall *misfit.*'

A thirty-eight-year-old woman battling anorexia for twenty-six years wrote, 'The past 13 years have been my worst. I have no friends. (I have never experienced a close personal relationship with another human being outside my family.) I reside with my parents in their home, and essentially exist in a surreal state of apathetic anonymity.'

Their habits become abnormal including the excessive hours devoted to exercise and food preparation, the odd mealtimes, and the frequent trips to stores for laxatives and/or diuretics. The whole focus of their lives becomes the illness.

Moreover, the more friends and supporters victims have, the more likely they are to be detected. The Negative Mind will not allow that. Detection goes against its instruction. It demands isolation to protect its secret. A recovered young boy wrote, 'I was withdrawn and isolated from my family and society; I couldn't trust people and was terrified of life and people. I felt completely unworthy of love and friendship because I was a failure as a person and could never be good enough or live up to the unrealistically high expectations I placed on myself and that I perceived were placed on me by others.'

'This whole thing has been so hard for my friends to observe that I have pushed them all away,' another young person wrote. 'My family does not understand what is happening to me and they do not know how or what to do to help me. I have alienated everyone around me. Therefore, I am all alone and going crazy.'

And an acute patient in the early stages of recovery at

our clinic wrote in her journal, 'My family came up to see me a few times over the weekend. I don't like seeing them at all. I wish everybody, my family, friends, and everybody else that knows me would just leave me alone. Let me live the way the ANOREXIA has driven me, towards HELL!'

A distraught father wrote, 'Caroline is dying now as she said she had planned to do all along. I live in Miami and Caroline lives somewhere in Colorado. I don't have her address or phone number. She had been living with a man but she got so bad she had to move out. . . . Her boyfriend doesn't even know where she lives now.'

If acutely ill victims do find 'friends,' they often come from therapy groups. Misery loves company. These friends often compare notes with one another. Commiseration is an important concept. This is not a situation in which girlfriends get together to talk about boyfriends or compare prom dresses.

Alexandra had been in eating disorder programs and in hospitals for five years and had amassed seventeen like-minded friends. Immediately before her arrival at our clinic, the entire group had conspired to conceal themselves in the attic of one of their homes so they could all waste away together. Fortunately, Alexandra dropped clues that enabled her parents to intervene.

In the acute stage, victims become asexual beings for biological and psychological reasons. The same biochemical imbalance that halts menstruation also impacts sex drive. By the same token, the Negative Mind shuns any close relationship because it might provide a helpmate. Intimacy with parents and loved ones is the first to go. Moreover, victims feel disgusted by their bodies and are not allowed to give themselves the pleasure of an intimate relationship.

Victims stay in school until they collapse, but they do not participate in social life there. They use studying as an isolating strategy. Recall the young girl whose journal I quoted in Chapter 3. She ran track before and after school and did homework during her lunch break and studied until 2 a.m. In her quest for 'perfection,' what time did she leave herself for socializing with such a relentless schedule?

Finally, unlike cancer or AIDS patients, acute victims do not have a constituency of support precisely due to the social isolation their condition engenders.

FEEDING THE BODY BUT NOT THE SOUL

The feeding phases of existing traditional intervention methods can provide relief for the moment. Patients are temporarily physically healthier. Their weight gain has assuaged their parents' anxiety, as well as their body's physical pains. But the internal mental pain never ceases and with feeding, it can become intensified because the Negative Mind insists on weight loss.

One young man wrote to me about his dilemma. 'I have been struggling with anorexia for 4 years. I am 16 years old. I have been hospitalized 8 times in the last twenty months. It is just so hard because I have gained 43 pounds in one year, but the program that I'm in is doing nothing for all the terrible things that go on inside of me – what I call "The Angels and The Devils" inside. . . . I just can't talk to my doctor. I feel he doesn't have a clue what I'm going through. Everything is centered around weight gain and I never get a chance to talk about what's really wrong with me.'

When the origin of the condition, the CNC, is not

corrected, feeding programs will fail and the disorder will persist. In Part II, we will look at how one can effectively address CNC and the Negative Mind so that these sensitive and giving, yet afflicted, individuals are no longer held hostage to this insidious condition.

PART II

Addressing
the
Negative Mind

5

Reversing the Negative Mind

The Negative Mind is nasty and uncouth and is the antithesis of the gentle nature of the Actual Mind. Alarming in the shocking, base language it uses, it holds the patient in helpless horror at its effectiveness in alienating others.

Imagine that we are engaged in the highest level chess game with this parasitic mindset. The Negative Mind will use every trick, every gambit to gain the advantage and destroy its victim, prompting her to starve or otherwise harm herself, to undermine treatment, to shun all help and affection, to hurt and drive away loved ones with offensive and bizarre behavior. It serves to be two moves ahead of the Negative Mind, aware of all of its possible countermoves.

Very rarely does the acute patient speak for herself. Her Negative Mind is always conniving methods for mayhem and will do almost anything to achieve the demise of the Actual Mind unless we prevent it from doing so. Thus, as the Negative Mind proceeds with deceit and deception, so must we find ways to fool it into loosening its grasp on its victim.

Clearly, there is no shortcut to reversing this condition. This is truly a challenge for the patient, her loved ones, and those charged with her psychological and medical care. Yet there are some principles and strategies that we have found not only helpful but highly effective in subduing the Negative Mind and bringing about the reinterpretation of the patient's identity and healing. I would like to share these with you in this chapter.

As you read, remember that though this condition is painstaking to work through, it is reversible. The difficulty notwithstanding, if the patient has the courage to undergo the process, how can we deny her our support?

RECOGNIZE THAT THE PATIENT IS DESPERATE FOR HELP

Since the eating disorder neither knows logic nor entertains reason, it would seem remarkable that any person afflicted with it would be unable to outsmart it. The victim's Actual Mind wants help, or she would not search for it relentlessly.

It is easy to detect the split between despondence and hope in the letters we receive: 'I want to go back to work, get my own apartment, and be a responsible human being that works hard and doesn't rely or need other people to take care of me. I'm doing nothing except sitting around getting in everyone's way and getting fatter and fatter. Suicide is looking better and better. . . . I am desperate for help and would appreciate any suggestions.'

Another victim wrote, 'I am now convinced that nothing will help. It seems there is no "cure" for someone as damaged/broken as I am. Try as I might, I cannot stop this horrible binge-purge cycle. It controls my life. I find it difficult, if not impossible, to hold a job, go to school, or commit to a meaningful relationship. My life has been on hold for the last 14 years! I am desperate. If I don't get some help, I will die. Please help me.'

In the same breath – my case is hopeless; please help

me. I want to kill myself; I want to be independent and productive like everyone else.

Sadly, victims find it difficult to reach out; they gather more courage to do so when they know that others are speaking their secret language. Therefore, we must be attuned to their muted cries for help if they are to be rescued.

SEPARATE THE CONDITION
FROM THE PATIENT

In dealing with a person who has an eating disorder, we must be constantly aware of the dual mindset. It is essential to separate a victim from her condition, placing anorexia or bulimia on one side and the individual's uniqueness on the other. We do this so the person understands that the illness is not who she is, but merely an imposition, a parasite she is hosting.

The victim is not anorexia or bulimia, but because of the relentlessness of the Negative Mind, she may believe that she is. She may abuse, degrade, or mutilate herself, or alienate others because the Negative Mind orders her to do so.

To help the acute anorexic, we must recognize the negative mindset and create an alliance with the victim against it. At the clinic we use several techniques to separate the condition from the patient. If her behavior seems abusive or bizarre, we might say, 'Honey, I know you didn't mean that; it was your head talking' or 'I know your head is giving you a rough time. It is making you do this.'

Patients may respond, 'But it is so hard. The voices are so mean. I am so embarrassed' or, through tears, 'I don't know why that happened. I would never hurt anybody's feelings.' We also ask patients to paint pictures of their condition (see Chapter 4) and to write down what the Negative Mind says. Here is one young woman's Negative Mind in action: 'No one can help you because you're psycho, and no one can deal with you. You're not worth it anyway. Everyone HATES you; you only cause trouble. There's nothing you can do right. Things will never work out for you. You'll ALWAYS be miserable. Everyone knows you're shallow and two-faced. Even strangers HATE you. You make the world miserable. You should burn in hell. You're not the victim, you're the evil one.'

Another acute patient begged her Negative Mind to leave her alone: 'I need to be loved by my own being. Please do not punish me for the years that I was so destructive. Please! Let me live and be happy with myself and my body. Don't hurt me anymore!!!!' And then she wrote, 'I hate you to the ends of the earth. Anorexia leave me alone, surrender. You are the enemy and there is no place for you in my life.'

As a part of their treatment, we also ask the patients to write what the Negative Mind ('Condition') tells them in one column of a steno pad and the response of the Actual Mind ('Me') in the second column. This is so they can identify the negativity more clearly and therefore fight against it. It follows then that given that the Actual Mind is logic, they use it to question negative comments and reason themselves away from them. This strengthens the Actual Mind.

Here is an example of Mindy's dialogue with her Negative Mind. Since she was still in the very early stages of recovery, her Negative Mind had much more to say to her than did her Actual Mind:

- Don't buy it! She is only trying to get you fatter. What makes you think she is any different than anyone else? Why would she? What do you have to offer anyone – only ugliness and boredom. Look at you – disgusting, selfish pig. You eat all day every day – Such a loser.

- I have to trust someone. Why would she want me fat? What is it to her? How can she benefit? I want to believe she cares.

- I don't deserve to be helped. I can never do anything right. Nobody could possibly care about me. I am demanding and selfish and mean.

- I'm not going to listen to you. You are nothing but cruel all day long, every day.

- I shouldn't be here. I shouldn't eat.

- I don't choose to be here. I am alone and should isolate myself from people around me. I am too fat.

- I have no control over that. Peggy promised me she wouldn't make me fat. He will be with me forever and no one can make him go away. I should live like this forever. Why won't he fuck off and leave me alone? Peggy said it would. In time it will.

- I am a bad person because I can't fight him myself. I can't believe in people here and shouldn't trust them. Why can other people believe and I can't? I wish I could believe. I ruined my family's life. I have to do everything he says or he will punish me. Peggy and the other people

135

here say he can't do those
things that he says. Why
won't people give up on me?

Mark's journal in the acute phase of his illness is a
typical expression of the relentless negativism of the
condition badgering the victim.

CONDITION	ME

- Embarrassing – she must really
  be grossed out looking at you
  work out. Feel like such a nerd.
  Wish you looked normal –
  Eyes down, don't look around.
  Hate rooms – so embarrassing
  and feel so sick. So inept at
  sports. He must really laugh
  at you. Wish you could play
  like him, and be so in proportion. You're awful. That
  cloud is shaped just like you;
  totally out of proportion. The
  careworker is lying. He's just
  trying to be nice. Fat. Ugly.
  So disgusting; look almost
  pregnant.
- You're such a pain, such a   • It's just his job. He needs to
  free-loader. You're a burden.   keep you safe.
  Everyone hates you. You're
  useless. They are pushing you
  too much; won't let up. They

want too much; you weigh enough. Don't let them make you do it. Too many choices, too many types. Too much in the basket – return some – return it all. Leave. Go home. You don't belong here. Those people are staring; your shirt is too damn tight and you're grossing them out. Hurry and get this over with and leave. The careworker must think you're a real idiot – a real nerd. Sweating like crazy. Even getting dizzy, you idiot – stop breathing. Put the basket down and leave. Do it tomorrow.

- You're bothering all the other exercisers. You're never thinking of others. You're a jerk. You're so unsociable, so boring and self-centered. They must all laugh at you when you leave. They must think you're such a nerd. Why can't you be normal?

- Don't think about it – close it all out. Don't panic. Calm down. Peggy won't lie to you and you need all this stuff. Just keep going and leave. Trust.

- You were really stupid talking to that lady/mother on the phone. You should have been more professional and less excited. She likely

- Calm down. Ignore all that.

thought you were a salesman
of all things. You likely
scared her off. Peggy will have
to do damage control, thanks
to you.

- That earring lady looks at
you as if you're nuts. What's
she thinking? Must really be
disgusted. Why doesn't she
look at the careworker like
that? Stop. Do it here. Don't
drag him back to the first store.
They won't hurt you. You
shouldn't have put in that earring. You're so vain. It was a
dumb idea. Rip it out. It
makes you look even worse.
You're so ugly, such an idiot.
Why did you do it? So huge.
So bloated and out of proportion. Must be the food. Three
hot dogs. Good grief. You've
said something wrong. You
never think before opening
your mouth. Better shut up
or you'll screw up again.
Wish you'd watch your big
fat mouth.

- Nothing fits. Nothing
covers you enough. You
must be gaining. You must
be. Should be being useful,

- Mom and Dad might freak,
but it's done!

- Apologize; say sorry. It
might help.

should be doing more.
You don't fit in here.
Everyone knows what a
bore you are. What a jerk.
You shouldn't have had so
much protein; you did nothing
all day and remember what
you looked like this morning.
This will just make it worse.
Ask to go to the end of the
beach; this isn't far enough.
Go up the road and back;
don't stop walking; it's not
long enough. Too much food
the rest of the day still. What
if it rains and you can't get
out? You're boring the careworker. If you weren't such a
pain he could be with someone
else, having fun instead. So
ashamed and embarrassed.
You are so ugly. Pray he
isn't grossed out.

- Too much food, so many
people. So busy. Leave.
Get out of here. Must get
out of here. Too many
people running around,
too many types of yogurt
and tofu. You idiot. You're
such a pig. Such a fat, ugly,

- Don't worry. You don't want
to lose weight. Have to try
harder. Trust and eat more.
It's okay. Be patient.

CONDITION	ME
boring pig. They must be shocked that you eat so much. How could you? Damn you. So dull, so afraid. Imagine how the fat will pile up. No one eats three hot dogs. Crazy. You fat pig.	
• You are such a jerk. Why didn't you phone him? Now the careworker called you – exactly opposite. Can't believe you – you should have phoned and left a message – he must think you're an inconsiderate, uncaring idiot. You are. Why'd you wait? Even a message. Damn you. Could have eaten later – no rush. Too much food. Won't go away, won't leave. You never see the other careworkers anymore. Should keep your mouth shut, as if you should be talking. Look at you.	• He wanted to call you. It's OK. He really does want to talk to you.
• Imagine how everyone feels about you. They are stuck with you. They have no say. And neither should you. You're a jerk. No one wants to be with you. They're so	• Wow! They said 'I hope you're not planning on leaving soon!!' Wow – they even meant it! Right on!!!

uncomfortable and uneasy.
You never say anything
right – you just upset
people. And here you are,
ruining everyone else's pros-
pects and future – who are
you to talk? Hypocrite.
You're complaining of others
when you are no better. He's
trying so hard. It's impossible
for anyone to like you. You
shouldn't criticize him.
You've ruined everything.
At least he was friendly,
and happy and in-
teresting and caring.
Look what he must think
of you. He's stuck with you.
He has no choice. You are
no-good, useless, inept.

- That clerk is staring. Better
not get the pants. He knows
you'd look ridiculous in
them. Besides, you don't
deserve them. And they
don't fit you. You can't wear
them. Why can't you be
normal? Damn you.

- Forgot to thank Peggy for
the chest, you jerk. She must
really think you're an inconsid-
erate, unthankful idiot. Why

- No one notices. You're too
self-conscious.

141

can't you remember simple things? Where's your brain?

- Those people are wondering why you're in McDonald's and not having anything. As if you should. That burger is huge; imagine the calories in that. And he's in charge of telling you what's appropriate sizes? Look how huge that is; it's enormous. Afraid you'll gain weight like crazy if you listen to his ideas of food amounts. You are such a pig, such a fat ugly pig. Why did you eat that hot dog – that was so stupid. You totally overate. The care-worker must be the one that's wrong. He's the one who ate at McDonald's without any guilt.
- The careworker must think you're a real idiot. You should act your age for once. People will discover what you're truly like and you will lose everything. It will all disappear and you will be lonely again. You'll

- This burger is not going to make you fat. It will be okay. Trust. No one will let you get fat. Hey – maybe you really are getting somewhere.

lose everything.

- I wish I was normal. Wish I was less boring and looked better. You're such a nerd. You act so stupid.

- Trust Peggy. She doesn't lie.

- You idiot – you jerk. The careworker's going to kill you. How could you say such a stupid, insensitive thing. Why don't you think before you open your mouth. So embarrassing. He's going to think you're a real jerk. He's going to be upset when he hears your message. Explain what you really meant. You should never have called him. That was stupid. Your mouth is always spewing off and insulting and hurting. He'll be really shocked. How could you have said it that way? You're forever getting flustered on the phone and when you talk to people – damn you. I hate you I hate you. I hate you so much – go to hell. You never think of

- Call him back and leave a message to clarify what you said. Simple as that.

anyone but yourself.
He'll wonder how you
could have said it. He'll
know what a jerk
you are. He'll stop wanting
to work with you and be
quiet and more curt when
you're around.

- Go to bed. Go straight to
  bed. Forget it. Ate too
  much today and you're
  fat enough as it is. No
  more food. Just sleep and
  start a new day tomorrow.
  Don't eat any more today.
  Keep eating so much and
  it will get worse. Just call
  it a night.

- No, don't use this as an excuse. Just one hour. Stay up
  and try to finish. Ignore
  how you look; it's all in
  your head. Eat one more
  thing. It's okay – you can
  handle it.
  Trust Peggy and try hard.

- You're not important
  enough to have so many
  sessions. She's bored with
  you. You are wearing
  her out like all the other
  doctors. You aren't
  working hard enough.
  She doesn't really like you
  – she's pawning you off on
  someone else. You're not
  worth her time. She isn't
  so eager to be with
  you; you're boring.

- Give it a break. She's very
  busy. The other counselor is
  excellent and you are so
  much better. She knows
  what she's doing. It's really
  only one less session per
  week. She likely feels you
  can handle things on your
  own more.

- Look at you. You're huge.

- Trust Peggy. You've got to.

CONDITION	ME
Peggy's lying to you. You're the ugliest, most revolting thing. You're eating too much.	It's your eyes.
• Oh hell, way to go, you idiot. You forgot about the meeting. You never even thought. They must have been upset. Where was your brain? Only thinking of yourself.	• Okay, so you forgot. Apologize tomorrow – it wasn't on purpose.
• You look so disgusting, so revolting. Find something else to wear. Don't wear that shirt. Cover up more. Gross. Peggy must be wrong. There's no way you can look like this.	

As the patient moves further along toward her recovery, the Actual Mind becomes stronger and more adept in its arguments against the Negative Mind. The following is Darlene's journal:

CONDITION	ME
• No one cares about you.	• People love you.
• Dying is a welcome prospect.	• Life in its true form is worth living.
• You will always fail.	• Life has ups and downs.
• You don't deserve good things.	• You deserve goodness.

Faith's journal shows the progress she has made. As her Actual Mind engages in logical discussion, it is clear that she now has vision toward her eventual recovery:

CONDITION	ME
• My body is too big. A lot of it is probably fat. The more I look at it, the more disgusted I get.	• I have been told time and time again that my eyes aren't seeing things the way they really are. I am looking at my body through the eyes of anorexia so therefore I cannot rely on my own perception. Instead, I have to trust in what Treena has told me which is: My weight is at low normal. I am not 'too big.' I more or less look like a teenager rather than a 21-year-old woman.
• I am bigger than all the other girls at the house. Most of them are allowed to maintain an anorexic weight and they don't have, as I do, to accept their body at such a high level.	• Once again, my perception of the others I'm comparing with isn't very accurate. I always look for things and, course, I'm going to find them one way or the other. It's a very twisted game in which I can never 'win.' But mostly, it doesn't matter what weight anybody else is at because I'm me and they're them. That's the

- I have gained a lot of weight since I've been put back on a food plan. It's also been a very fast process. Probably only 2 weeks to dump at least 10 pounds on me. . . .

bottom line. I can strive all my life to be like this person or that person. All that's going to do is take away from my own self. It doesn't accomplish anything! I want to do something with my life, not let it go by, wasting my time envying everybody else.

- I really have no way of knowing numbers as facts. I may feel as though I've just been fattened up big time but I have to remember that my feelings are strongly influenced by the condition at times. Trust is really the key. . . . I've been promised that I will be comfortable with my body in the end. . . .

Paula's journal indicates that as she progresses through treatment, her negative thoughts become less specific, more diffuse and ineffectual. She also gains enough objectivity to notice the changes, strengthening her resolve to move ahead.

CONDITION	ME
• obese	• probably not
• something is wrong with my body	• trust counselor
• i am gaining too much weight too fast	• trust counselor
• i am a bother	
• i am a mean nuisance	• anorexia is mean
• i am being punished and i deserve it	• no one deserves anorexia
• i look pregnant	
• i am so swollen my legs are going to explode	
• i am a failure	
• there is nothing good about me	
• i have no talent	
• i have no worth	
• i am an embarrassment to my family	• they love me unconditionally
• no worth	
• no talent	
• i am crazy	
• i hate me	
• i am ugly	
• i can't do it	• i don't have to; Montreux can do it.
• i am too disgusting to be hugged	
• i am an evil sinner	• anorexia is evil

CONDITION	ME
• i am doing better than i deserve	
• i am too fat to be here	• it doesn't matter if i think that i am too fat to be here because i am committed to be here until i get better
• i am a bother	• i am supposed to ask for help. It is part of complying with the program.
• i can't do it	• i do not have to do it. i just have to trust Montreux and let them do it.
• intake is my choice	• intake is not my option. i am being good by trusting and complying.
• i am bad	
• i feel guilty for asking for help and bothering my workers	• it is my job to ask for help; it is part of the program.

The voice has shifted. It used to torment me with very negative, specific thoughts, but now it is just a mass of negative confusion in my head. Instead of a voice it is more like a resounding gong or a clanging cymbal. Before, I could combat a negative thought with a positive one by telling my careworker what it was saying and having them respond. Now, however, there is nothing specific to combat.

CONDITION	ME
• i can't do it; it is too hard	• i am supposed to be here. It is part of a bigger plan. i will stay as long as it takes. This pain is nothing compared to what the past few years have been. I will have my life again.
• i am scared	• anorexia is scared
• i do not deserve a happy life	• i hate anorexia and want to have a happy life. i want to be able to go out to eat and enjoy life.
• i will always hate myself	• i cannot finish the program and still hate myself. When I get through the program I will like myself. Liking myself is part of the program.
• something is horribly wrong	• Trust counselors
• i am miserable	• this bad feeling will go away. Everyone goes through it. The others made it.

THE NUMBERS GAME

Given that the Negative Mind uses all it can against the victim, we must be aware of the material that we present it. One of the best ways of offsetting the Negative Mind is to refuse to play the numbers game in order to weaken its effect.

For instance, hospitalized anorexia patients have often been told their weight and threatened with having to maintain a target weight. To the Negative Mind, this will translate as a weight to reach, albeit reluctantly, in order to effect release from the hospital. Once on its own, the Negative Mind will have free rein once more and will command its victim to stop eating. I believe this is one of the reasons why recidivism is so high among anorexic patients soon after hospital release!

Many patients hospitalized in traditional programs refer to gaining weight temporarily to appease their doctors and therapists as 'playing the game.' One of my patients called her hospital weight-gain program 'Anorexia University.'

Scales can also give the Negative Mind a number to use against its victim. Usually, it commands her to weigh less than the weight recorded each day. However, denied that number, the Negative Mind has less clout and nothing to go on. Its threats become, of necessity, more scattered and obscure – and less effective. Faith's response, for instance, that she has no way of 'knowing any numbers as facts' when her Negative Mind asserted that she had gained ten pounds, underscores how this can be helpful. Unawareness of her weight gives the victim some protection from the Negative Mind's hectoring.

It is for this reason that at the clinic, we weigh our patients backward. They are never told how much they weigh (the number is simply noted silently on their charts), nor are they given a 'target weight' to achieve to obtain release.

Another way of circumventing the Negative Mind is to present food in a way that is not as fear-inducing to the patients. Small nutritious meals or snacks presented six times a day serve the mind and body well without grievously offending the patient.

Smaller portions at one sitting are less threatening than three large meals a day. If the patient finishes a meal and stops eating before she feels full, she is less inclined to feel the need to purge or exercise. We are aiming for a slow, steady process that encourages gradual weight gain for physical safety and physiological balance. Force-feeding huge quantities of calories to a patient with an eating disorder is extremely unkind. Ultimately such a strategy is counterproductive and physiologically dangerous. It is gentler to body and soul to encourage slow, safe weight gain that allows the patient dignity and time to adjust emotionally.

Giving the patient her own individual plates and dishes, provided for her on coming into care, makes her realize she is not a number and gives her confidence and structure. Indeed, even the style and color of dishes are important in that they indicate respect of individuality and consistency – cardinal principles of the Montreux program. Every day she will eat from the same dishes until she no longer feels the need to focus on any of the utensils she uses. This is another marker of her recovery for at that point, food will no longer be the center of her life.

In the acute patient, feeding has to be justified often mineral by mineral, vitamin by vitamin until the Actual Mind subsumes the Negative Mind. Sometimes for the satisfaction of the patient we have to analyze and explain the reason for eating almost every bite.

'Why am I eating a banana, Peggy?' I am asked. 'Why should I eat papaya? Why are they giving me yogurt?'

'Bananas have potassium to keep your heart strong,' I reply. 'Yogurt has the calcium to keep your bones from deteriorating, and papaya has enzymes to help your digestive system.' Everything must be justified.

COUNTERACTING THE NEGATIVE CHATTER
WITH UNCONDITIONAL LOVE

Through the whole term of recovery, eating disorder patients will spew negative chatter. Their heads are full of it. It is a decided challenge, therefore, for anyone to contend with. Nevertheless, we answer every negative thought with a positive one. It is essential to respond to every self-defeating outburst with unconditional gentleness and kindness. We offset every subjective comment with an objective one.

If the patient says, 'I'm worthless; don't bother with me. How could you even want me here anyway? I should give my bed to someone more deserving,' we will respond, 'You're very valuable to us and the world. There is a wonderful person inside you who is going to come out when the negativity is gone. You are deserving of all the care you get.'

Or if a patient says, 'I've just eaten. My mother is going to die,' she receives the response: 'Honey, that's just your head talking to you. Your fear has no basis in reality. No one is going to die. What has your eating to do with your mother except to make her happy?'

At the clinic we are firm believers in the benefits of unconditional love, and so we build an environment of unqualified support, responding to each patient with terms of endearment. Given that the patient is at the mercy of an onslaught of unrelenting negativity, showering the patient with unconditional love is necessary to create balance. Unconditional love counteracts the harsh voice of the Negative Mind as it teases out the possibility of reconnecting with the Actual Mind. It lures the Actual Mind into a place of comparison of stark opposites: the punishment of the Negative Mind and the caringness of unconditional love. The victim eventually allows the unconditional love because it feels so much better and is certainly more conducive to healthy living.

If a patient can goad a careworker to frustration, the Negative Mind has won. The careworker has 'proven' to his subjective patient that his caring is conditional. The patient in the acute stage will brood and pout and the careworker will have a difficult time proving himself truly caring. The careworker must then be removed from the case since the trust so critical to the healing process will have been destroyed. Remember, the Negative Mind hunts to confirm that the Actual Mind is useless.

Moreover, given that the CNC victim has highly developed receptors for everyone else's problems, we at the clinic must always appear calm and unruffled to the patient. Caregivers studiously avoid involving the patient in their own personal dramas. Of course, this can be very taxing to caregivers; they aren't permitted the usual ups and downs, hardly a normal existence. But we are dealing with an unrealistic mindset here which is so extreme that we must be as extreme in the opposite direction. Remember, as well, that the Negative Mind dominates only in the first two stages of therapy before the patient begins to achieve mental balance.

The CNC victim may continually test her boundaries to ensure her own safety. We find it mandatory, therefore, to stay close to the acute patient at all times. This is one of the reasons that we have such a high ratio of careworkers per patient (one to one or higher around the clock), especially during the early phases of treatment. The careworker's responsibility is to 'shadow' the patient from the time she comes into twenty-four-hour residential care to the time she leaves it and moves into partial care.

The carefully trained careworker provides unconditional support, caring, and a normal perspective to enable the patient to feel secure. Until she indicates a true belief in herself and begins to wish some independence, the patient will use this positive shadow as a reference point. Should she need to talk about her feelings, to have an explanation and interpretation of her internal dialogue, the careworker will be ever-present.

Careworkers prevent the Negative Mind from manifesting by gentle talking, being with the patients, and impeding them from exercise or any other destructive behaviors. They accompany patients on walks and keep a constant vigil beside their beds through the night. Such faithful attention is necessary because if a patient is able to fool a caregiver and manage to hide food or do anything counterindicative of care such as exercising, vomiting, using or securing laxatives, or even cutting herself, she will see the care as inadequate, feel unsafe, and become increasingly anxious.

Also anorexics are poor sleepers, and it is often comforting for them to find someone at their side with whom they can converse in the middle of the night.

Safe boundaries are imperative for healing. One patient came to us after hospital authorities had allowed him to vomit for one hour each day and to exercise for one and a half hours. As a consequence, his condition did not improve and the victim realized more markedly his aloneness. How could he put his faith in therapists who brokered compromises with his Negative Mind?

When caregivers bargain with the Negative Mind, the victim is always the loser. She feels misunderstood and helpless. In fact, any compromise strengthens the Negative Mind's position and weakens the victim. Even in an ideal situation, the battle to support the victim is a constant struggle. Given that in acute anorexia, the victim always believes she is wrong in her own mind, surrendering to the Negative Mind only reinforces those beliefs.

As other safety precautions, at the clinic, we also keep kitchen knives locked away; no razors are allowed in the bathroom. We keep vitamins and medicine locked up so they cannot be abused.

As I'll explain more fully in the next chapter, when a patient has enough focus and concentration to be able to sit through a session, usually in the middle of the initial stage, she will begin receiving counseling three or four times a week from one of three levels of counselors.

DISTRACTION

The goal of distraction is to keep a victim's attention external, to prevent her from disappearing inside her Negative Mind. Eating is such a frightening time for anorexics, because the Negative Mind will come out in force. Immediately after meals, victims will often feel extremely anxious. This is when distraction is most essential.

At the clinic we have found anything that encourages external focus and concentration, that keeps the person in the present, can be helpful. We use lively conversation, board games, pool, Ping-Pong, humor, art, writing, studying foreign languages, and other educational outlets. However, watching TV can allow a person to 'zone out' and give the Negative Mind an opening for silent abuse.

The first twenty minutes after feeding is generally the most difficult for the patient and she may become agitated. A skilled careworker takes it upon herself to go to extremes to entertain the patient because diversion through laughter really proves to be the best medicine.

Distracting questions give the Actual Mind another focus to reclaim the patient's attention. The Negative Mind has no way to process information that cannot be used to demean the victim. This can give the careworker the advantage for the moment.

ROCKING AND TOUCHING

Sometimes words are inadequate to express the depth of our caring. When we see a crying baby, our first instinct is to pick him up and cuddle him. When we see a wounded animal, we want to cradle it.

Children with eating disorders are wounded and extremely frightened. I think there is great therapeutic value in giving in to our natural impulse to soothe them with healing words and touch.

On several occasions, I have spoken to nurses in wards for children with eating disorders. The first thing I ask them is whether they have a rocking chair. Then I will say, 'Is it possible for you to hold that child in your lap and rock her?' The sufferers need the comfort and security to offset the terror of their mental state.

At the clinic, we try to find the connection that works for each patient. If it is not rocking, it can be sitting by the bedside, talking in a gentle tone. The words themselves may not even be that important, but the attitude is. We also take patients to massage therapists. One mother told me she would rub her daughter's back. The child obviously enjoyed it but told her, 'Please stop doing that because I like it.'

Remember that though the victim is an intellectual prize, her emotional maturity has been arrested at an earlier stage. She is in constant need of the reassurance and comfort we would naturally offer a young child.

WORKING WITH TRANCES

At the clinic, careworkers recognize the signs of a patient beginning to go into a trance and will call a counselor to attempt to prevent it. Anyone attending a victim in a trance must display absolute confidence in his or her ability to retrieve the Actual Mind from the clutches of the Negative Mind. The Negative Mind will seize upon any hesitancy or doubt betrayed by caregivers and use it to prolong its absolute hold over the patient.

As soon as we realize that a patient is in a trance, we sit on the floor or a chair, and gathering her into our arms, we rock her while holding her tightly. We speak soothingly, encouragingly, saying, 'We can do this. Anorexia is very frightened of us. He is nothing but a bully in the schoolyard. Even though he feels real, he is not. He is just a construct in your mind. We are much stronger than he is. You can come out now; it is safe. He will never win with us here.'

If we ask a patient, 'How much of you is here with us?' the initial response will be muffled and barely audible. Persistence on the part of caregivers, albeit extremely gentle persistence, will most often strengthen the Actual Mind and bring the patient back. Indeed, the level of preoccupation and the length of time it takes the acute patient to answer can indicate the degree of control the Negative Mind exerts.

We have also found that distraction is quite helpful when a patient is in a trance. If we ask her distracting and diversionary questions such as, 'How is your dog doing today?' or 'What is the weather like?' we can often bring her back quickly. We are giving her Actual Mind tools to circumvent the power of the Negative Mind because she feels she cannot tackle it directly. A question about one's dog, for instance, is neutral territory. The Negative Mind is not anticipating us to come back with such a question. Usually it would expect a query about well-being or food. The caregiver may need to repeat a question gently three times or more because the patient is so internally preoccupied.

Usually there are a few other people nearby, gently stroking the patient's forehead with a cool cloth, comforting her with terms of endearment and encouragement. How long it takes to bring a patient out of a trance depends on her sense of trust in her careworkers' words. It is unwise to let her stay in the trance, because the Negative Mind is given more time and jurisdiction.

Gradually the patient's eyelashes will begin to flutter, indicating that she is beginning to come back to consciousness. We make statements such as, 'See, your eyes are starting to flutter. We see you are coming back. You are starting to see us right now. It's all right.' As the patient comes out of the trance, she usually breaks down, sobbing uncontrollably, holding on to her careworker tightly, repeating any number of things that she has been instructed by the messages holding her hostage.

Usually extra staff members stay with a patient for a good half hour after she has 'come back.' Following much more reassurance and soothing talk, we put the moment into perspective for the patient. We tell her, 'You were in a trance. You're safe and it's over.'

Apparently patients are usually aware of the fact that they have been in a trance. They felt themselves slipping into it. They will then tell us what the voices told them to do: 'I'm supposed to run outside in front of a truck. I don't want to be killed.' We always then attempt to distract them. Only after we are certain that they are completely stabilized will we give them a change of scenery, usually by having them go arm in arm with two careworkers outside to the garden or to some other pleasing, distracting place. They are in a fragile state at this point; it is never wise to allow such a patient to go anywhere unaccompanied because she needs to feel protected and secure.

STAYING TWO MOVES AHEAD

In this dangerous chess game, caregivers must always be two moves ahead of the Negative Mind because the Negative Mind is always two moves ahead of the patient's Actual Mind.

One of our most useful tools is to hunt for ulterior motives in our patient's behavior. If a victim says, 'It's a

As part of their therapy, Peggy asks her patients to illustrate their relationship with anorexia. These are examples of their art.

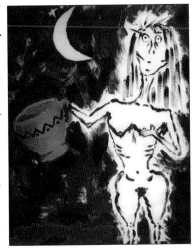

The victim is in a trance where it is forever night, pouring out her life's blood. She is not sure if she is fat or thin; part of her body seems fat and other parts look like bones.

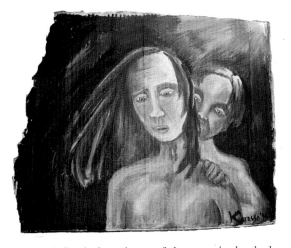

This painting is the epitome of the game in the dual mindset. The glazed, trapped gaze of the obvious Actual Mind is managed and directed by the insidious cunning of the behind-the-scenes Negative Mind. The Actual Mind becomes a mere puppet to play out the demands of the Negative Mind.

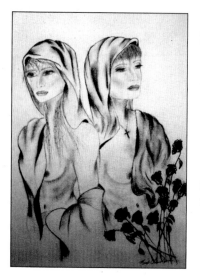

My daughter Nicole created this. She explains that it represents the dual mindset of the pessimistic (no-hope) Negative Mind and the optimistic yet (faint hope) smaller Actual Mind. The cross on the right figure shows the possibility of belief. The black roses indicate that most hope has died. The red rose indicates that the fire of life is still burning if anyone could fan its flames.

This victim describes herself in black worthlessness, primarily bad, ashamed, yet confused because she feels she has a good heart. It is significant that the heart is deep and out of view of the common perception, therefore not easily available to be helped.

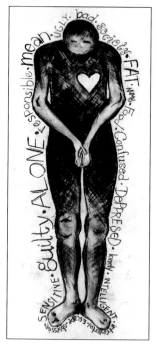

A very desperate case, this patient is convinced she is in the fires of "hell" being punished for all the bad she has supposedly done. When asked what these bad deeds were, she didn't know. Of course, she is guilty of nothing.

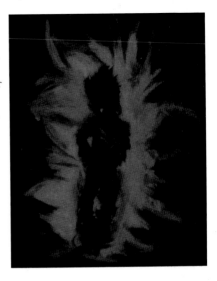

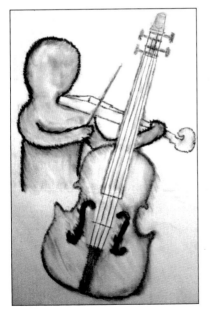

When this artist was anorexic, she was the violin in the background, totally controlled and dominated by the "black figure" who played her at will. In the foreground, the violin herself is now free. She is her own master now that she is "cured."

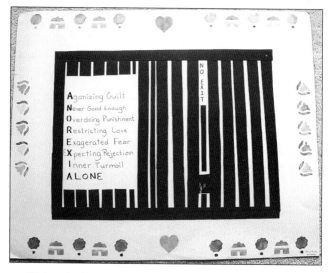

This artist is now cured of her twenty-year struggle with anorexia. She never thought it possible that she could ever enjoy a home, flowers, and life. She often said that she was hidden in a black jail with no means of seeing life except in other people's pleasure – something she did not deserve for herself.

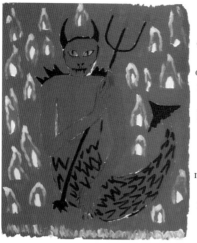

This artist has had anorexia since she was eight years old. She came to our clinic after years of unsuccessful treatment, in which she was blamed for noncompliance and hurting her family. When we received her, she painted this picture of what was raging in her mind, creating threats and unrelenting fear. She is now completely well and has returned to her wonderful family.

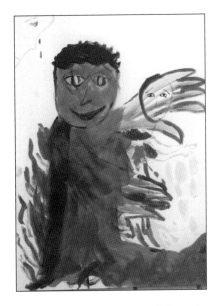

In the upper left corner, the ghost of the patient weeps as she watches her head being manipulated and thrust through with the negativity of the "monster" who comes from a source of such diabolical unkindness.

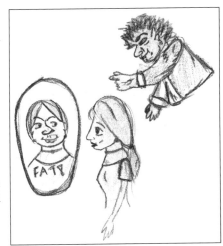

This thirteen-year-old artist depicted a girl being instructed by an ever-present negative force on how to see herself.

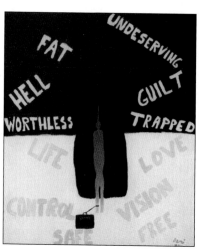

This victim sees herself paralyzed in the living of life – her feet can know no direction; they are locked in place. Her head is a hypodermic needle injecting itself into a black well of negativity – of no return.

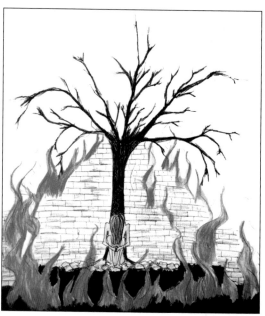

The artist sees herself as dejected and in darkness surrounded by flames – an inescapable barrier to the living of life. The artist struggled with eating disorders for over five years.

THE VALLEY OF HAPPINESS

AS OUR DREAMS ARE SHATTERED,
AND OUR HOPES ARE TURNED TO DESPAIR,
YOU STARE INTO OUR EYES, STAINED WITH
THE BLOOD-RED TEARS OF TORMENT.

YOU ARE FULL OF HEARTLESS MIRTH.
YOUR LAUGHTER IS EVILLY INTOXICATING.

WE CRY OUT IN SORROW AND IN RAGE,
YET, WE ARE HEEDED BY NO ONE.

WHAT HAVE WE DONE TO DESERVE THIS?
WE DID NOT REQUEST TO LIVE,
OR BRING IT UPON OURSELVES.

AWAY, FROM THIS WORLD,
OUT OF THIS LIFE,
WE WILL RUN TO ESCAPE THIS HATRED.

THE NEVER-ENDING SCREAMS WILL BE
WASHED AWAY BY THE RIVERS OF PEACE.
OUR ANGUISH WILL BE BLOWN AWAY BY
THE WINDS OF LOVE.
YOU WILL BE FORGOTTEN, AND FOREVER DEAD
AS WE LIVE FOR ALWAYS, IN
THE VALLEY OF HAPPINESS.

— Jen.

THE GREEN GRASS OF A FLOWER COVERED MEADOW.

YOUR SILENT SCREAMS ARE IGNORED,
AS YOU WALLOW IN YOUR SELF-CREATED
AGONY.
"LET JUSTICE PREVAIL," YOU SAID,
BUT YOU LIE, THROUGH GRINDING TEETH,
WHILE NOT EVEN YOUR HOLLOW, EMPTY
EYES, SHINE THE TRUTH.
WHAT CAN HAPPEN, OTHER THAN WHAT IS
DESTINED TO?
IS THERE NO WAY OUT OF THIS HELL?
YOU WILL BE JUDGED IN THE END,
YOU ARE RESPONSIBLE FOR YOUR ACTIONS.
MAY YOU BE RENDERED DEAD AND DESTROYED
IN A WAY COMPREHENDED BY NO ONE.
THERE IS NO WAY OUT,
NEVER, UNTIL YOU DIE AGAIN FOR ETERNITY.
IN A BLACK WOODEN BOX, YOU WILL BE
BURIED,
BENEATH THE GREEN GRASS OF A FLOWER
COVERED MEADOW.

— Jen.

A patient has lived eight years in the torment of her Negative Mind's hatred. She feels her only escape from this relentless tirade is to dream of a place beyond this life. This earth appeared to offer her no reprieve. She is well today and safely at home with her family, riding her horse across meadows with flowers and unending green.

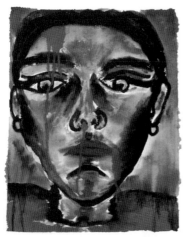

Typically, this artist focuses on the head as the center of her turmoil. According to this victim, the "voices" are draining the life out of her. She is staring and dismal as she is powerless to staunch the flow of blood from her head.

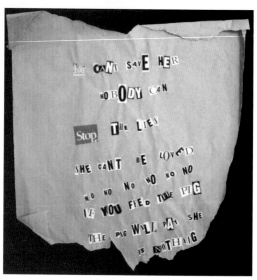

YOU CANT SAVE HER

NOBODY CAN

Stop THE LIES

SHE CANT BE LOVED

NO NO NO NO NO

IF YOU FEED THE PIG

THE PIG WILL PAY SHE

IS NOTHING

Oftentimes the Negative Mind refers to its subjects as "pigs" if they allow themselves anything or if they allow anyone else to give them the pleasure of food or kindness. When a patient accepts something for herself, the voices shriek at her, deriding her worthlessness. This is usually emotionally exhausting.

beautiful evening. I love walking in the rain. Would it be all right to go out for an hour or so?' we must question her motives.

And so we would ask, 'Who wants to go for a walk, you or anorexia?'

Frequently the child replies, 'Actually, anorexia does. I don't like the rain at all. It's wet and dreary.'

In understanding the child's motivation, we are creating an alliance with the Actual Mind. She then realizes that the battle is not hers alone to fight.

But immediately thereafter, we must create a distraction so the Negative Mind does not 'beat up' the patient. In that distraction, we are confirming the patient's security with us. She knows we can see past the outward behavior. That strengthens her trust and moves her ahead. She does not have to take the responsibility for making the decision.

If we had allowed her to go on that walk without questioning her motivation, on the other hand, she would have felt despondent that nobody had recognized she did not want to walk in the first place. Her Negative Mind was ordering her to exercise.

By staying two steps ahead of the Negative Mind we create a sense of security and deep trust on the part of the patient.

CHALLENGING THE SUBJECTIVITY

At the clinic, once a patient is no longer acutely ill and has a better grasp of reality (see Chapter 6), counseling that focuses on reversing the subjectivity of the Negative Mind helps her begin to put her life into a more tenable perspective. We are constantly challenging the subjective in order to do what we call Objectivity Training.

For instance, if patient Patty's mother seems highly emotional, Patty's subjective response would have been to take responsibility for her mother's moods. In counseling sessions, we might point out, 'Your mother says she's very unhappy and you believed you caused that, but it's your mom's issue. You didn't cause her unhappiness.' We explain that perception is not always reality and gently guide the patient to step outside the situation and see it as an objective observer.

In response, Patty might respond, 'I always thought the divorce was my fault, but now I understand that my mom has her own problems.'

Because the patient is subjective in so many areas of her life, this Objectivity Training becomes an ongoing part of treatment.

We also use role-playing situations to reinforce objectivity. We break down situations for the patient to analyze and carry out mini-dramas. One patient will voice the perspective of the subjective mind while another will speak for objectivity:

THE FACTS: Your brother is ill with cancer.

THE SUBJECTIVE RESPONSE: 'It's all my fault. If only I had done more for him, if only I were a better person, I would have spared him this pain and suffering.'

THE OBJECTIVE RESPONSE: 'Cancer is a terrible illness. No one is sure why some people get it and others don't. Heredity and environment are most likely to blame. I love my brother and will do everything in my power to help him, but I didn't cause this disease and I am not responsible for curing it. I'm only responsible for loving him and being there for him as much as I can.'

THE FACTS: Your mother has depression.

THE SUBJECTIVE RESPONSE: 'She's depressed because I've disappointed her. I've got to pull her out of it. I'm to blame.'

THE OBJECTIVE RESPONSE: 'Depression is a clinical diagnosis and requires professional help. Mom, Dad, and other adults have to get her the help she needs. Mom's depression has made her respond inappropriately to me. That's not my fault. If Mom can't get her depression under control, we'll have to adapt, but it's not my responsibility.'

We often do role playing with situations drawn from typical family or school interactions.

THE FACTS: Father comes home tired and agitated from work. Hannah asks him if he would go over some homework and he snaps, 'I've got too much on my mind now.'

THE SUBJECTIVE RESPONSE: 'My father doesn't like me. I knew I shouldn't have asked him for help. I never will again.'

THE OBJECTIVE RESPONSE: 'Poor Dad. He's had a hard day and he's tired. I should have waited till later. Now I'll get him a cup of tea and maybe I can ask him again later when he's more relaxed.'

We act out many situations such as these to help patients understand the difference between their subjective reality and objective reality.

Often, in our modern psychological world, patients are taught to blame or find reason for their disorder in other people's failures. This can prove counterproductive to the person with an eating disorder in the long run. It may teach her to not see herself objectively and this may prevent her from forming a too compassionate perspective on life.

As I've said, blaming parents for the condition might also cut off the sufferer's essential support. A parent will always be a parent and ideally will always be there for the child. It is better to strengthen the existing structure of a family than to weaken it by criticism. Since the anorexic's first interest is in the well-being of her family, the lesson she must learn is that the world hosts many differences and variables, and her family is no different.

That having been said, at the clinic we provide residential care for patients without their parents. This is not meant as a criticism – far from it. The patient realizes that to get through the condition, she needs to concentrate all her efforts with the group supporting her. She knows that her parents are not the best people to do that at this point. Putting distance between the patient and her parents is often misconstrued by the well-meaning public and can be terribly distressing to parents if not properly understood.

Nevertheless, some innate sense seems to direct the victim to perceive that the staff understands her needs better than her family does. The analogy that comes most easily to mind is that of a woman in labor whose need is temporarily more for a doctor or midwife than for her parents or husband. In no way does that belittle her love for her parents or spouse. It makes sense that a person whose job involves itself in obstetrics may be more objective than anxious loved ones.

Many parents are concerned that their caring of their child was inadequate. Nothing generally is further from the truth. But in order for the victim to fight her battle to wellness, she cannot also have the responsibility of her parents' worry about her. She must be temporarily relieved of this and other responsibilities until she can put things in the proper perspective. The child's need is so great, she must for the interim not perceive that her loved ones have any needs, lest she divert her energies toward helping them rather than healing herself. Obviously, that is all but impossible in most settings in which parents come into contact with their children. Parents, siblings, and other loved ones are so emotionally involved that they may be incapable of delivering unconditional love unemotionally and without fear, or masking their understandable anxiety.

When families and loved ones try for months and sometimes years to accommodate the unrealistic situation they are facing, they can be nearly destroyed. But as victims in care become confident that their structure will be intact until it is no longer needed, they are more and more capable of responding to their loved ones. We also counsel family and friends to help them understand the youngster's condition and how triggers in the home may contribute to her CNC.

The patient's progress toward wellness will define how parental visits are structured. In the early stages of recovery, the careworker will accompany parents on outings during the time of their visits. This comforts both parents, who are unsure about how to be with their child at this point, and the victim, as she is beginning to find herself but does not yet always know how to interpret comments without being subjective.

The victim will venture slowly back into the world when she decides it is safe to do so. And she will do so when she is armed with the objective perspective that people do the best they can within the limitations of their own humanity at that moment, that whatever they do depends on myriad variables, many of which they never had any control over and never need to feel any guilt or responsibility about.

6

The Five Stages of Recovery

We have found that most patients with eating disorders experience recovery in distinct, defined stages. As you will see, each stage of recovery presents its own problems, possibilities for backsliding, and triumphs. Each stage demands its own breed of security, gentle prodding, and persuasion for the patient. Each demands a solid platform from which the patient will spring. Each demands the hope of eternal possibility.

Interestingly, the stages of recovery can be compared to a crash course in the normal development of a human being, from the utter helplessness of infancy to the self-confidence and autonomy of adulthood.

THE MONTREUX LIFE
WELLNESS SCALE

The Montreux Life Wellness Scale is our way of clarifying a patient's progress. It encompasses the five stages that eating disorder patients experience as they work their way toward wellness.

This is a percentile scale as well as a human developmental stage scale. The percentages refer to the degree to which the Actual Mind is in control. The lower the percentage, the more dominion the Negative Mind holds over its victim's life. After working with many patients,

I have arrived at these numbers intuitively, and they explain perfectly what goes on during recovery.

The Montreux Life Wellness Scale

THE ACUTE STAGE: Infancy. This is the stage of total dependency. 1 percent to 30 percent.

THE EMERGENT STAGE: This stage is equivalent to the development of a young child. It is one of investigativeness and limit testing. 30 percent to 50 percent.

THE REALITY STAGE: This is the adolescent phase of treatment. It is a time when the pendulum swings from dependency to a false courage and the new identity begins to coalesce. During this stage, the patient moves into partial care. 50 percent to 68 percent.

INTERACTIVE STAGE: This is equivalent to young adulthood – the beginning of maturity and objectivity. It is a time of moderation. She becomes an outpatient. 68 percent to 80 percent.

ENVIRONMENTAL INTEGRATION STAGE: This is the final stage of recovery. The patient returns to her home environment but makes three to four assessment return trips within twelve months and has a five-year follow-up. These assessments determine the patient's ability to reintegrate and adapt to adult life. 80 percent to 86 percent.

Generally it takes the patient the same amount of time to traverse each stage of recovery, though this depends on how soon and how well the patient can grasp the concepts that the counselors and staff teach. How closely the patient adheres to and understands these concepts depends, as well, on her inherent courage and confidence to try new things.

The Montreux Life Wellness Scale serves as a marker of recovery to victims and their families. To the victim, it gives a road map to understanding how her disorder can be reversed each step of the way. To the family, it provides a greater vision of their supportive role and helps them achieve greater tolerance of their child in her emotional journey. Watching a child or loved one disappear into an eating disorder without adequate recourse or explanation can make a parent go mad. The Scale provides a sense of order and purpose in the recovery process.

To ensure against relapse, treatment should not be interrupted until it is completed. Consider the analogy of building a house. Weather will destroy the interior unless a roof is put on. You might then think of the basement as the Acute Stage, where only the builder or architect rather than the owner can visualize the potential completed house. Someone uninvolved in its construction can only assume and respect that the architect has made plans to follow.

A basement is not a house. Neither are three or four months of treatment a cure. It is simply the essential first step that establishes a platform for building upon. So refeeding a patient is a necessary first step in the treatment of an eating disorder. Physical stabilization must occur before one can work with the mind. If a patient is agitated and distracted by inadequate nutrition, her concentration will be scattered.

However, physical stabilization does not equal cure. Otherwise, all of the patients released from traditional hospital settings which merely focus on refeeding would be 'cured' after having reached their target weight. In fact, we can almost surely predict relapse or failure in many cases if treatment is interrupted too soon. An acute eating disorder has taken a long time to develop; it can require up to two years and sometimes longer to reverse.

Of course, each person's recovery depends upon the individual and her inherent predisposition to trust. As well, each patient will adapt to treatment differently, depending on:

- the length of time she has been enslaved by the CNC (although not necessarily the degree of severity of the eating disorder).
- the degree of inherent sensitivity.
- the guilt and trauma she may have felt over time in hurting those around her whom she loves.
- what nurturing is available to her when she returns to her home during the Environmental Integration Stage.
- how her relationship has developed with her family and friends throughout treatment.

Each individual will take her own time for recovery. As with any growing child, one can predict the normal time for each stage of development, yet allow for variation depending on individual makeup. This is also true for the eating disorder victim. Each person will interpret her world in her own way as her identity emerges. Each child will determine her own schedule of recovery. It is inadvisable to push a patient more quickly than she indicates is possible because the work to that point could become partially undone.

THE ACUTE STAGE: 1 PERCENT
TO 30 PERCENT

The acute anorexic or bulimic patient believes she is responsible for everything. Just the opposite is true in treatment. The Acute Stage of treatment is synonymous with infancy. The patient needs to be totally without responsibility either for herself or for anyone else in order to begin growth.

It would seem the only way to correct an eating disorder and ultimately CNC is to enable the patient to start with a fresh interpretation of life. Therefore, the Acute Stage must allow a patient's total dependency until she no longer needs or desires it. Just as an infant needs twenty-four-hour care to protect her from herself and minister to her needs, so does the victim of an eating disorder.

Ideally, the patient must live in this unreal environment until she feels protected enough to emerge and begin to fight back for her life. Trusting in that environment is mandatory to initiate effective treatment. The patient is so subjective that the staff must be trained to be on top of the Negative Mind at all times.

It is therefore imperative during this stage to reiterate ad infinitum that the individual means much to the world and that she is cherished by her loved ones and the clinic staff. The victim will repeatedly deny her worthiness on one hand, yet demand attention and love on the other. Her needs are basic and all-consuming. Constant, loving care and reassurance accompany her return to physical stability.

The victim must necessarily have her physical self restored. At some level, she is aware of this, though she cannot yet admit it to herself or others. Neither is it essential that she admit it until later, when her mind has eased into an acceptance of her need to eat and she is able to argue with logic against the Negative Mind.

Once a person has been put under care, she is able to begin to relax into letting go of the negativity she has constructed against herself. Though she is still quite fearful of her mind's agility in attempting to trap her and trick her, she wishes to believe she is safe.

In twenty-four-hour care, the patient begins to test her boundaries (she hides food down her sleeve rather than eating it, for instance) gently and warily, hoping everyone is aware of her incredible need for protection but not yet quite able to voice it because of the trouble her Negative Mind will give her once she makes that need known. It may not allow her to read, to sleep, to drink, to lie on a bed, to use a pillow, to be kind to her parents or friends, to eat with other children, to play with them, to laugh, to talk, to sing, to complain.

At that point, the onus is on the careworker to let the patient know she is good enough to sleep on a bed, to use a pillow, to sing, to laugh. She has the same rights any of us has as a human being.

It is also important at this stage to create a structure of support for the patient to grow from. As the structure of careworkers and activities forms around the patient, she will begin to rely upon it. This is an interim, though a terribly important, stage. What appears as dependency provides a bulwark for the Actual Mind to defend itself from the persecution of the Negative Mind. This is the key to unconditional support. If we fail to give the Actual Mind the correct ways in which to enlist our alliance, the patient will be in grave danger.

Ideally, the patient will have the same staff team throughout her first stage of treatment because this helps fulfill her need for stability. When keeping the same staff team is impossible, the patient may have to be reassured that a particular staff member did not move elsewhere because of her. The patient is at a very subjective stage of her development, and she may interpret any change as a reproach against her.

We create a food list/mini-menu for added structure. The patient, who at the Acute Stage doubts everything about herself, suddenly can see that her meals are the same every day, served two and a half hours apart. This structure, again, gives her a platform of consistency to grow from. Both her food and her weight are no longer her responsibility. Not having to think about her meals because she needn't think about her weight leaves her freer to begin learning that she is valid.

Still, during the Acute Stage and early on in the Emergent Stage, the patient inevitably pretends to resist some efforts to feed her in order to save herself from being unduly beaten in her mind. There have been times when it has taken three hours, immense concern, and reassurance in order for the victim to brave a small bowl of beans, after which it took more hours of rocking and talking to assure her that she does not need to exercise frantically to burn off the just-consumed calories.

We don't change a patient's meal plan until she begins to become impatient with her existing one. This will indicate her need to move on in the program.

Initially, the patient will be relieved to feel 'safe,' to be at a place where she is absolved of responsibility for her own well-being. Simultaneously, however, she will become more anxious because at this point her condition will realize it is trapped and increase the negative activity in her head.

Now, as the Negative Mind becomes desperate and

begins to lose control of the Actual Mind, the 'civil war' will deepen. Her Negative Mind issues increasingly intense orders, instructing her to refuse food or supplements because she is unworthy. It commands her to run into traffic, cut herself, or exercise any calorie from her body. Her Negative Mind tells her to take too many pills or to put poison into her food because she does not deserve any unadulterated form of pleasure.

At this critical stage, the careworkers are constantly alert and ever-conscious of the devious nature of the Negative Mind. At times the patient will become agitated and may wish to act on the Negative Mind's orders, thereby lessening the mental pressure. This behavior is usually apparent only in the first few months of treatment.

As the victim begins to feel more comfortable in her surroundings, she will verbalize what her Negative Mind is saying to her and accept her careworker's dissuasion of its importance. Slowly thereafter she begins to experience some hope.

At twenty-two, Catherine had weighed forty-one pounds when her doctor contacted us. She weighed sixty-six pounds when we took her into the clinic. This is what she wrote at her sixth week of treatment.

Dear Spirit:

After 12 years of torment, turmoil, and never-ending sadness, I feel like I am slowly surrendering or rather my Anorexic counterpart is slowly getting tired. I am petrified, however, to live my life free of a familiar entity. Years of starving myself, vomiting the little I did ingest, haunting thoughts of fear, anguish, despair, and thoughts of self-hatred paralyzed my being. . . . Fear houses itself throughout my soul. However, despite indescribable fears associated with living 'Life' and being 'Free' from this terrible separate identity, I persevere.

THE EMERGENT STAGE: 30 PERCENT TO 50 PERCENT

As the Acute Stage begins to give way to the Emergent Stage, the eating disorder victim becomes more mentally available. Because of the physical stabilization that occurs during the Acute Stage, serious counseling can now begin. The Actual Mind can listen for short periods of time, and careworkers will note that the patient is able to concentrate on events in the external world. This stage is basically a bridge between the Acute Stage and Reality Stage. It consists of confirmation of positivity and reiteration of worth.

The battle that was primarily between the patient and her condition now shifts noticeably to a battle between the condition and the staff. The patient hands over the problems in her head to staff members more readily and easily. At this juncture, she has gentle assurance in her own mind that she is sometimes worthy to be loved.

During the Emergent Stage, the patient is still dependent but now hunts desperately for an identity. She begins to question her values and everyone else's. The search for self begins, and it's not unusual for patients to experiment, 'trying on' different personalities as they struggle to find their essentialness. Brian came to the program wearing a woman's wig. He was acutely anorexic and was not expected to live past adolescence. His voice was high and quiet. In the following six months, he changed his outward appearance as many times. When we asked what he wanted to be when he was older, he said, 'I want to cure people who are sick in the world.' His external identity was that of a caregiver. Beyond that, his personality was all confusion, and remained so for several months until he began to sense and embrace his core self.

Depending on the patient's level of emotional stability on any given day, she begins to attend three-hour class sessions in our afternoon Educational Program. During this time, a patient will participate in class discussions. This reflects her sense of individuality. Students' opinions and comments are always valid and encouraged. As a patient lends her self to a group, her identity becomes more defined to herself. School becomes a microcosm of the macrocosm of society. It is also an opportunity for patients to discover and 'own' their own interests, motivations, and passions, rather than assuming those they believe the world wants for them.

At this delicate stage of self-construction, caregivers must avoid deciding who the patient is to become. Therapy is not about creating a person – that individual already exists – but rather about allowing one to develop with unconditional guidance and caring.

This stage can prove confusing to the unschooled because the patient will continually be looking for behavior to copy. Therefore it is essential that caregivers are as emotionally stable as possible to ensure that they are in control of themselves when working with such fragile minds.

The mind of the patient during the Emergent Stage is extremely receptive to suggestion. Given the patient's old habits of adhering to others' needs, the caregiver takes pains to present nothing but kindness and compassion in dealing with every subject matter. Victims sort out their life philosophies based upon their own observations; they must not borrow these philosophies from their care-givers' opinions. When asked their opinions, caregivers are apt to reply, 'Tell me what you think. I'm interested,' or use other such gentle encouragement. Indeed, care-givers must keep their personal lives confidential, sharing only happy or humorous anecdotes.

Though the patient is still tentative and desperately in need of her boundaries, she is necessarily demanding during this stage. Soon, the 'terrible twos' appear. The patient has found herself surrounded by unconditional loving attention. In order to prove herself worthy of being so loved, she tests the staff daily and subjectively for motive. Initially, she suspects ulterior motives are behind the acts of loving kindness. She may throw tantrums if we do not give in to unreasonable requests but we must remain steadfast for her security or she will start to lose ground in her support system and begin to regress, as would a two-year-old.

She begins to make her identity known. She wishes variation in her food plan; she asks for some new workers; she wants changes in outings and direction in activities. The patient is creating her own identity within a safe structure. Her actual self is beginning to evolve and emerge. Selfishness is a natural and welcome part of that growth. While the staff cannot seem to jump high enough in the Emergent Stage it also must gently provide guidelines and reassurance.

This is a time when a patient becomes curious about her world, a welcome development because it means she is turning her focus outward and taking an interest in other things for their own sake. It is a time for learning by trial and error. One young girl apologized to me for a tantrum she had during this phase. 'I'm sorry I acted so immaturely,' she wrote, 'I want to be like a normal thirteen-year-old and normal thirteen-year-olds don't get so upset if they can't go for a walk.'

Then she went on to say:

> I know that you can tell the difference between me or my head, so I listed the reasons why I want to go on walks and why my head wants me to. The reasons why he wants me to are:
>   I'll gain weight if I don't keep going.
>   I need to burn more calories.
>   I'm lazy if I don't go.
>   Everyone including clients do way more than me.
>   I must do the same amount of activity that I did yesterday.
> The reasons why I would like to go on a walk are:
>   I'm 13 and like to get out and do things.
>   I love to get fresh air and be outside.
>   I have a lot of fun looking in stores.
>   It's summer and the weather is getting warm and sunny.
>   It really distracts me and takes me away from most of my problems into the real world for a while.

As the patient comes to trust her surroundings, she gives clues to the counselor about what is going on in her head. If the counselor is trained to interpret the secret language of the Negative Mind, the patient will be relieved and will lean more heavily on him.

For instance, we had given a food list consisting of six eating times in a twenty-four-hour period to an eleven-year-old boy in the Emergent Stage. Tim's Negative Mind had instructed him not to comply. His caregiver phoned me and asked how to address this situation.

I spent time on the phone with Tim, who asked, 'Did you say that there was no option to eating this yam?'

I knew that I had never made that statement, but I quickly realized Tim needed me to insist on it.

'Yes,' I replied. 'There is absolutely no option.'

Tim said, 'I thought so. I was just checking.' He wanted the yam but could not bring himself to eat it without permission from an authority figure. He was not yet at the point at which he felt he deserved the food and his Negative Mind was strongly disallowing it.

Tim was prohibited from expressing his desire for the yam because if he did, the increased negativity would be unbearable. He could only hope that he would be understood and I would respond as I did.

The patient's outward behavior may not indicate what is really happening at this stage. She is eager to allow someone to side with her against the condition. But until she comes to this point, there are severe ramifications from the Negative Mind for cooperating with the caregivers. So it is indeed an exceedingly brave thing for the patient to ask for help.

Distraction continues to be the best way to offset the ceaseless negative chatter the patient must endure immediately after eating. Telling stories or playing board games such as Scrabble and Monopoly that require a redirection of the patient's concentration are great diversionary tactics. Before the Reality Stage (see page 181), the patient's concentration is at best sporadic. However, most of the time, distraction serves to bring the patient past the hardest moment.

In the Emergent Stage, a victim's relationship with her parents (if she is on twenty-four-hour care) is tentative. She is so conditioned to feel pain vicariously that she uses her best virtue – her sensitivity – against herself. She may wait for any nuance of projected need from loved ones. The internal mental battle waging inside the patient's head is difficult to objectify and understand for parents and family who love their child and are ever present to her emotional needs.

Parents often do not understand why their children do not want to see them, though they can easily communicate by phone. As I've mentioned in the last chapter, the reason is obscure but valid. Parents are the people who mean most to the victim and whose opinion is paramount to her. Victims generally love their parents so much that they feel guilty for allowing themselves to eat in front of them. They still see themselves as unworthy and find it extremely difficult to permit themselves any pleasure since they have surely not protected their parents from all earthly ills, and in fact have brought them anguish by becoming ill.

It seems selfish to patients to admit openly that they are allowing themselves to partake of life. They still believe they have disappointed their parents, although generally, parents have not encouraged their children to think this way.

Patients may display much anger in the Emergent Stage, lashing out at times, and then immediately becoming repentant and self-abusive. It is imperative for caregivers to respond kindly and supportively, explaining the behavior to patients with no sense of judgment or reward and punishment. The Negative Mind will use any reproof against its victim. Further castigation is counterproductive since it confirms the CNC mindset.

Patients may swing from despair to hope as the Actual Mind begins to emerge from the shadows. As Marci wrote in her diary at this stage:

Life sucks and then you die! This is the saying that keeps running through my mind continuously every day now. It's getting harder. I'm having a very hard time right now having to accept the changes that are going on. Sometimes I feel like I'm ready to quit this fight but I know I can't give up because I have quite a long life ahead of me and I feel like I have a lot that I could offer to others. It's the day-to-day struggles that are difficult and hard to face sometimes, but I know that I'm going to make it, and I'll be happy and stronger because of it.

THE REALITY STAGE: 50 PERCENT TO 68 PERCENT

The Reality Stage begins at 50 percent on the Life Wellness Scale. At this point, the Actual Mind is equally as strong as the Negative Mind. And though the patient generally continues to hear a voice, albeit subdued in her head, as often as not, she has the strength to veto the negative mental activity.

As the patient continues through the Reality Stage, she will grow more accustomed to trying new things in the world. As she realizes she is capable of these small maneuvers, her confidence and identity grow.

Somewhere between 50 and 60 percent, the patient is likely to change her demeanor. The tentative, anxious mood will become assured and generally happy. The patient will be able to talk of her attitudes and perceived issues without as much subjectivity. The world will no longer seem an unfriendly, frightening, and foreign place. The patient will no longer perceive her past to have been in vain and her future impossible. This is a glorious thing to see. Witnessing a person's wonderful uniqueness emerge from the dampened spirit that first entered the clinic is simply amazing.

Though patients will be on care for most of this stage, the constant monitoring will ease radically and they will experience some planned free time. Now, they look forward to parental visits and even enjoy them.

The patient is beginning to respond normally and is gently able to put the world into perspective a better part of the time. She starts to enjoy small parts of life without too much guilt. Even desires and wants can be discovered and fulfilled successfully.

One patient wrote to me, 'I just want to let you know I'm so happy being in my new room. It's great. Life is almost a bed of roses. There are just a few odds and sods, and a few weeds to be dug up. Every day is a learning experience. Last night I went on my first big major solo voyage to town. It may not be the best sightseeing spot, but it was like the Bahamas to me. . . . Well, I must go now. My snack is calling me.'

Many victims have lived in fear for so long that they are used to being anxious. Soft and firm encouragement, always with unconditional support, lends them a structure to fall back on if they attempt to move forward sooner than they are able.

During this period patients begin to venture out for one of six or seven daily snacks. They will make these restaurant visits initially with counselors or team leaders who are completely aware of how to interpret every nuance or innuendo patients suggest. The staff is well-schooled in eating disorder behavior and therefore adept at averting any of the patient's negativity.

A careworker and I accompanied Abbie to a restaurant. It was the first time she had eaten a normal dinner in a setting outside the clinic. The careworker and I ordered the identical meal of salmon, vegetables, and mashed potatoes. After Abbie had ordered, she became increasingly agitated waiting for the food to arrive.

Suddenly she leaned over in her chair and whispered quietly to me, 'When the food comes, please insist that I eat it, no matter what I say out loud.'

The waiter brought our meals, and almost on cue, Abbie announced forcefully, 'I'm not going to eat that. You better not try to make me.'

I replied firmly yet gently, 'Yes, you are, darling. There's no argument here.'

Abbie gratefully ate her salmon, her eyes swimming from the success of the battle.

The courage to appear normal by eating in a restaurant poses two problems for the tentative patient. The first is that she is afraid that others will see her as being recovered. She will appear physically well before her head has joined her. She is afraid that if others perceive her as cured before she is able to accept responsibility, she will feel overwhelmed, less protected, and will crash again. A patient will generally give many indications whether she needs care or is 'safe' without it. At this point, she is able to verbally and physically ask for help.

'Safety' depends on whether the patient is able to effect her will without the instructions of the Negative Mind overriding it.

One of the main focuses during the Reality Stage is to continue to help the patient develop her identity. The Negative Mind robs the patient of her ability to make decisions about likes and dislikes. Now she begins to ask her careworker for help in choosing among options. The careworker need only guide and perhaps reinforce likes or dislikes of the person he sees emerging by throwing the question back to the patient. 'What would you like to do?' he might ask, or 'How does that feel to you?'

The Reality Stage invites reason. Finally the emotions keep pace with the intellect. One of my patients wrote to me as he was reaching the end of this stage: 'Montreux is all about challenges, yours as well as mine. It is no small task that you've set yourself, and you must have hard days as well as good ones too. But as I am learning daily, nothing valuable in life comes easily or without work.'

The patient becomes much more responsive in counseling sessions. It is during these sessions that we begin to focus on the Objectivity Training and role-playing that I described in the previous chapter. We might discuss how the patient can put a parent's divorce or other stressful trigger into the appropriate context. The preoccupation that formerly existed with the Negative Mind is subsiding. Between 55 and 65 percent of the patient's Actual Mind is present enough to begin understanding her own preferences and choices. She starts taking an interest in her clothes. Rather than the layered look, which patients wear in the Acute Stage to avoid detection of the seriousness of their illness, clothes begin to have a style, an identity, a definition, a color.

As well, other tendencies for honing one's personality will appear. Michelle likes the piano and tennis. She is doing it for the sheer enjoyment of it, no longer chased into 'having to.' Robin is taking a veterinarian course at the local college. 'Animals are more dependable than people,' she says and grins impishly. Sophia is a poetess and actress of the best order. Chuck plays violin. Andy skates and makes pottery.

Everyone loves art – and what these patients create is

amazingly observant and representative of the human condition. The Reality Stage is exciting because the patient's personality is beginning to emerge and establish itself with more than a hint of independence.

As this stage progresses, the individual's confidence increases (as in adolescence) until it grows to a false sense of ability – a confidence necessary for emotional establishment different from whatever the status quo indicates as imperative. The patient rebels. She chooses anything different than what is the norm. She is trying her wings, her independence.

This pendulum swing (at 65 percent) is a wonderful sight to caregivers and counselors, who can have a hard time comprehending that this manifestation could occur within the same year and in the same body that offered no hope earlier.

If the patient is not actually a teenager, the pendulum swing lasts for no more than two or three months – a relatively short period for adolescence. If she is, it seems (though there are many variables involved) the teenager has no need to engage in extreme normal teenage behavior, such as breaking rules. It is possible she feels she has already 'done it.' Of course, this is not true of all cases.

There is an interesting point to be noted at this juncture concerning parental attitudes when a child is released to them. Before the manifestation of anorexia, parents generally had a view of their child as being incredibly agreeable all of the time. Remember that most patients have spent their conscious pre-anorexia hours in consideration of others. Unconsciously, parents may take this attitude for granted and assume the extremely cooperative individual they knew before will come home again in exactly the same way, minus the eating disorder symptoms. In some cases, particularly when the patients are children, this will not be the case.

However, if parents think about it, they will realize that all they really wanted earlier was a healthy, normal, sometimes selfish and rambunctious teenager. What they had to endure was a living nightmare. It sometimes comes as a shock to them that the effects of 'curing' an individual necessarily result in her becoming 'normalized.' In other words, the recovering anorexia patient will become a healthy person and occasionally an unreasonable and demanding one. Though she will always be caring of others' needs, she will allow her needs to take precedence some of the time.

This is as it should be. Balance is sanity.

During the first two stages of therapy, it is important to maintain the consistency of whatever caregiving team was in place when the patient arrived. As the patient moves into the Reality Stage, it now becomes productive to change counselors and even careworkers. These new people bring a refreshing vision and avert dependency, both for the sake of the patient and the counselor.

Before any change is made, however, the intermediate counselor gets to know the patient so that the transition is smooth and nonthreatening. He does this by joining the acute counselor in some session work at the end of the Emergent Stage. By the time the patient lets go of the acute counselor, she is generally eager to move on and confident that her former counselor will never close his door to her should she have a concern or a question.

The Reality Stage requires a quick mind in the intermediate counselor. He becomes an instructor and teacher of the first order. He has different guidelines than that of his previous colleague, but he need be at least as alert.

The patient, though she will be feeling her own way, will be looking for approval or boundaries. The counselor is in the same precarious position that a parent would be at this stage – guiding wisely, gently, yet firmly if it becomes necessary.

Because the counselor must prepare the patient for the world, his will be a trial-and-error role. The patient will need and want the safe structure of a reference point as she ventures to test her identity and her world. Given that the Negative Mind still has a healthy portion of control, it behooves the counselor to persuade the patient away from it. She will quickly accept his advice because she is not as frightened of the negative voice. She can now regard the Negative Mind more as a nuisance.

The danger during the middle of this stage, roughly around 60 to 65 percent, is that the individual may feel a false sense of courage, as does an adolescent, and may strive to be off care before she is capable of doing so. Again, we can compare her behavior to someone who is fifteen or sixteen, still needing guidelines yet eager to try things in the world.

If the patient continues to insist, 'I am fine and can deal with everything now,' then we may give her a trial period to prove whether she is correct.

The danger of stopping treatment is obvious. The Negative Mind could gain ground, and the patient might regress. Erring on the side of caution leads to a quicker recovery in the long run.

This is a time when positive self-esteem or 'self-regard' – self-acknowledgment and acceptance of who one is – begins to develop. However, 'Who I am' may not be at all what the family, loved ones, or even the patient expect.

Ironically, most of my patients discover that at a time

when they are truly able to appreciate their external achievement – good grades, trophies, awards, which they had previously garnered only to please others – they find that their achievements do not matter as much to them.

One acute patient had qualified for the Olympics as a runner. When she got better, she stopped running entirely; it was no longer important to her. Another, who had set herself on the path of gymnastics, discovered after her recovery that the sport did not interest her.

THE INTERACTIVE STAGE:
68 PERCENT TO 80 PERCENT

By the time the patient moves from the Reality Stage into the Interactive Stage, she feels as if blinders have been lifted from her eyes. One of the comments I hear frequently now is, 'I feel as if I am conscious, living again, whereas I was in a surreal daze before.' In the Interactive Stage, Marci wrote to me:

> I'm so happy today. While I was on my way to my session, I felt like I was going to burst because I was just so full of happiness. I had just come from my interview and was thinking about what I said and how far I've come. And I just felt like Yes! Look at me now. I'm so proud of myself and the person I've become. Basically you could say that I'm Lovin' Life. This feeling is amazing. I'm high on life. . . .
>
> The person I've become, or should I say, the person that was never let out is also amazing. I feel so energetic inside. I'm more outgoing and less self-conscious or worried about what everyone else will

think of me. There are still things that I am working on but it's like a lot of things in life. They take time. Besides, I had been sick for as long as I could remember.

This, from someone who just a scant few months earlier had proclaimed, 'Life sucks and then you die!' The Negative Mind has little jurisdiction at this time. Indeed, as we can see from Marci's letter, at this stage, the Negative Mind has mostly seeped away, and certainly the eating disorder manifestation is gone. Another patient said to me, 'It's not about anorexia now; it's about learning confidence.' At its worst, in the beginning of the stage, the CNC has a little less than 35 percent clout.

Even so, the patient still needs support. There are things to work on. We cannot regard the fact that she is doing well in her battle against CNC as a sign of complete safety. As CNC grew initially, then subsided, so could it grow again without proper attention. The patient has a better chance to outwit CNC now that she has the tools of understanding to work with. However, after all that labor, why take the chance?

The danger is of course, now that the patient feels as well as she does – probably better than she has in her lifetime – she is eager to surge forward without help. If she does this prematurely, she is risking everything she strove for. In order to prevent a relapse, the counselor must teach her as much as she can learn in the time allotted.

One of the counselor's main goals is to help her understand her options in the outside world and the consequences of her choices. She is learning how to live responsibly. Like a young bird learning to fly from its nest, the patient wants to step away from her safety net a little. She is exploring with her counselors exactly what this may mean to her.

The patient learns to understand motivation from an objective, rational, humanistic perspective. She can then accept varying points of view, without being self-righteous about her own. As one patient wrote to me, 'I've come to learn, for instance, patience. By learning that patience, I am a lot more content inside and with others.' The patient will spend this period of time researching her personal needs in an effort to comprehend what brought her to the eating disorder manifestation.

The counselor will ask the patient, 'What do you think you might be afraid of? Who will your friends be? How will your family react to your wellness?' Though the patient is familiar with her home environment, she will eventually be facing it with a completely different interpretation of herself in it. This thought can be at the same time exciting and alarming. Confidence of her 'new' identity will take time and testing.

Fears about how to be in the world will be addressed in many ways. Gentle discussions of rationality will be the subject of many sessions. If a patient is concerned about her interactive skills – after all, the eating disorder may have stalled her social life for a long time – the counselor can place her in an atmosphere of her choice, to work on them. Often this involves volunteer work outside the clinic. At other times, it can be doing puzzles with or reading stories to people in the Acute Stage. These interactions depend on the individual's nature and desires.

One patient who became involved in helping others at the clinic wrote to me, 'Work has been a great experience for me. I don't even like to call it work, because I don't feel like I'm working. I just feel like I'm being a friend who is giving support to a friend in need.'

During this period of intensive learning, an adult patient becomes a 'residential outpatient.' Although she still lives mostly in the clinic, as she reaches the end of the Interactive Stage, she moves out. She is encouraged to live with one or two other adult patients in the same stage of care in an apartment near the clinic. She learns how to exist in the community and how to make her own choices without fear. She develops as many friends outside the clinic as within.

Many outlets become available to the patient at this juncture. The Educational Program classes of afternoon school are usually about subjects the patients-students do not learn in the normal school setting. Comparing societies and their value systems, for instance, teaches patients not to take any one society too seriously. Studying habits that explain other peoples and societies as well as the microcosm of their personal circumstances teaches patients not to take themselves so seriously either.

Patients do amazing project studies and submit reports. They are remarkably wonderful students who are leaving their negativity behind them and reaching out with a curiosity unhampered by worrying about what everyone thinks. By this stage, patients can have extra tutoring with specific help from home if they want to continue with studies that may have been interrupted by illness.

Patients in the Interactive Stage sometimes study an instrument they enjoyed while they were on full care in the program. They study art, opera, museums, or architecture if that is their wish. One or two patients decided to write a play on the anorexic condition. Other patients joined outside poetry classes and put their art into displays. If patients are of age, they are able to get driver's licenses. Some take classes at a local junior college. By this time, each person indicates her personal interests, and we support her as much as possible.

The interactive patient must prove to herself and her counselors that she is ready for almost anything. The body language and gentle confidence of this stage are wonderful to see. From the once desolate, fearful patient has emerged a courageous, self-assured, aware individual fully able to take her place in society. Her gait is no longer downcast with humility. She makes eye contact with no hesitation and walks with assurance.

During the Interactive Stage, the patient spends much time forming and honing her identity. Toward the end, she often expresses a wish to try short visits at home to prepare for the final phase, that of Environmental Integration.

The patient will spend much session time with the companionship of her family, studying and explaining points of similarity and differences in family members' attitudes and deeds, past and present. For this session work, parents come to the clinic. Before the patient goes into the last phase of therapy, she will theoretically have figured out a way to live compatibly with her family. The theory will be put into practice once she gets home.

It is important, though, to remind parents that their children are returning to them as they would and should have been, had they followed their natural road to development. Surely, then, they will not be perfect. We would not want them to be.

THE ENVIRONMENTAL INTEGRATION
STAGE: 80 PERCENT TO 86 PERCENT

As the patient readies for her home trial period, the last part of therapy, she feels both excitement and trepidation. She has built up home in her mind and despite how wonderful it may be, it is almost always initially anticlimactic to get back to reality. The first month or two are anxiety-ridden for families, who struggle to absorb this 'new' individual into their conception of the way things are.

Counselors instruct parents and siblings in sessions, in front of the patient, not to walk on eggshells around her but to have gentle understanding that her world is as new to her as she is to them.

Usually the well-being and acclimatization of the individual depends on the character of her home environment. Ideally, she will return to a supportive, positive environment. Ideally, family and loved ones realize the deep journey the patient has just made and are prepared to gently accommodate her first year at home where she will glean more stability in her environment. This can be likened to a convalescent period after a long hospital stay. Or one might compare it to bringing home a new baby. It takes a while for everyone to get used to the new arrival. Parents who have returned from the edge of the abyss will naturally be worried, and they are bound to misconstrue some of the signs when they see their child acting in normal ways – being a teenager, for example. Teenagers typically magnify the degree to which others notice and criticize them. A teen's lament that 'Everybody in school hates me' need not prefigure a relapse into an eating disorder.

While the recovered patient is not the emotionally frail person she once was, it is nevertheless important that families seek appropriate therapy to resolve the stressful situations that act as barriers to caring.

After two months at home, the patient returns to the clinic for her first last-phase assessment, the duration of which will depend entirely on her stability during the time that has elapsed. Generally she will discuss things that did or didn't create problems for her on the home front.

If the counselor deems his patient safe to continue her home phase, she will return home after eight or twelve days of daily double sessions. If, on the other hand, the patient seems unprepared for the Environmental Integration phase, then she will continue her objectivity training as an outpatient at the clinic. This extension can last anywhere from two to three months except under unusual circumstances.

If things go well, the patient will return home after a normal assessment period to continue her second phase of adjustment, which lasts four months unless otherwise indicated. At this time, the patient generally makes a remarkable positive leap ahead and sets aside all wariness. She begins living in full swing.

Generally there is great variation in what happens after this point in therapy. During the whole time that the patient has been home, she can phone the counselors as needed, who will troubleshoot any problems as they arise. It is usually a shock to families to find that their children are establishing their needs, sometimes, necessarily, before those of their parents. However, most families are delighted with their child's growth and desire to grow, and interactions with siblings are a great relief, even if they involve 'normal' squabbles.

After the first two visits back to the clinic for assessment, the patient is eager to get on with her life and would rather keep in contact by phone even though the program asks that she come back again in six months. In roughly half the cases, the patient returns on the six-month visit period merely to prove, with a grin, that she needn't have. This visit provides her time to catch up with patients who were just entering the clinic during her assessment times. The time is enlightening to all and much fun.

Some of the patients who entered the program at the same time as others ask to schedule their return assessment times together for an 'old home' week. They compare tales as any normal graduates would. One of the most gratifying experiences is that they always want to encourage the patients new to the program. The interactions between new and former patients bring tears to many eyes. The former patients are, after all, proof of incredible potential, patience, and humanism.

It generally takes a year in the home environment for the 'patient' to feel comfortable and at peace with her new identity. During that time, she is getting used to her new sense of self and may be more vulnerable to disturbances around her such as a parent's or a friend's divorce or substance abuse, or an upset at school or at work. She may well find it helpful to work with a therapist at home in order to come to terms with any such issues.

Patients in the process of recovery discover their actual, potential self, what some might call their true self. They achieve what humanistic psychologist Abraham Maslow referred to as 'self-actualization.'

Self-love and acceptance appear to be a natural evolution in development. When a person realizes her self outside of what she perceives the needs of others to be, she finds it very natural to love and take joy in living.

WHY 86 PERCENT AND NOT 100 PERCENT?

Readers will note that our Montreux Life Wellness Scale ends at 86 percent, not 100 percent. This underscores our core philosophy at the clinic: our stress on human limitations. No one can ever be 100 percent anything; nor should we strive to be. Every aspect of this therapy stresses acceptance and compassion for our imperfections. How better to arm anyone for the hurdles of life than to teach her to ask nothing from others except mutual respect and kindness. Understanding this concept allows objectivity and compassion.

The very nature of the percentile scale indicates the imperfectability of mankind. Eighty-six percent allows for 14 percent imperfection. Eighty-six percent represents that this is as perfect as we can or ought to be. To quote Robert Browning:

> What I aspired to be,
> And was not, comforts me.
> . . .
> Ah, but a man's reach
> should exceed his grasp,
> Or what's a heaven for?

No matter how deeply or thoroughly we strive to understand ourselves, we still have our human moments. Learning how to be objective, how to see the good of life rather than what is not wonderful will help the journey.

I clearly remember one of my first lessons. One hot summer day when I was a child, I had fallen off my bike; a very sweaty woman had hugged me; and I had lost my silver locket in the stream ALL IN THE SAME DAY. I was crying when a wise man I knew stopped to ask me what was the matter.

I answered, 'Not one but three bad things happened to me today, and I don't know that I can bear it.'

'Bear it! Three things! Only three?' he asked incredulously, shaking his head. 'Here, wipe your tears, and when twelve things happen in your day that aren't pleasing to you, come to me, and cry.'

Twelve bad things have never happened to me in one day. No day has ever been that bad, and that was a long time ago, several lifetimes, I think. Life is, finally, only pertinent in our translation of it.

Our program is about teaching objectivity: seeing the world as it really is rather than as it appears. That is its essential component. Objectivity allows a 'no-fault,' 'no-blame' situation. Its purpose is to allow a person to reinterpret the world so that she can appreciate what motivates others' behavior rather than seeing herself as the cause or blame for it. Her attitude will naturally then become one of understanding and caringness in a positive way.

CNC victims are naturally frightened of the world because it presents to them negative responsibility. Patients who have recovered have learned not to take things personally or demonize those who seem to harm them. They do not lose their sense of caring or compassion for others. They do not lose their essential kind nature; they are merely able to put it into better perspective. They are more able to create a balance between themselves and others.

An acute anorexic stands like a willow wand buffeted by the winds of others' needs, blowing back and forth in accordance with what she perceives others demand of her; this is naturally an exhausting process. When she has recovered, she finds that she can stand anchored in place, able to reach out and choose for herself what she needs and how she wants to respond to the needs of others. She has more energy to respond to those needs because she has more physical wellness, emotional balance, and a secure sense of self.

7

On Love and Healing:
The Challenges at Home

How do you know if your child or loved one is on the road toward developing an eating disorder? How do you recognize the warning signs? What can you do if your loved one develops anorexia or bulimia? Can you prevent the condition from becoming acute? In this chapter I will attempt to answer some of these important questions.

But first a few caveats. If you suspect that your child has a predisposition for Confirmed Negativity condition, it may be possible to prevent it from developing into an eating disorder. However, bear in mind that I am not fully convinced it is always possible to do so, even if parents and loved ones do everything in their power. I am reluctant to provide the opportunity for parents and sufferers to shoulder any more blame than they have already experienced.

I want to reemphasize that as a parent or loved one, you are not to blame for the sufferer's condition. However, I need to draw a distinction between exemption from blame and responsibility.

As parents, you are responsible for your child while she is in your care. You did not cause your child's condition, but you have the responsibility for helping her get the right help. More than anything, you can offer hope, love, and optimism, if not understanding. When your child realizes that neither she nor you are to blame and that you are willing to understand what she is feeling, that in itself helps relieve the terrible pressure feeding her Negative Mind.

Allow me to offer some guidelines that may help sensitive children and their parents, friends, families, and other loved ones face the challenges at home.

DETECTING THE CNC PREDISPOSITION

There are certain character traits that may help us determine whether a person has a predisposition toward Confirmed Negativity Condition.

Often CNC dispositions become apparent at an early age. These young people develop a sense of responsibility well beyond their tender years. As I explained in Chapter 2, most parents tell me they knew almost from the beginning that something was different about their child. They recall how she was worried, concerned, or overly responsible at an unusually early age.

Also, in Chapter 3, I mentioned how highly sensitive CNC-predisposed youngsters are. They overreact to the slightest family squabble. Here I do not mean to minimize the misery caused by truly 'dysfunctional' families, which certainly do exist and cause damage. But I am drawing a distinction between genuine dysfunction and how a child with CNC perceives the world.

Amanda, for instance, appeared outwardly cheerful and sociable. All during her childhood, however, she grew up listening to her big sister, Eileen, complain about how Amanda received favored treatment at her expense. I did not find this demonstrably so, but apparently

Amanda accepted her sister's interpretation of events. She later developed anorexia and moved out of the house so that Eileen 'could have it all.'

As I mentioned in Chapter 2, many have suggested that eating disorders develop in children after they experience some stressful or traumatic event. I have found it far more common, however, for sensitive children in these situations to be affected by the stress and trauma that befall their loved ones. They worry much more about others than they do about themselves.

Although I believe these children will perceive a crisis where there is none, real crises can cause the CNC to manifest itself as an eating disorder that much more quickly. A parent's or sibling's physical ailment – and the child's inability to cure it – are obvious triggers. Tricia's mother had cancer; Claire's father had heart surgery; Meg's sister had been in a car accident. One little girl watched her two older siblings go into intensive care because of physical crises; she held her breath searching her parents' faces for a sign of relief indicating her siblings might survive. Three years later, at age eight, she developed anorexia. Another anorexic girl I treated asked me, 'How is it that my being born caused my mother's cancer?'

These children all responded to crisis by trying to parent their parents. In their caringness and kindness, they immediately made themselves responsible, equally, at least to their parents – and vulnerable.

Children with a predisposition to CNC also seem to find doom everywhere. Of course, in our society, it's not hard to find: Think of the headline news on the radio and TV and in the newspapers – death and destruction everywhere. It seems not to be a coincidence that so many of my patients have been exposed to soap operas. Here they ingest a steady diet of betrayal, rape, and even murder in the afternoon. But what appears as escapist fare to us is the stuff of nightmares to them. These children work diligently trying to offset the pessimistic view of life gleaned from such shows by attempting to make their own families that much safer.

Most parents describe children with the CNC predisposition as uncommonly selfless, altruistic, and sensitive. They are deferential and compliant toward others to a fault. They live with their antennae alert to everyone around them even as, it seems, they cannot receive transmissions of their own needs.

Thus, CNC may evolve into an eating disorder after some traumatic event in the family when subjectivity has the upper hand.

PREVENTING AN EATING DISORDER FROM DEVELOPING

As I explained earlier, it may be impossible to prevent an eating disorder from manifesting. However, there are some precautions parents can take with their CNC-predisposed youngsters that may help.

Insist That Kids Be Kids

It is perhaps too easy to allow a competent, intelligent child to take responsibility when it is actually inappropriate for her to do so. If it makes our busy, stressful lives easier, how can we turn down her heartfelt offers of help?

Nevertheless, we must. It is imperative for parents to be parents. A child should not take on adult roles and responsibilities even though she may – in fact, probably will – possess extraordinary capabilities to do so. Nor should we unwittingly allow her to become our confidante. Our children are not and must not be our best friends, therapists, or marriage counselors. The CNC-predisposed individual will assume need if parents ache, and will naturally try to fix any problem that she perceives. But in so doing, she may set aside her own developmental needs and in her mind necessarily become a full-fledged counselor. It sounds like such a cliché, but it is vital to let our children be children. It is helpful to encourage normal childlike behavior and discourage adult behavior such as taking undue responsibility.

Seek Outside Help for Family Troubles

Families with marital strife or other anxieties and tensions would benefit from seeking appropriate counseling from qualified professionals or friends and adult extended-family members. This serves several purposes:

It provides families the help they need.
It relieves the child's anxiety and distress about the family's troubles.
It takes the responsibility for 'fixing' the problem from the child's hands.
It demonstrates to the child that her parents are in charge.
It sends the message that it is okay to get help when it is needed.

A vulnerable person with CNC will use family strife to feed her Negative Mind. And while these triggers do not cause an eating disorder, they add to the victim's stress, and they will impede the progress of her recovery. They are more fuel for her self-consuming fire. As a parent or loved one, it is imperative for you to take a searching look at your life with the victim and identify those triggers. I say this with trepidation because I do not want parents to waste their precious energy blaming themselves instead of giving a victim the help she needs. Here again, it is important to draw a distinction between the laying of blame and the responsibility to change a harmful situation. That responsibility is yours. The challenge of addressing an eating disorder is great enough without putting more impediments in the way of healing.

We are all human. We have all made mistakes, advertently or not. As you'll see, it is a parent's role to teach his or her child about the imperfectability of human nature. When your loved one has progressed to a stage at which she can judge the situation objectively, you and she will most likely need to work through the issues with the help of a qualified therapist.

Encourage Your Child to Accept Imperfection

In addition, we must allow our children the imperfections of childhood. We can point out often that we are all human, while we remember to have patience with their mistakes. When we teach CNC-predisposed youngsters that childhood and adolescence are a necessary time of trial and error, we can help them let go of some of their overwhelming sense of perfection and responsibility.

When your child makes a mistake and is upset about it, gently remind him that it's okay to make mistakes, that you love him no matter what, that no one can or ever should try to be perfect. Encourage your child to try things for the love of it. Many children with CNC are reluctant to try something if they can't do it perfectly from the start; for them it's all or nothing. Try to coax them gently from a world of black and white to a rainbow of grays. If a child seems dead set on achievement, discuss with her what she finds meaningful in the effort and help her realize that you don't have any expectations of her. I would be concerned about a child who frets constantly over grades, who overstudies for every exam, and who is crushed by anything less than an A+.

Set Respectful Boundaries

Children also need to know that their parents will rationally and respectfully provide structure and boundaries. Extremely sensitive children benefit from households in which the adults have set reasonable rules rather than having everything decided by committee. The parents of CNC-predisposed children should be mindful of their offspring's greater need for security in the form of adults' respectful authority. These children need a firm platform, even if it is not the one they ultimately choose. In fact, healthy growth can include a child's opposition to the status quo, whatever it may be, simply for the sake of establishing her own identity. Moderation comes with maturity, not necessarily adulthood.

Children and youth need the encouragement of being believed in despite their differences in personality from their parents. Children also need to believe in their parents' strength and the stability of their circumstances, even in today's age of divorce and anxiety. The more adult friends, family, and counselors who support parents through the stumbling blocks of life, the more relatives who provide other perspectives that can influence the child, perhaps the more able the child will be to grasp an objective reality.

Put Problems into Perspective

Because the CNC-predisposed child is so sensitive to trauma and crisis, it is crucial not to blow up small problems into big ones. Parents can make clear to their child that life's annoyances are, after all, just annoyances. We can say, for example, 'Oh, well, we missed the bus. We'll just wait for the next one,' rather than 'Oh my heavens. We missed the bus. Now what will we do?' It may also be helpful to point out that the pessimistic news that grabs the headlines may not be an accurate reflection of reality. Discuss with your child how the media use negativity to capture our attention. I am not advocating that you sugarcoat the world's woes, only that you give your children a context for understanding them. Always make it clear that these are adult problems requiring adult solutions. For those children too young to appreciate the context (recall the preschooler I counseled who absorbed daily negativity from TV news coverage while sitting on his mother's lap), I would recommend keeping the radio and TV off while the child is within earshot.

Help Your Child Cope with Life's Issues

If we address 'issues' with optimism, hopefulness, and objectivity, the CNC-predisposed child will have fewer long-lasting effects than if she were convinced that she has been wronged and she lives with the fear that life is out to get her. A person with CNC will enlarge her problems to include whatever her parents did not do for her when she was young, whether it be buying her enough clothes in high school or concerning themselves adequately with needed orthodontia. Such 'wrongs' will sometimes border on the ridiculous.

Intervene When Your Child Puts Herself Down

When you hear your child making self-deprecating remarks ('I can't do anything right'; 'That was a horrible drawing'; 'I'm the worst batter in the whole world'), step in and gently try to correct your child's perspective. Don't let your child blow up a single specific incident to a global indictment of himself ('I'm always screwing up'). Say things like, 'Well, you missed that pitch, but that's no big deal. Everybody misses sometime. If it's not fun, why not try something else?' Encourage her to focus on the positives about herself instead of beating herself up for perceived or even real flaws.

Encourage Your Child to Explore Her Interests – Not Yours

If a CNC-predisposed child shows interest in any given subject, it is important that parents work with this interest in a moderate way without giving the youngster the idea that they have expectations about her level of attainment. It would be helpful to repeat, 'You're fine the way you are.' I would be watchful for children who pursue something with the hope of pleasing you rather than themselves.

Be wary of presenting an expectation to excel. If a child guesses that her parents have high expectations – 'We want you to be the best' – she will do her utmost to please them. Indeed, I even become nervous saying to one of my own children or patients, 'Good for you; you make me so proud.' I prefer, 'I really enjoyed looking at that. Thanks for showing it to me.'

Many of us were raised to believe that one should finish what one starts, that quitting is failure. I have seen many people with CNC doggedly pursue perfection in a field, regardless of how truly interested in it they are. It may help parents to remind their sensitive children that they should feel free to drop something if its pursuit doesn't bring them real pleasure, that they should follow their true passions, lest they be seduced into fulfilling the perceived expectations of others.

The consistent message should be 'Whatever you do is okay by me, as long as it is done with respect to yourself and others.' However, there is a fine line here. When a patient asks me, 'Are you proud of me?' I always reply, 'It's not my place to be proud of anybody. I am me and you are you. I love you no matter what you do or don't do. You're not living for me.' I do not want to buy into a patient's living to please me rather than herself.

This is not as easy as it sounds. Sometimes parents work very hard not to create expectations of their children, yet sensitive youngsters perceive them nonetheless. The parenting that works for children of normal sensitivity may not accommodate the needs of hypersensitive children. A thoughtless remark from a parent ('I expect better from you' or 'Why can't you try a little harder?') might be shrugged off by the first child, while the hypersensitive one would take it wholly to heart and dwell on it for months.

Myra and Jonathan, two loving parents who were highly successful in their careers, brought their daughter to my clinic and said, 'We love Stephanie just the way she is. We don't care what she does. We don't care if she's rich or famous or adheres to our values, as long as she's alive.'

'Tell her that,' I replied. 'Perhaps you have never felt you had to, but she has developed expectations of herself, based not on what you've said to her, but on who you are, your professions. She believes you expect the same of her without your having said a word.'

Naturally, we wish our children well in the world and will encourage them in their natural talents, but while we do this, we must explain to them that if following their talents into a career is their choice, that is wonderful, but if they do not choose to do this, but wish to choose an alternative profession or lifestyle, it is just as wonderful. And we have to mean what we say.

If your child fails to get a part in the school play or a spot on the team, you might say, 'It doesn't matter. Did you have fun trying out?' I would even be wary of statements such as 'Don't worry. You did your best.' These set up an expectation that the child has to do his or her best for you or that her best was not good enough.

I counseled one family whose son had been sick for many years. I told them, 'Jeffrey is going to be a wonderful person. I can't tell you what his likes and dislikes will be. I cannot tell you who he is going to be; I can only tell you that he is going to be terrific.'

After eight months, as Jeff's marvelous and unique personality began to emerge, his parents started to express plans for their son, what he was and was not allowed to do, and so on. They were both creating expectations and putting conditions on their love. This was counterproductive because Jeff could be only who he was meant to be.

The only thing that saved Jeff was that he had learned enough objectivity by then to understand his parents as people with their own fallibilities rather than as authorities of anyone else's direction.

It is imperative to accept our children and let them exist on their own terms, no matter what their values, sexual orientation, beliefs, or preferences. These need not match ours. We cannot assume that our own values are the only right ones or impose them on anyone else. Our children are not our property; we have merely the right and the responsibility to guide them and interact with them. Ultimately, they are who they are. In the words of poet Kahlil Gibran,

> They come through you but not from you,
> And though they are with you yet they belong not to
>   you.
> You may give them your love but not your thoughts,
> For they have their own thoughts.

WARNING SIGNS OF EATING DISORDERS

A child with Confirmed Negativity Condition is set up for an eating disorder before he or she ever manifests it. Sometimes the signs are obvious; sometimes they are subtle. As I explained in Chapter 4, not all anorexics or bulimics are underweight, so family and friends must be attentive to other signs.

Many parents are understandably concerned when their children go on diets, particularly if they are a normal weight to begin with. But how does one distinguish between a child's 'normal' – if misguided – attempt at weight loss and the manifestation of an eating disorder? After all, eating disorders are common in teenagers and people in their twenties, particularly among females (although I see many patients in my clinic, male and female, well past these ages), and every magazine and bestseller aimed at them trumpets the latest miracle diet. Does someone caught up in the enthusiasm of the latest diet fad necessarily have an eating disorder?

Look at the history of your child. The sensitive child will be affected by everything and will try to adhere to the norm. If the norm around her is that everyone is on a diet, she will go on a diet and be the best at it. If she has CNC, she will always take it to an extreme. A 'normal' child will stop when she feels she is thin enough; a CNC child will not.

As a parent, I would be wary of any child who always seems to be on a diet, regardless of his or her weight. Take note if your child begins to fret excessively about fat content, calories, and the like. I would be sure never to have diet products around the house, although I would keep the cupboards stocked with nutritious foods. Diet drinks are a particular problem. It has been suggested that some artificial sweeteners in them cause hyperactivity and other mood alterations in children. Many patients I see are literally addicted to them and experience acute anxiety when withdrawn from them. I would also be on the alert if your child begins making excuses to avoid mealtimes, constantly suggesting she ate too much at lunch and wants to skip dinner, that she ate at a friend's house, and so on.

A child with an eating disorder will generally manifest other signs beyond the dieting itself. I would be particularly alert if your child, always so deferential to others, becomes increasingly indecisive. Simple decisions about what to eat, what to wear, what movie to see become torturous. What may have evinced itself previously as kindness to others becomes an imperative for all action.

When asked what she wants to do, the child may seem abject. 'I don't care, what do you want to do?' might be her response. Or 'It doesn't matter what I want. What do *you* want?' These are warning signs that should be heeded. As I mentioned earlier, take notice if you hear your child continually putting herself down. I realize in retrospect I had done that myself as a child. When my mother heard my self-deprecating remarks, she would say to me, 'Peggy, charity begins in the home. You have to love yourself more than other people.' And I thought, 'How can I love myself?' Attitudes such as these are important to watch for if we suspect an eating disorder.

SIGNS OF BULIMIA

One need not be thin to be bulimic. This makes it a doubly devious condition because it often goes un-detected. Yet, as many bulimics die from chemical imbalances and suicide as do anorexics.

Bulimics who are purgers seldom eat a comfortable amount of food at the dinner table and then stay for conversation. They will generally make a trip to the bath-room immediately following the meal to get rid of what they ate. They may turn the shower on to drown out the sounds of vomiting.

Many bulimics abuse laxatives and complain to the doctor of constipation in the hope of getting a prescrip-tion for the strongest possible preparation.

Some bulimics have scars on the backs of their fingers from scraping them on their teeth as they stick their fingers down their throats. They may have poor gums, sallow complexions, and pitted, yellow teeth eaten away by stomach acid.

Many bulimics exercise constantly (basically, another form of purging) to burn off the pounds and pounds of food they can eat at a single sitting. They gradually exclude friends and family and spend more and more time on their single-minded quest for food. Groceries and money disappear from home; there may be reports of kleptomania as the bulimic searches out more supplies for a binge-and-purge.

Bulimics generally appear constantly physically agitated.

SIGNS OF ANOREXIA

Anorexics generally have strange eating habits. Many refuse food outright. Others consume it in a ritualized, almost robotic way. It is common for anorexics to be deeply anxious while eating or shortly afterward. They often disguise the fact that they are eating at all, going to the refrigerator at night when no one else can see them. I believe this is an effort to fool the Negative Mind. When my daughter Nikki was sick, she would pretend to be writing, then sneak a piece of food.

Anorexics are generally obsessed with food, even if they are not getting enough of it. They might prepare grand dinner parties, not consuming any food at the time, but allowing themselves leftover table scraps once the guests have gone. Eating out of garbage cans is common. Sufferers believe they are unworthy of good food, but worthy of any illness they might pick up by eating spoiled, discarded offal.

Anorexics have a marked pallor and black pools under

their eyes; their fingernails are cracked, and their skin, particularly on their hands, often becomes dry. They experience a profound insomnia, and have difficulty concentrating and making eye contact. (See Chapter 4.)

There are other secret clues that people in the throes of an eating disorder might leave, awaiting translation by those aware enough to detect them. In Chapter 4, I mentioned that evocative artwork and tiny handwriting provide such clues.

I also find that depression goes hand in hand with an eating disorder. This can come as a result of the nutritional imbalance and an unhealthy emotional focus on food. Imagine not being able to do anything else but focus on food. As one sufferer described it, 'Food is my only friend, but it's also my enemy.' I find that such people are generally listless and apathetic, unable to take any joy in their surroundings. They have what psychiatrists might call 'flat affect.'

Given their intense mental suffering, it is not surprising that bulimics and anorexics will often mask their pain with alcohol or substance abuse.

I would seek professional help as soon as you suspect a loved one has an eating disorder. Take your child to the doctor for an evaluation. Do not attempt to treat the condition yourself. You will need all the help you can get.

WHAT TO DO WHEN SOMEONE YOU LOVE IS DIAGNOSED WITH AN EATING DISORDER

If your child has been diagnosed with an eating disorder that has not yet reached an acute stage, her situation cannot be ignored. Just because this is not an emergency, it does not mean that you should not take immediate action. Be aware of your child's growing subjectivity. If she becomes exceedingly negative, her condition will only worsen without appropriate intervention. The severity of her condition depends not on her weight but on the entrenchment of CNC – something that cannot be as easily measured. While the severity of the eating disorder lies on a continuum, I believe that we must combat the underlying CNC in the same way for both an acutely ill person and one who is only at the beginning of the slide. Both people must traverse the five stages of recovery; the difference lies in the relative ease with which someone with greater access to her Actual Mind can absorb the recovery process.

Moderately ill eating disorder patients can be helped with outpatient therapeutic care, as long as their families participate in a loving manner. But first we must get these people into care. At this earlier stage, they may have more of their own 'head space' intact – the Negative Mind may still not predominate. In that case, parents or other loved ones can explain to victims where they are now and what could happen to them if there is no thera-peutic intervention.

You might say to your child, 'I know you are trying to manage a difficult situation in your head and that you are afraid you are ruining the family. We love you and we know this isn't your fault. It's happening because you're such a good, kind person. If we don't get the right help now, the problem will just get worse. We're all going to get through this together. We are going to get a therapist for you so you won't have to worry anymore.'

The key here is early intervention. Remember, no matter where a patient is on the eating disorder continuum – in the early stages or acutely ill – the steps for recovery must adhere to the guidelines and principles

I have set forth below and in Chapters 5 and 6. We must always begin to reverse the confirmed negativity from the bottom up.

Eating disorders are insidious and difficult to treat once they become acute, and they can become acute alarmingly quickly. Reversing them requires a high degree of commitment, understanding, and training that is beyond many. The firmly entrenched Negative Mind is determined to sabotage every attempt of a helping person.

Once a person manifests an acute eating disorder, the circumstances which determine its progression are much more difficult to control. As I discussed in Chapter 2, at this point the victim takes a highly subjective and negative view of life, and will work overtime to translate any event or circumstance in a negative way.

From this juncture, it is not impossible, but certainly difficult, to reverse the Negative Mind without appropriate intervention. A victim's Negative Mind will be confirmed much more easily than not. As she heads toward self-destruction, her Negative Mind grows in importance and magnitude. As Julie wrote to me early in her illness, 'I hate myself all the more and I feel more alone (rightly so) than ever before.'

The victim's mind does not allow her to ask for help, as badly as she wants and needs it. And she cannot be treated by the ones who love her most and whom she loves because of the added burdens of guilt and sense of responsibility to care for her parents. Julie writes of this terrible dilemma: 'It pains me to torment my mother so and despite all requests of me to speak, to divulge my thoughts, it is too dangerous for I increase my burden upon her too often. So many times I speak without regret and further aggravate my own mind. And too many times my wordless tears bring on her tears. And so the terror and pity, sorrow and hatred intensifies within me. Each utterance I make is done with overwhelming trepidation. I engage in a vicious cycle in my head, pleading for my silence, praying for her peace, knowing only death as an answer.'

In a perfect world, every victim of an eating disorder would have full access to a treatment facility that could treat not just the symptoms of the disorder but the patient's interpretation of her role in life, thereby restoring her sense of self and worth.

However, I am all too aware that access to such facilities are few and far between, or beyond the reach of most people. Many lack the financial resources, and unfortunately, insurance companies have been slow to appreciate the severity of the disorder and the length of time required to treat it fully; they therefore do not offer the kind of full coverage many families need to have a loved one treated effectively.

Other families may have access only to treatment programs that they have either tried and found wanting or that they intuitively recognize will not meet the needs of the sufferer. Still others may be unable to convince a loved one that she needs help.

What, then, can families and friends do to help the victim of an eating disorder? As a first step, I feel it is essential to ally yourself with a caring medical doctor and other health professionals to work as a team, a united front, to help your loved one.

As you have read in the last chapter, the care offered by our clinic is not something that one can readily replicate at home. I wish I could lay out a linear, step-by-step program for helping your loved one; I wish it were that easy. Critically ill people with eating disorders are in dire danger; their bodies are almost completely depleted and they are often suicidal.

You need help getting your loved one through this acute stage and on the road to recovery. In the next chapter I will offer some advice about seeking professional help. Here I can share with you the guidelines that I have found so helpful in my practice. I hope that you can use them as you work as part of a team with medical professionals to help your loved one.

I applaud you for your bravery and tenacity.

TAKE RESPONSIBILITY FOR RECOVERY FROM THE VICTIM

As is clear by now, sufferers of eating disorders cannot take responsibility for their condition. They have already taken responsibility for much of the world and have been exhausted by their failure to make a significant difference. They desperately need for you and the rest of the health care team to take the burden from their shoulders.

I generally tell my patients, 'Imagine a place where people worry about you and you don't have to worry about anyone. Can you think that maybe it's time you had a turn to be first? I know that you want help. I know that you can't ask for it. I am going to give you what you need without your having to ask for it.' The patient needs to be relieved of this crushing burden.

You might tell your loved one that you and the doctors will be fully responsible for her recovery. You will make all the decisions for now. Your loved one will no longer have to worry about preparing or eating meals. You will schedule doctor's appointments. You will take care of food.

At this point, sufferers are usually both enormously relieved and terribly frightened and anxious. They will protest continually, 'I've got things under control; I don't need your help,' 'I'm not worthy of your help.' 'You are going to make me fat.' 'I don't deserve to live.'

You may answer each time by saying, 'I love you and I know that you deserve to live. I am not going to let you go until I know you are better. I am not going to let you get fat; the doctors and I are going to get you well. You can trust me. I am in charge and I'm going to take care of you.'

OFFER UNCONDITIONAL LOVE AND SUPPOERT

When our children are infants, it is easy and natural to love them unconditionally. We do not blame them when they cry or keep us awake. We know that they are not responsible for the hard work required to raise them. We love them no matter what.

You need to recapture that same sense of unconditional love and support while helping a person with an eating disorder. It might be helpful for you to see the victim as an emotional child. That may be a way to connect with the feeling of unconditional love and support you would naturally give a baby.

Why unconditional love? As I explained in Chapter 5, unconditional love counteracts the harsh voice of the Negative Mind and allows the possibility of connecting with the Actual Mind.

In the early as well as the acute stages, the patient must be bathed in unconditional love. A harsh word should never be spoken because the Negative Mind will seize on it and use it against the patient. Not reproaching the victim can be extremely difficult, especially if the victim is behaving badly – cursing, throwing dishes, or having a tantrum. In these instances, draw a firm boundary between the person and her bizarre and distressing behavior. Instead of punishing or rejecting, I always say in a soft voice, 'I know you're frightened. Can you sit by me?' Your challenge is to love your child no matter how upsetting her behavior.

Always treat your loved one with respect. From my experience, it stops the behavior more quickly than any other response.

Giving love as a reward for only good behavior actually reinforces the Negative Mind. Don't try to encourage someone to eat by saying, 'If you loved me, you would try some of this.' It is saying, 'You are worthy of love only if you comply. There are terms to my love.' This gives the Negative Mind leverage to explain to the victim her unworthiness. It might say to her, 'See, they don't love you or they wouldn't have punished you.' As the patient recovers, a healthy, realistic balance begins to establish itself between these polar opposites.

Sometimes our unconscious actions imply conditions on our love. Think about your own reactions toward the victim. Might you be praising only those efforts you consider to be her best? Are you more responsive to her when she behaves the way you want her to? Do you react negatively when she does something you find objectionable? Such actions might send signals that tell the victim your love is contingent on her meeting your expectations. You are striving for consistent, positive, loving support all the time – love and respect that depends in no way on how the victim behaves, but in honor of who the victim is.

While some people believe that 'Tough Love' may be

effective in moderating or controlling certain adolescent behaviors such as drug use, shoplifting, and so on, we have found it to be entirely counterproductive in treating eating disorders. Tough Love basically says, 'My love for you has many conditions. You can't rely on me.'

Using this approach, doctors might tell parents to set limits on their child – for example, to remove every source of pleasure for a child unless she agrees to eat. Here is a typical letter describing the failure of this approach:

> The psychiatrist told us that they were 'going to make Jane's life miserable until she chooses to eat.' His behavioral approach of punishing Jane for not eating literally shattered our daughter's soul. She said in this hospital you have to eat to get love; she would not be able to see us unless she ate.
>
> After a few weeks of hospitalization, where her phone calls were monitored so she could not confide in us, she was discharged having gained only a few pounds. She was returned to us and for the next several months, we began the work of repairing the damage they had done. . . . Needless to say, whatever sense of herself that she may have had before this trauma was gone.

DO NOT TAKE BEHAVIOR AT FACE VALUE

It is essential to separate a victim from her behavior. Remember that the child is plagued by the Negative Mind. She may become abusive, or she may engage in degrading, self-mutilating, or bizarre activities (see Chapter 4).

This negative behavior is not your child. When it

occurs, attempt to ally yourself with your child against the Negative Mind. If you blame your child for that behavior or act repulsed by it, you are reaffirming and supporting the Negative Mind and confirming and strengthening the condition.

At this stage your child is extraordinarily suggestible and will twist everything you say into a negative to feed the condition. If you throw up your hands and say, 'I can't take this anymore,' the Negative Mind will have won. If your child tosses a dish at you, understand that she is doing it out of fear. She is operating on negative instructions to alienate the ones who love her the most. Indeed, the ones who love her best must be the first target.

How should you respond in the face of all this horrifying behavior? What I instinctively do is to put my arms around the patient, first to take away the fear, then to comfort her, to attempt to persuade her with logic, and most important, to convince her that I am stronger than the condition. I must convince her that I am not vulnerable to the pressure of the Negative Mind, and I am not going away, no matter what.

You might tell your child, 'I know that wasn't you throwing that dish. I know the condition made you do that. No matter what the condition does to try to push me away from you, I'm not going to leave you. I'm here to stay.'

Referring to the condition as a separate entity helps your child draw a distinction between that negative part of her and her Actual Mind.

Explain to your child about the Negative Mind. Tell her that she is not crazy, that what she is thinking and feeling is common among people with eating disorders. When you tell her that you know that she may be experiencing negative thoughts, even voices, music, or loud noises, that she is bound to be bewildered yet compelled by them, she knows that you understand, that she is not alone. To take away the stigma, liken it to a broken leg or pneumonia, except that it is an emotional condition rather than a physical one. Explain that you and she are going to be allies against this condition.

DON'T EVER JUDGE THE INDIVIDUAL

As an eating disorder wends its way to acuteness, parents and friends become increasingly lost about what to do. The horror at their helplessness only accentuates the plight of the victim who is becoming aware of her own inability to control or remedy her situation.

Within their fear, parents can react, usually against their child. Desperation persuades them to shout, demand, and lay on guilt. It seems inconceivable to them that their youngster is truly incapable of what is a most natural fact of living – eating. But remember, the victim of an eating disorder believes she is not permitted to eat because she has failed to save her parents or the world, and therefore does not deserve to live.

I cannot emphasize enough how easy it is to reconfirm the negative condition at this stage. The child already believes the worst possible about herself. Parents must be excessively kind. It takes great self-control to never react in the negative. It is unwise to tell a child, 'You have a problem.' Rather, say, 'We have a problem, and we're going to fix it together.'

BE PREPARED FOR IRRATIONAL
OR 'MANIPULATIVE' BEHAVIORS

I've put 'manipulative' in quotes because these behaviors are often misconstrued as a child's attempt to control others. In fact, they are the consequence of the Negative Mind controlling the child. As the Negative Mind attempts to control the child, so it attempts to control us through the child.

These children are terrified and confused. They intuitively know that their parents are their first source of help. Imagine the victims' turmoil when the Negative Mind tells them to push their parents away even as they pull their parents close.

It is helpful to regard these behaviors as the outcome of fear or the Negative Mind's internal manipulation, not the desire to control for its own sake. The child is loath to disrespect anybody.

Irrational behaviors in particular can appear as 'control issues.' Sufferers often attempt to structure their eating or sleeping habits based on illogical fears that harm might come to loved ones if they do not adhere to the Negative Mind's dictates. The Negative Mind threatens dire consequences to the sufferer's family members if she does not obey. 'If you eat this, then your mother will die,' it may say, or 'If you don't run around the house a hundred times, your little brother will be harmed.'

One patient could only prepare food between one and three in the morning. Another would not let her parents sleep together in the same bed; she kicked her father out so she could sleep with her mother and keep her as physically close as possible because she was afraid something would happen to her mom if she didn't watch her all the time. These behaviors are naturally exasperating to parents.

Kathleen had bought her daughter quart-size containers to store her food. Later she casually asked Mara if she had bought the correct item. Mara responded by sobbing uncontrollably, 'What I really wanted was the gallon size.' Mara acted as though it were the end of the world.

On the surface, this seemed like a bizarre overreaction, but it was a major crisis for Mara. She had desperately wanted the gallon size, but she was so grateful to her mother for purchasing any containers at all, she did not want to impose on her further. There was nothing she could do to redeem herself for not feeling utterly grateful and satisfied for the quart-size containers. She felt unworthy being asked to express a preference for herself.

EXPECT TO BE TESTED

Parents of children with eating disorders find that they are tested at every turn. If they are unaware of the workings of the Negative Mind, the destructive behavior will win, and the child will become immediately more agitated because she will be more fearful.

Your child might be hurtfully rude to you, and you may be tempted to break down and cry, a temptation you should do your best to resist. She might hide food she was supposed to eat to see how astute you are in finding it. (Some of my patients told me they have purposely hidden tidbits to see if I was smart enough to figure it out.) Conversely, a child might pretend to be overly cajoling or compliant so you will give in to something. 'Well, I've eaten most of it,' she might say when you are concerned about her nutrition. They may jump up and down in place doing exercise to see what you will do. In all cases, it is best to respond with distraction instead of anger. 'Come, let's work on a puzzle together' or 'Let me tell you about a funny thing that happened to me at work today.'

Victims often present an illogical logic that draws parents in. 'I need to exercise because it relieves my stress,' they might say. Or 'Yoga clears my mind.' In Chapter 4, I presented many of the tricks the Negative Mind will use to further its condition. Victims will almost certainly know which foods have the most water, fat, and calories. And they may resort to hiding uneaten food or exercising in secret.

If you find your loved one engaging in these deceptive behaviors, it is important to refrain from anger, disgust, or resignation. Instead, you might say, 'Hi, honey, I know your head is giving you a rough time. I know your head is making you do this. Come on, we will figure it out together.'

The victim will usually be embarrassed and relieved at the same time. And you are proving that you can determine the difference between the person and the condition. My patients, once cured, generally laugh at how creative and inventive they were while in the grips of the disorder.

USE LOGIC TO COMBAT EVERY
NEGATIVE WITH A POSITIVE

Anorexia knows no logic as we understand it. Redirection of the child's mind depends, then, on re-iteration of logic. It is therefore essential that you respond to each negative statement with a positive one.

IF YOUR CHILD SAYS: 'I'm a burden on society.'

YOU MIGHT ANSWER: 'No, you're not. You are wonderful. You've never done an unkind thing in your life. If you were a bad person, you wouldn't worry about being a burden. Selfish people don't worry about being a burden.'

IF YOUR CHILD SAYS: 'I'm so selfish. I don't deserve to take up your time.'

YOU MIGHT ANSWER: 'If you were selfish, you wouldn't care about that.'

Challenge subjectivity with objectivity. A victim will translate anything said, no matter how positive, into a negative. If you say, 'Your hair looks so lovely today,' she will think, 'Oh, it must have been a mess yesterday.' If you say, 'Good morning, dear. Thanks for cleaning up the kitchen counter so well,' the victim might translate this as, 'The kitchen counter . . . the kitchen counter . . . didn't I do a good job dusting the living room? Or scrubbing the bathroom? Does she mean I didn't do enough? Or maybe she's just saying she liked the job; she doesn't really mean it.'

Your child's words reflect the Negative Mind; your reply will be what her Actual Mind will one day be able to tell her objectively. If she says, 'black,' you say 'white.' In many ways, this resembles the split-page journal exercise and the role-playing our patients do at the clinic (see Chapter 5).

Your messages should convey unmistakably that you will always be there:

'I will always listen to you if you get upset and cry.'
'You aren't supposed to be perfect.'
'You are not crazy, and you won't always feel this way.'
'I have to know how you're feeling in order to help you, but if you can't tell me right now, I have a good idea anyway.'
'Let's talk about it and work it out.'
'I am nice to you because I love you a lot.'
'Nothing you say or do could ever make me love you less.'
'One day you'll be strong enough to be nice to others.'
'I won't let your head hurt you.'
'I know what I'm talking about. You can trust me.'

DO NOT COMMENT ON BODY APPEARANCE

Anorexics will try to maneuver you into commenting on their appearance. This is the Negative Mind's attempt to collect more ammunition to use against the child. If you say they look fine, they will think they look normal. They will then think they have to lose weight to prove they are subnormal and unworthy.

If you say, 'You look great,' the normal dieter will feel a sense of satisfaction. But the person with the eating disorder will feel unworthy. The Negative Mind translates such a comment as, 'You look fat and therefore unworthy.'

If your child asks, 'Do I look normal?' an unaware parent might respond, 'You look just fine.' The victim will translate this sadly as, 'Now I have to lose more weight.'

It is hard for any parent to 'win' at this game; there is so little neutral territory. If you must, comment on hair or eye color.

DON'T PLAY A NUMBERS GAME

Parents or practitioners have been known to threaten anorexics with statements such as 'If you lose seven more pounds, you'll have to go back into the hospital.' Ironically, this is in fact giving the victim permission to lose six pounds, fifteen ounces. Numbers are best left unsaid.

Take the scale out of the house. Insist that your doctor weigh your child backward so she cannot see the result, because her Negative Mind will use any number, no matter how low, against her to lose yet more weight. Get rid of measuring cups because to the patient they are yet another means of determining her worth ('I'm only allowed to have two ounces of juice').

DISCOURAGE COMPETITION

Ideally, it is absurd to expect us all to compete with one another because we are all unique individuals. Yet society advertently and inadvertently demands that we do. Any concept that demands that some people be superior and some inferior has no place in a humanistic society, and certainly not in the home of someone with an eating disorder. This will only aggravate the condition; these children are already competing to make the world the best place for everybody else.

If possible, send your child to a school that gives written evaluations, where every child is an individual, instead of a letter grade. It would be hurtful for her to be in a position in which she would be ranked or measured, which again would measure worth. Refrain from bragging about your child in front of her, because you are sending her a message that you value her not as an individual but for her achievements. Avoid displaying artwork and essays that you or the teacher believe represent the child's best efforts. Consider talking with your child's teachers or principal about what they can do to reduce your child's pressure to compete.

Tell your child over and over that you love her for what she is, not just for what she does.

ENCOURAGE SELF-EXPRESSION

I would encourage self-expression that is individual and that by its very nature does not demand perfection. Painting, poetry, creative writing, and journal work are excellent tools. These are also a wonderful outlet and a way to enhance communication. You might discuss your child's creative output with her to gain a better understanding of how her mind works. Rather than impose your own interpretation, you might say, 'Tell me more about this.'

In fact, you might say, 'I know your secret. There's someone inside telling you what to do, telling you to hurt yourself.' It can help your child to let the Negative Mind out into the open because she will be reassured that the onus is not hers alone to bear. The enemy has been found out. It is imperative, however, not to ask your child to agree with you. In so doing, the Negative Mind will punish her.

If there is another adult the child respects, invite interaction with him or her too. Allowing your child other opinions will increase her ability to be objective.

FOOD AND YOUR CHILD

Work very closely with your doctor to design small, nutritious meals and monitor your child's progress. As I explained in Chapter 6, six small meals a day are less threatening than three large ones.

You might also ease the stress that follows eating with distraction, rocking, and holding to help your youngster accept the food and prevent her from disappearing into the Negative Mind.

There will be times when the dinner table seems like a battleground. Do your best to stay calm and supportive. Although proper nutrition is obviously vital to a victim's recovery, keep in mind that the focus should not be on food, but on helping the victim reinterpret her world.

HELPING SIBLINGS COPE

Siblings can make a confusing situation even more so. A normal family setting often involves rivalry between sisters and brothers. But it is difficult for children to make sense of something that makes no sense to adults. Suddenly, almost before they know it, parents start catering to everyone.

The parents' role is to ensure the well-being of their children. When they cope with a child who has an eating disorder, their energy is naturally focused toward that need. Because of this special direction of their time, the other children in the family may take on different roles. Some siblings have been the first in line to help, others have desensitized themselves to the problem in order to survive. A teenager in the family is likely to resent everything with little encouragement. A teenager with a sibling who has an eating disorder can become very resentful indeed. Some previously 'well' siblings may even compromise their own development because of their anxiety.

Siblings are naturally concerned about the sufferer. To prevent their anxiety, it would be helpful to teach them that they are not to blame for their sister's condition, that she is in an illogical place, and that they should not judge her abnormal behavior or show anger toward her.

I would take all my children to a therapist, involving the entire family for two reasons: The children will realize that the family is a whole and that their parents are committed to maintaining that whole, and they will see that the problem is being addressed by the adults and it is not up to the children to mitigate their parents' frustration or anger.

Some siblings will be resentful that all the attention is sucked away from them, but in my experience, it is more often true that the 'well' siblings are more concerned about the intensified emotions they see in their parents.

At the clinic we talk to siblings and allow them to express their feelings. They understand that the condition is not their responsibility, they did not cause it, but they can be part of the solution by not judging the victim's behavior. They must also realize that this is an interim time – that wellness will return to the sibling and balance to the family.

I often say, 'The left arm is broken, so we have to pay attention to it. It doesn't mean that we don't value the right arm or the legs. It's just that the body will work best when every part is healed.'

It is imperative that all is done with patience and with no blame. If you tell a sibling, 'Can't you see that your sister needs my help now? Don't be so selfish,' it can be damaging because the onus of negativity will land on that child. Moreover, if the victim sees her siblings suffering from what appears to be rejection or anger, she may feel more guilt as well. Remember, the eating disorder victim loves her whole family and would like nothing better than to have it work. Your goal is to try to achieve as much balance in the family as possible, discouraging siblings from stepping into adult roles.

COPING WITH BURNOUT

There can be nothing more frightening than the belief that your child might die. When my daughters were ill, I felt as if they had been kidnapped but no body could be found. I had the frantic sense that there had to be something I could do, but I did not know in which direction to run. I was terrified and at times immobilized with fear.

Never knowing which day might be their last was utterly draining. Would death come from heart failure or suicide? I weep inside when I remember the relentless fear of the not knowing.

The player of a potentially lethal chess game, you may have to be two moves ahead of your child's Negative

Mind, aware of all of its possible countermoves. Such hypervigilance can also be exhausting.

As a parent, you may find yourself on an emotional roller coaster with no scheduled stops. I can empathize with the pain and courage you feel when your child is ill. For your own sake, remember that you are not to blame for your child's illness. This is a time when many parents set aside their own needs entirely and risk burnout. Be reassured that the time for balance will come later, but there are some things you can do now.

Support groups for parents, family members, and other loved ones can be helpful in avoiding burnout. Build a network of friends. You need to draw on anyone you know who is kind. Do not isolate yourself in shame or fear. Look to family and friends for support. Seek respite from the necessary intensity of the condition. You need adequate sleep to maintain your stability. Find a safe place where you can express your feelings. If you take better care of yourself, you will be a more effective caregiver for your child.

To hold your center, learn to not take CNC personally. It will pass. You cannot be the perfect careworker. Some people escape into their jobs. Find your spirituality, even if you are not necessarily religious. This will encourage faith, courage, and direction.

It is possible to work within your community to find the help you need. In the following chapter, I provide some guidelines for advocating a new kind of care for your child. Although finding the right kind of help may be difficult, I know from experience that well-intentioned caring professionals do exist who want to do all they can to help victims of eating disorders become well again.

Last year a family from the eastern United States

dropped in unexpectedly, hoping their child would be immediately admitted – an impossibility. However, given that the fourteen-year-old was so weak, we established communication with her doctor and her extended family at home. Together they are successfully bringing this child through her condition by fax contact with us. As the caring network of physicians who appreciate the role of CNC and the Negative Mind expands, I hope that all facilities will work with one another to help these victims.

8

Finding the Help You Need

Some people with eating disorders will, through luck in the form of inadvertent intervention and/or the attentiveness of others, find the help they need and reverse their condition before they have reached rock bottom. Those who are in the grip of acute eating disorders are in a potentially life-threatening situation. At the time they most need help, however, they will seldom be able to ask for it, much as they wish it. It will be up to family and friends to insist on that help. The acute victim must be kept safe until the crisis is over. Practically speaking at the present time, that means hospitalization.

If your loved one is not in immediate physical danger of collapse – something that only a medical doctor can determine, since physical appearance is not the only determinant of the health of someone with anorexia or bulimia – you may find it necessary to confront her with the need to get outpatient help. Explain to her that she must begin meeting with medical and/or mental health professionals. You might say, 'We're concerned about you. We want you to get the help you need. This isn't your problem, it's our problem, and we'll all work together until you're better.'

Remember, the victim is embarrassed at being a burden, so she will insist she is all right. If you know she is seriously ill and she appears adamant about wanting no care, you can be assured that the Negative Mind is in control and you must be strong for her. Her life may depend on it. Sometimes a dire situation demands that I feed a child when she refuses with almost anyone else. Even though she may resist feeding before I start, immediately afterward, she begs me not to let her go and insists on me convincing her she is not bad.

If your loved one is acutely ill, your first step must be to inform her that she needs help, and that she will have to go to a hospital to begin treatment. The victim is likely to react with anger, denial, or refusal. Perhaps she will tell you that she is worthless and does not deserve help, that no one can help her, that nothing will work. These protests are the work of the Negative Mind.

In response, it is helpful to say firmly but gently, 'I love you and know you need help. I am going to see that you get the help you deserve, and we will all work together until you're well. You don't need to worry anymore; we will take care of everything for you.' Reassure your loved one that you are not abandoning her by putting her in the hospital; you will be there for her no matter what her condition makes her say or do.

Given that an acute patient is more in the grip of the Negative Mind than the Actual Mind, she will typically react in two ways: the small Actual Mind will be both relieved at the possibility of help and terrified at the impending onslaught of unkindness that the Negative Mind will assail her with. When the status of the Negative Mind is threatened, it responds with horrifying determination to maintain itself.

The priority of acute hospital care is physical wellness, which comes down to feeding the patient to get her to a safe weight and rebalancing her electrolytes. We must save the person's physical life before attempting anything else. Normally, a patient in an acute care hospital is fed by means of a gastric-nasal (GN) tube inserted through the nose into her stomach. This is hardly pleasant, and it is not surprising that patients react to this first step in their hospitalization with anger, tears, fears, or depression.

Explain to your loved one that her body is so depleted that the GN tube is the only way to help her body for now so it can heal. Reassure her that this is a temporary measure.

The idea of feeding and weight gain is frightening for most patients, yet it is a necessary first step in acute care. Unfortunately, however, feeding can be such a battle and focus that the patient's emotional needs and the root of her problems – CNC – are often inadequately addressed in hospital care. As one person wrote to me, 'Any program I've been in was a stop-gap measure. . . . I'd put on weight that I'd immediately drop as soon as I was released.' Family and friends have a crucial role here, one that can make a big difference in a victim's recovery. Your loved one needs your careful and thoughtful intervention and advocacy on her behalf.

It would be difficult to overestimate how terrifying and overwhelming hospitalization can be for an acute patient. The letter below expresses this so eloquently. Reading it will help loved ones appreciate how crucial their support is at this time.

There was no way out. . . .

The room was cold and white, spotlessly clean. I sat on the edge of the window seat, alone. To my left stood the small, untouched, sterile chest of drawers, in front of me was the huge white pressed bed. To my right a vast television screen bulged out from the corner – empty and blank. The wardrobe was big, wide and bold. Everything – white. The door was shut tight. I listened and strained to hear a voice but there was nothing, just a buzzing electrical sound which seemed to become louder and louder as time went on. My bag leant against my right leg. I daren't move. Behind me the window was black. The curtains were drawn open. Outside I could see nothing but myself and again the same cold, hostile, white room. The smell was unlike anything my nostrils had ever come across, I kept sniffing. I was certain there were people outside looking in, watching every twitch or move I made. I was scared and ready for attack. As the fear built up and up I could almost hear it grow louder. The voices in my head were calling out as loud as they could but nobody was there. Why had they left me here? Was this my punishment? I had screamed and cried all the way in the car, partly with fear but also with the pain, my whole body ached. As I sat in the stillness I wanted to move, to get out, to escape it all, but what would the nurses say? What would they do to me? What was I allowed to do? Nobody had told me anything, I'd just been told this was my room. My room? This cold, empty, silent room, was mine? There was no time, no clock ticking, nothing, just a deafening silence.

I stood, quickly, turning and saw my reflection. It wasn't me at all. I looked and studied the figure, as she did too. Her eyes were dark and hollowed out, her cheekbones had tight white skin stretched taut across them. She wore a huge woolly, green jumper on top of two other jumpers beneath, which poked untidily out at the neck – just like mine did. She looked drowned and hidden inside the many layers of clothes. The strange, emaciated girl turned with me as I looked down at my hands. They were raw and unfeeling, numbed with harsh, penetrating cold. What nightmares lay in front of me? The insecurity and uncertainty of it all were too much to bear. Despair, hopelessness and the prospect of eternal loneliness which lay before me were intolerable. I had been left, abandoned, isolated, deserted without anyone or anything. Although with these feelings there came the inevitability, a sense that it was deserved, a justified torture – but what for? – I did not know.

I was 'killing myself' they had said but I hadn't cared. But now I had been caught and imprisoned. Strangely resigned to my fate, there was no way out. My control and power had been torn away from me. My coping mechanisms were to be stolen, and I'd be left vulnerable and open, naked. They would be able to do anything they wanted and there was nothing that I could do about it. Yes I was here in this isolated white cell but even worse, mentally I was condemned to the timeless void that was 'treatment.'

Having a good liaison with the doctor is imperative. Consider that you are building a care team. You might say to the head physician, 'Our goal is to work with you as closely and as effectively as possible. We have insights into our daughter that we think will really help.' Ideally, the doctor will be open to your perceptions.

Perhaps you can share a copy of this book with the doctor so that he or she will appreciate your approach and accommodate you wherever possible. You might wish to explain CNC and the Negative Mind to the medical personnel so they will understand that the victim is not 'insane,' noncompliant, or truly wishing for death. You could say, for example, 'We feel very strongly that our child needs and wants help, but that a large part of her mind is preventing her from asking for it. She wants to comply, but the negativity in her makes it very difficult. We believe she wants very much to survive, but emotionally she doesn't feel she deserves it. We don't want her to be blamed as being uncooperative if she cannot follow through on your orders. She is simply not able to take responsibility for getting better; we need you to do that until she is strong enough to do it for herself. She needs positive reinforcement, no matter what. Here's a book that explains our viewpoint. Can you support us on this?'

It is also important for the physician to appreciate that while your child may be attempting to push you away at this stage, it is most likely because she does not want to be a further burden to you and already feels horribly guilty about putting you through this ordeal. It has been my experience that any reluctance disappears when CNC is reversed.

Ideally, at this stage, patients will receive twenty-four-hour care. Unfortunately, most hospitals are not set up for such intensive attention and will not provide it unless the family insists strongly; even then, it may be impossible. If a hospital does permit round-the-clock care, practically speaking it generally falls to the family members to fill in the gap themselves, although many hospitals may not allow this because of liability issues involved in family members coming and going or interfering with hospital routine.

Families need to be particularly vigilant at this point. I have come across many facilities that recognize that acute stage anorexics need round-the-clock care, but put the patients in five-point restraints because they do not have the manpower to offer one-on-one attention. This can prove devastating to patients, though it is unfortunately sometimes necessary if hospitals are short staffed and there are not enough family members or friends to help.

Saving the child's life is the immediate imperative. However, saving the child's spirit is imperative as well. Reiterate gentleness in everything you say and do.

I think that it is easy for us to underestimate the powerful effect that hospitalization can have on victims of eating disorders. I've received countless letters from parents detailing how their children felt traumatized or demoralized by the use of feeding tubes or restraints. Many of these children viewed their hospitalization experience as confirmation that they were worthless and misunderstood. They saw medical treatment not as a life-saving measure but as a punishment. In these cases, I believe we need to do much more to change patients' perception of the hospitalization experience so that they don't divert so much of their energy to fighting it instead of working with health professionals toward a common goal. The key is better communication between parents and the health care team before, during, and after treatment.

Ideally, patients and their families will work with a staff that understands the Negative Mind, even if they don't identify it as such. When they do not, the consequences can be dire. I've had reports of desperate children running away from hospital programs and cutting themselves off from needed support.

In discussing your child's case with the medical personnel, be sure to explain which treatment approaches are totally unacceptable to you. You might say, 'Punishing our daughter by withholding privileges if she can't follow orders will only reinforce her belief that she is worthless and unworthy of being helped. We also feel restraining her unkindly will have a terribly negative effect.' You might then discuss how the staff should handle situations in which they would normally punish or restrain the patient. What will they do instead? I have found that people always respond eventually to unconditional caring.

As we have seen, the Negative Mind will make every attempt to foil treatments like gastric-nasal feeding, especially in the absence of one-on-one care. Patients sometimes pull out the tube, as Emma did, empty the gastric-nasal bag down the toilet or into a plant, or dilute the nutrition with water. They may also exercise through the night when the nursing staff is reduced. One patient pushed her gastric-nasal bag on a pole around and around the nurses' station, burning off every calorie she absorbed; another used the break between feedings to go up and down the stairs incessantly. The caregivers, so well intentioned but understaffed, simply could not keep up with these ploys.

Parents might want to ask the nursing staff for particular help. You might explain to them all the strategies your daughter might use to outwit them and all the bizarre requests she might make. You can say, for example, 'Please understand that Mara's behavior is not her; please don't blame her for her actions because she can't be responsible for them until she's well.

We believe that positive reinforcement and lack of blame are absolutely crucial for her recovery. She thrives on physical contact. Would you be able to rock and distract her after mealtime? If you're overburdened, may we come in and do that?' Most professionals who treat eating disorders are eager for any assistance in the task of saving lives from this tenacious condition, once they realize it can be productive.

Many hospitals make the mistake of giving patients a target weight and telling them that once they make that weight, they will be released. The patients' Negative Mind lets them put on the weight because its long-term goal is to get them out of the hospital and out of the reach of wellness, but once released patients usually go right back on track. The hospitals obviously must feed these critically ill patients; the task is to do this without letting the patient know any numbers.

Similarly, programs that specify a time limit for the patient, telling him or her, for example, 'You'll be out of here in three months,' can be counterproductive. In my experience, the patient dutifully 'does time' in the facility, pretending compliance as she waits out the days until the Negative Mind can get back to business. As Camille, a twenty-eight-year-old woman wrote to me, 'I have had an eating disorder for more than twelve years. I've been in and out of hospitals for this over eleven times. Each time, I just did what "they" requested in order to get out and ended up right back where I was before I went in.'

I prefer to tell my patients, 'You will graduate to the next level of care when I know that you're not being directed by your Negative Mind.' I am very clear with them that moving ahead does not depend in any way on weight or a number. I never give them a specific time line because each person progresses at her own pace. One must not give the Negative Mind a structure to work with. Although my staff and I will have that number or structure in mind, the patient's Negative Mind will never be privy to it. This is a great relief to the patient's Actual Mind, because the Negative Mind has nothing to work with and cannot issue instructions based on it.

Consequently, it would be helpful for you to ask the hospital staff to weigh your child backwards and request that they refrain from revealing her weight to her, no matter how many times she demands to know it. Moreover, there should be no discussion with the victim regarding the length of her stay in a particular program.

In addition to the advocacy I have suggested, your chief role in this stage is to reassure your child and soothe her anxiety. Reassure her that she is not to blame for her illness, that you love her no matter what, and that you will stay by her for as long as it takes for her to get well.

Spend as much time by your child's bedside as the hospital permits, as long you are sure not to transfer your anxiety to her. At our clinic, parents stay away initially because their presence can cause the patients too much guilt and anxiety. After all, children generally have managed to *not* get better in their homes, so they don't initially know that their parents can help them. If parents are part of a 'caregiving team,' they can make a positive contribution to their loved one's healing.

If you find yourself incapable of handling this emotional burden, send other loving people in your child's life in your stead. She needs to feel positive that you are not abandoning her, and that you have a confident vision that she will recover. Where allowed and possible, I would use comforting touch, words, and rocking to soothe your child.

It is particularly important at this stage to distinguish between your child's needs and the demands of the Negative Mind. Children will typically ask their parents, 'Tell them to stop putting so much food in my tube' or 'Tell the doctors I need more medication.' Parents naturally want to respond to their children's distress calls, but in this case, they need to realize that these requests are not in the child's best interests. They are coming from the Negative Mind. Explain to your loved one, 'I know that the real you wants and needs help. I love you and you can trust me to work with the doctors to get you better. You don't need to worry; let us take care of you.'

Depending on the nature of the acute care facility, patients who act particularly irrationally or suicidally – patients who are not 'compliant' – may be put under psychiatric care. There are many different approaches: group therapy, one-on-one sessions with psychiatrists or psychologists, psychopharmacology. Some patients do very well under such care.

Ideally, patients and their families will have the opportunity to work with a professional who understands the Negative Mind, although they may use other descriptive terms for the concept. In reality, there are not yet enough therapists who realize that someone in the acute grip of an eating disorder is generally incapable of coming out of it without a very specific kind of help and support and so the course of treatment can be difficult. If you find that the doctors and nurses at the hospital are obviously uncooperative and unresponsive to your concerns and requests, you will need to look elsewhere for help.

THE ROLE OF PSYCHOPHARMACOLOGY

When most patients arrive at our clinic, they are generally on four or five psychoactive medications. They start out being prescribed one. Then the doctor adds a second to compensate for the side effects of the first, and a third to compensate for those of the second, and so on.

I do not want to stigmatize anorexia patients who are on medication; they bear enough stigma as it is. There are important reasons for acute patients to be given medication to treat their symptoms. Without twenty-four-hour care, they can be suicidal, and the drugs can help mitigate that deadly impulse. People with eating disorders who live at home are acting out continuously and may be suicidal. Drugs can help moderate their behavior and keep the household together. In an outpatient setting, medicating is understandable, because the doctor must keep the patient safe while dealing with her mind.

Antidepressants are commonly prescribed because depression comes along with anorexia and low nutrition. I have never seen a happy anorexic! People with eating disorders do respond to medication, but I would suggest that it is mainly their symptoms that are being addressed; the medications do not treat the underlying reason for the condition.

I believe that to correct the CNC, I need access to a person's unhindered mind. I am concerned that medication can mask or alter a patient's symptoms and behaviors, thereby reducing the effectiveness of psychotherapy to effectively treat the condition. In twenty-four-hour residential care as we provide it, in order to ascertain the severity and direction of the mindset in the patient, the fewer drugs used, the better.

We work very closely and carefully with a number of medical doctors who make the decision to decrease the drugs depending on what they deem safe and necessary. When a negative mindset urges a patient to throw herself off a balcony or in front of traffic, sedation has an imperative role.

If patients indicate the need of medication for disorders other than those connected with eating disorders, our doctors will prescribe it. However, I would say that in well over 90 percent of the cases we see in our clinic, the symptoms for which the medication was initially prescribed disappear as we reverse the Confirmed Negativity Condition. We chart our patients' progress closely; if after two or three months it becomes clear to the doctor that the patient has been fed to the point that depression symptoms should have been abating but have not, and an antidepressant would be medically recommended, the doctor will involve it in her therapy.

A recent study suggests that Prozac can be effective in reducing occurrences of relapse, although it does not address the underlying cause. In our program, patients whose CNC has been successfully reversed are not likely to relapse. However, you may want to investigate the use of medication for this purpose.

As their children enter treatment programs, it is important for parents to discuss with their doctors whether they are considering prescribing medication. Hospitals have their own rules and reasons about these matters. I would ask about them, make sure I understand them, and state my preference. If children are already on medication, gradual, supervised withdrawal may also be an option worth exploring. But I cannot emphasize strongly enough that no one should *ever* withdraw from any medication unless under the close supervision of the prescribing doctor. Sudden withdrawal may have serious consequences.

It is also imperative to note that if, after a patient's CNC is reversed, he or she has another disorder that is not related to this condition, medication may well be necessary. This has been true of patients I have treated in my clinic. For example, our doctors discovered that a patient's underlying hormonal imbalance was contributing to her difficulty in keeping her emotions under control. In such a case, it is necessary to stabilize the hormonal imbalance before working further with the eating disorder.

OUTPATIENT THERAPY AFTER HOSPITALIZATION

After a patient has regained what the hospital considers an acceptable amount of weight, she is usually released. At this stage she appears physically well, but in fact she has taken only the first step toward total recovery. It is quite common for people with anorexia to leave acute care wards and immediately lose every pound they have gained, as in Camille's case. Most of the patients we see at the clinic have had multiple courses of unproductive treatment in acute care hospitals – sometimes dozens and dozens of visits. Remember, though, we are in the unhappy situation of seeing mostly worst-case, 'tried everything' patients.

I do not want to denigrate the quality of care in such hospitals but I believe that treatment there usually has not been taken seriously enough because it has neither understood nor focused on the true nature of the underlying condition. This is what comes of defining eating disorders as primarily a medical problem whose cure is physiological repair or focusing on a single issue as 'the cause.' Many parents have written me that while they appreciated the caring efforts of the hospitals that treated their children, they felt the programs weren't getting to the heart of what compelled these victims to behave in such self-negating ways. Ideally, your enlightened advocacy and intervention will render hospital treatment more effective. I also believe that most hospitals and treatment centers fail to appreciate how long it takes for a patient to feel completely secure even after emotional healing. Recall that it took my daughter Kirsten over a year before she felt wholly at peace with her sense of self.

After hospital release, patients typically begin outpatient work. Outpatient psychotherapy can also be helpful – and necessary, I believe – for people with eating disorders who have not yet reached an acute stage.

Your first task should be to find a therapist or clinic that believes in and practices total recovery, not maintenance of the condition. Again, just as you allied yourself with the care team at the hospital, it would be helpful to take a team approach with the outpatient psychotherapist. Once more, it would be constructive to explain CNC and your frame of reference vis-à-vis the Negative Mind. You might explain that your child needs and wants help, but that the negativity prevents her from asking for it or complying with recommendations. Reiterate that she is unable to take responsibility for her actions and thus should not be blamed or labeled uncooperative. Insist on positive reinforcement and unconditional positive regard. You might suggest that the therapist read a copy of this book to better understand your position.

However, be forewarned that the magnitude of the

Negative Mind is almost more than one would wish to believe. Its reversal can be more taxing than most people are prepared or willing to lend themselves to, even committed therapists. It is imperative that the battle of the loved one's life become your battle for the duration. If you embark on this mutual journey, keep focused on the destination in mind, expecting and accepting the waves and storms that will occur.

To effectively rid herself of the Negative Mind, a victim must feel protected all the time. The Actual Mind of patients who are acutely ill or who are long-term sufferers is already feeling so beaten and so exhausted from fighting that an outpatient situation can be counter-productive if not approached effectively. The patient feels guilty for money spent on her and for taking up the therapist's time. Or she feels needy for having had a touch of caring squeezed into a narrow time slot. She must then go home with her Negative Mind and be berated for her obvious selfishness.

The Actual Mind knows that to survive it must take advantage of any kindness extended to it. However, given the victim's incredible need, the Actual Mind must prove that the love and kindness is unconditional. Expect your loved one to test the therapist, and prepare the therapist for this. That means the victim may engage in bizarre behavior such as abusive language, throwing things, and other acting out in an attempt to alienate the therapist. Unfortunately, at this point, few people who do not understand the source of this need will cater to what they perceive as immature and irrational behavior.

It is imperative, therefore, that you find a therapist who understands that the onus of recovery cannot be placed on the patient, who will help the patient separate her Actual Mind from the condition, and who will offer unconditional love despite disturbing behavior. The treatment approach should be grounded in the conceptual framework of humanism rather than behaviorism.

Humanism is based on compassion, optimism, and positivity. Behavior modification techniques such as offering rewards (for eating) and imposing punishment (for not eating) are based on the idea that you are what you do – your actions are you. 'Good' actions are rewarded, 'bad' actions punished. By extension, the patient is perceived as 'good' or 'bad' depending on her responses. This is the antithesis of unconditional love.

Behaviorism may be effective for treating many conditions, but I do not believe it works for eating disorders, since a victim's actions are very much *not* who she is. One father wrote to me about his daughter's experiences with a 'state of the art' cognitive/behavioral program:

> This program DOES NOT WORK FOR Amy. Amy weighs 72 pounds and is 5 feet 3 inches tall. Her nutritionist and physician are both telling me today that Amy must be admitted again to the hospital's eating disorder unit. When Amy was discharged from the hospital the last time, I told myself that I would never admit her to a program again. When Amy is hospitalized she loses any sense of dignity that she has. She tells me, 'Just shoot me now and get it over with.' I'm afraid that if I do admit her, she'll find a way to kill herself.

I am not surprised that programs based on behavior modification are generally ineffective since the behavior they are designed to address is merely a symptom of the underlying condition, not the problem itself. If you are more or less saddled with such an approach because it is the only one available to you, make your preferences known that encouragement for 'good' behavior is acceptable but there can be no punishment for 'bad' behavior.

Unfortunately, there are many other approaches that I believe you must be wary of, as well. I recommend, for example, that you avoid programs that seek to explain the cause of the condition in terms of a single trauma, like sexual or physical abuse. While trauma *may* be a precipitating factor in an eating disorder, as I have explained in Chapter 3, it is not the underlying cause. Certainly, 'issues' and their consequences need be addressed, but with a positive attitude to the continuing work toward reversal of CNC.

Similarly, from our experience, twelve-step programs that can be highly effective for drug or alcohol abuse may be ineffective in producing total recovery from CNC. At the core of this approach is a belief that eating disorders are 'addictive behaviors,' and the patient must remain constantly vigilant lest she 'fall off the wagon.' While this approach may indeed improve the victim's quality of life, it essentially reaffirms and maintains the condition, thus obstructing the path to full recovery.

As a middle-aged anorexia patient, a mother of three children, wrote to me, 'I have been in therapy and have been to eating-disorder twelve-step settings. I've learned a lot, I think, about what it is . . . but frankly, it keeps getting worse.'

I would also be wary of a treatment approach that blames parents and other loved ones or excludes them from the process. As I have said, most of the parents I have worked with are loving and dedicated to their child. Ill-intentioned parents are the exception, not the rule. When their attitudes make it evident that parents' first interest is *not* the child, nevertheless, of course, the child must come first. The situation must be tailored to serve the child's best interest. But blame of anybody or exclusion must not enter the equation verbally, lest the victim use it to feed the Negative Mind or the parents use it to exacerbate the situation.

Parents are their child's best support and source of structure. When therapists exclude parents, I worry that the Negative Mind will use either the therapist or the parents against the child. For example, if a mother tells her child, 'You need to eat this meal,' the child can reply, 'Dr. Brady says I don't have to.' The excluded parent, still in a position of having to care for her child, has lost all authority. When she calls the therapist to ask what's going on, the therapist may say, 'Any communication between me and your son is private and confidential.' This plays right into the hand of the Negative Mind, which sets up one adult against the other, to the demise of the child. The child needs a united front, a solid team. He has to know consistency so that the Negative Mind cannot play games.

Furthermore, excluding parents is unfair because they will eventually continue the therapy that has gone on before, once the therapist's role is over. If they are not a part of the treatment plan from the beginning, how can they continue it? And you surely do not want to find yourself in a situation in which you are unable to evaluate whether the therapist is the right one for your child.

If you are not happy with your child's therapist, continue to search for a therapist with a positive attitude. Remember, what the child needs to learn to survive the Negative Mind is a compassionate objectivity that will arm her against the eventual plights in life, of which there will be many.

I have found that support groups for victims may be detrimental if they consist of other victims alone. In such a group, I am concerned that sufferers will compare and reinforce notes of negativity. I would worry that each patient will try to 'better' the next at being unworthy, whether it be at weight loss, number of times purging, hours of exercise, use of laxatives, and so on. Even if a positive leader monitors the group, that person might be overwhelmed by so many Negative Minds in one setting.

Group therapy situations can also be counter-productive. One girl said of them, 'I was offered group therapy with other anorexics, but declined because I know they would be thinner than me, and then I'd feel even worse about myself.'

In our clinic, we do not allow a dormitory situation for just this reason. We avoid putting two emaciated anorexics together. In those rare situations in which patients share a room, we will put an anorexic and bulimic together, and stress to them how their situations differ. At the same time, we emphasize that their one-on-one caregivers are an arm's length away if needed.

Many of my patients have grinned when talking about hospital programs where they exchanged 'trade secrets' in their support groups on being better anorexics. They delighted in being able to outsmart whatever strategies the hospitals used. Small wonder that the word 'manipulative' is so often used to describe the eating disorder victim.

A mixed support group – some members with eating disorders and some with other problems – can be helpful if it is positive. It can show the patient that other people have problems too, but the danger is that the patient will worry more about others than herself. Eating disorder patients automatically give themselves to other people's pain and therefore can tread water in such a group instead of progressing. I feel it is more than useful to have patients around healthy individuals as much as possible until they are better.

These are my observations based on my clinical experience. They are generalizations. Your loved one is very much an individual. If a program I am cautious about is working for your loved one, she should stay with it as long as it is effective. Whatever the approach, however, it is essential that victims know they are not alone. Parents and caregivers need to remind them of that again and again.

BE WARY OF LABELING

At the risk of denigrating the fine work of many reputable, well-intentioned mental health professionals, I must advise parents to be cautious about accepting diagnoses of mental disorders. Scores of patients have arrived at my clinic diagnosed variously as obsessive-compulsive, agoraphobic, schizophrenic, manic-depressive, and so on. Worse yet are the vague labels such as 'borderline personality' and 'undifferentiated schizophrenia' that could mean nothing or everything.

I do not in any way mean to suggest that any of these are not genuine conditions. However, in my practice, I have found that very few of the patients who come to me with these labels attached to them actually have these conditions, even though they may have had symptoms that matched them. As we treat the underlying condition of Confirmed Negativity Condition with love and respect, the symptoms fall away.

If your child receives such a diagnosis, you will obviously need to pursue further medical evaluation, but I would be careful not to discuss the diagnosis in front of her. The danger of emphasizing labeling to the eating disorders patient, even if it exists, is that she will further resign her worthiness, and it will arm the Negative Mind with the additional tool of stigma to use against her.

Instead, emphasize and celebrate your child's unique individuality as she begins slowly to describe it to you in moments of gentleness and truth. Ask your child what she is feeling, what her impressions of what is happening to her are, how her head is talking to her. Keep asking gently until she responds. As she comes further through the condition, she will be able to share things much more comfortably. If she tries to label herself or uses a label bestowed on her, you might say, 'I'm not interested in labels. That's not how I see you. Let's talk about what you think, not what others do.'

Say what comes from your heart. What works for me are terms of endearment. These are heartfelt and heart-meant for me and serve to soften the distance between me and my patients. Given the gentle, sensitive nature of this population, it comes naturally. You will find your own words as befits your character and ability.

It is imperative, however, not to appear anxious or nagging. Be unconditionally supportive and strong. Do not be afraid to lose your pride. Pride and ego have no place here; the road to recovery is a humbling journey.

BE WARY OF AUTHORITY
FOR AUTHORITY'S SAKE

As parents, we sometimes ignore our internal compass and cede our authority to the experts because we feel they must know better than we do, especially when we find ourselves in life-and-death situations. Parents inadvertently hone themselves to society's order, sometimes without question. But you know your loved one better than anyone else. Perhaps we should not honor authority for authority's sake alone, but consider what we intuitively feel in balance with it.

I feel saddened when I hear of what I consider atrocious behavior presented under the guise of Tough Love. Parents weep about how they have physically or mentally abused their child because it had been advised to them by an 'authority.' If I succeed in doing nothing more in this book than convincing you that your child is not in charge of what she is doing, that you must not abandon humanism for the sake of an unaware authority, that you must not follow the herd because it is there to follow – the path of least resistance – then I have not written it in vain.

I have heard from many parents who had terrible misgivings about the mismatch between a specific treatment modality and their child's needs. All too often, they went ahead and put their child in such a situation anyway, to disastrous results:

- One patient told me, 'I was screaming because the windows were covered so I couldn't see my father in the parking lot. My father came in, saw the therapist actually sitting on me to get me to stop screaming, and said, "Oh, okay," and left again, shutting the door. I knew that my father, who knew me better than anybody except my mother, had decided to give up on me, that I was truly alone. I felt so betrayed, and never so frightened. I didn't know what was happening in my mind. I only knew that it was out of my control. Now my father had turned against me as well and I would have to find the answers myself or die.'

- One therapist advised a couple to restrain their boy in a chair and force-feed him. They reluctantly did so, but when the boy's mouth began to bleed, they phoned the therapist to ask her advice. She responded, 'Keep feeding him.' These parents were frustrated with their child's resistance and could not understand that their child would not listen. They did not comprehend the dual mindset.

- Another therapist encouraged a mother to hit her anorexic child when the child refused food.

- A father was told to carry out a tough love intervention with a ten-year-old boy who had anorexia. If the child did not eat, the father was instructed to punish him, deprive him of all his pleasures, including all toys, games, stuffed animals, and books in his room, and keep him in his now-empty room until he 'complied.' Needless to say, the Negative Mind had a heyday – here was more confirmation than the boy needed that he was entirely worthless – and the child got sicker.

- An anorexic child was placed in solitary confinement in a mental institution because she would not comply with the program. Incredibly shy, she finally found the courage to knock on the door and request a trip to the bathroom. The

orderly made her wait another hour before
releasing her.

Parents are always apologizing to me for 'knowing better' but allowing their children to be treated in inappropriate ways anyway. If this has happened, please do not blame yourselves. Rather, proceed with the task of seeking out appropriate help.

Parents, listen to your hearts; do not forsake your children. Insist that your child be treated with respect and humanity. It will always continue to be my belief that man is inherently good. If all evidence shows an 'authority' figure to be without compassion, do not inflict his or her insensitivity on your child. Search for a viable alternative.

I know that alternatives do exist. I am in the position, at this point in time, of having doctors and nurses worldwide contact me for advice. Most medical people in my current experience are eager to help this patient population which continues to baffle most of the contemporary world. They are searching for answers anywhere they appear to be available. You can help provide some of those answers.

AVOIDING RELAPSE

Relapse becomes a nonissue if CNC no longer exists. The 'patient' has learned a different perspective on life and now has a mental road map to follow. She has more opportunity to make things happen, rather than have them happen to her. If ever her condition had been an issue of control, she is now in control as much as any mortal ever is. The many recovery stories in Chapter 9 will show you that full recovery without relapse is possible.

If your loved one's CNC has not been reversed, she is susceptible to relapse. If you see any of the warning signs, seek help immediately. You will need to begin again. Do not lose hope.

A TIME FOR PATIENCE

When we bring up any young child, we are tolerant of her fatigue, her hunger, her small fears of new things. We understand that to be gentle and to slowly explain life to a child is more conducive to her learning and her eventual adult mind than to be impatient and abrupt. Certainly there are moments in anyone's life when this does not happen as well as one may wish it. Nevertheless, it appears obvious that most parents care about the long-term results of their parenting.

Helping the anorexic victim is like bringing up a small child. The victim's emotional development has been arrested, so she may be an emotional infant. At some juncture, her subjective perspective and self-loathing culminated with the illness and immersion in total turmoil and confusion. She has lost her way and requires gentle redirection.

Society's response to the family's needs can cause either unity or disruption. When their child has an eating disorder, many families suffer enormous trepidation with no clear end in sight and are made to feel guilty without obvious reason. Many parents are told their child will never get better. This common societal dictum can only further paralyze their badly needed efforts to save their child.

It helps parents to remember that it took time for their loved one to develop Confirmed Negativity Condition; it will take time to recover from it. In my experience, it can require anywhere from six months to two years after a patient's physical condition has been stabilized for her to achieve total recovery.

One might naturally assume that someone who has had an eating disorder for only one year will 'turn around' more quickly than someone who has had it for five years. Surprisingly, however, in my experience, recovery does not depend on how long a person has had the eating disorder, but rather on how long the person has had CNC and on how severely confirmed the condition is.

If you keep in mind the reparenting model of recovery I explained in Chapter 6 – that your child will move from infancy to toddlerhood through adolescence and maturity as her condition improves – it will be easier for you to be patient with your child's recovery and to recognize the stages as she progresses toward wellness. Regard your child's reach for recovery as but one more way to prize her uniqueness and individuality.

9

The Poetry of Healing

*M*uch to my dismay, I found out years ago when trying to cure my children of anorexia that the eating disorders as I had studied them in psychology books bore little resemblance to what unraveled before me. Years of relentless research have revealed that a much more sinister, malevolent, and predatory mental construct somehow coexists in and directs the minds of some of the most caring, gentle individuals in our society. The horror of the depth and complexity of this powerful negative mindset is daunting to its victims and families alike.

However intimidating this mindset is, it has proven to be completely reversible. Although it is a difficult and sometimes arduous task, with patience, compassion, and unconditional caring, loved ones and therapists can reverse the negativity and restore the self.

I have had the privilege of working with and talking to hundreds of victims of eating disorders. Some have lived four to eight years in mental institutions. They were told they were lost causes and could not get better because they did not want to. Others have had electroshock treatments in the hopes of changing their thought patterns. Many others, nursing a Negative Mind, have lived years in sedation, merely existing rather than living.

Some of my past patients wanted you to know what

they *now know – that life is worth living; that you can become well again completely and forever. I hope their words will help your healing.*

Have courage and believe you are worth it – we do.

*   *   *

I was 20 when anorexia first manifested itself in me. Now I am 41. Half of my life (20 years) has been robbed from me. Anorexia is a lying thief that keeps you [chained] in a silent isolated prison. The years of my illness were like that.

Besides the obvious of denying myself food, everything else that was in the least way pleasurable or luxurious I could not allow myself. I wasn't 'allowed' to listen to music, watch TV, use the air conditioner, have friends or fun. Life was serious and discipline excessively strict. Necessities were allowed with strict restrictions: 1 roll of toilet paper a month, use the shower only once a week, can't drive car more than a ridiculously low number of kilometers per month.

I could not allow myself friends. I wasn't good enough to be loved, though I craved it. If someone gave me a hug that I desperately wanted, I would stiffen and slither from their grasp. I didn't deserve it. I would keep the phone unplugged, then cry and cry out of loneliness. I *existed* for 20 years but didn't live.

Changes came about slowly, often unrecognized. Then one Sunday about 6 months ago, I was singing a hymn in church with the words, 'My chains fell off. My heart was free!' It was at that moment I realized that I *had* happened. How did I know? I wasn't obeying that cruel taskmaster, anorexia, anymore. I no longer had all the rules to follow. I could drive my car as much as I wanted; I can use my shower as much as I wanted; I no longer have to put the 'company' toilet paper out if someone comes over. I have bought myself 'luxuries' that I quite enjoy – TV, VCR, CD player, microwave.

I guess my self-denial was pretty obvious. I was told about a remark made by someone who had visited my apartment here. 'Stacy is normal now. She has a TV, VCR, answering machine!' And I have friends. Friends that love me for the person I am and I am able to accept that love. I am able to accept myself. I have become aware of areas of strength and talent in myself and am developing them. They are a better definition of who I am than the number on the scale. My confidence has increased 100%. I am more decisive and can stand up for myself and what I believe. I don't have to agree with everybody to gain their approval. Exercising no longer rules my life. Relaxing is a welcome part of my life now. People have become more important to me than my diet, exercise, and housework.

I have had my mind changed from hearing everything that's said sifted and rearranged into an 'I hate Stacy; everything is Stacy's fault; Stacy is a failure' message. That's what caused such inner torment. Listening to the accusing, hateful, punishing, destructive voices all day and night was killing me. Now the messages are what is actually said. I can hear and accept words of love, encouragement, compliment, and even correction. It has brought peace of mind to me. I am enjoying life now. I have fun and laugh. I have an active social life. I have much more compassion toward others.

The recovery process has not only changed my life but given me a broader understanding of others which has definitely enhanced relationships with family and friends. I now see what a beautiful gift life is. I have been given the chance I thought was lost forever – to live that life.

* * *

I don't really remember a time in my childhood, adolescence when I didn't have an eating disorder. At age six, I remember looking in the mirror and thinking I was too fat, and so I began eating less and less. Severe food restrictions, obsessive exercising and vomiting were constants in my life. By age sixteen, my weight had dropped to 65 pounds. It is difficult to put into words for someone who has not been there, what it feels like to exist in this state. I wanted more than anything to be free of my eating disorders – I wanted to die. By age eighteen, I had gained some weight but inside me, nothing had changed. I attempted suicide, ended up in the hospital and was told by 'professionals' that I was more or less a hopeless case.

I met Peggy later that year. After years of hearing therapists tell me I was 'incurable,' she was the first person to assert that I would in fact get better. Of course, I did not believe her. I insisted she did not know how 'crazy' I was – I have to admit that I did not want to get better at first. My identity, the way I related to the world were all centered around my eating disorders. Stripped of those, who would I be? Through her continual patience, perseverance, and support, a slow change began within me. I see this as the beginning of my 'living' life.

I have been out of 'therapy' for about five years now. Each year I become increasingly healthier. I am far from the person I used to be and I have faith in my strength. I am happy. I have purpose. I have passion. I am alive.

*   *   *

I remember being suspicious and intimidated at every turn; I was hesitant and almost incapable of relating to anyone or anything. There was a time when I frantically looked up different psychological disorders and illnesses hoping to find a clue as to what could be wrong with me, and nothing in any book at that time alleviated my terror or my feeling of aloneness.

As a child, on the surface, I was very outgoing socially and a leader amongst my friends. I was always initiating new ideas and open to trying new things. I felt I had to be this way all the time to be noticed or acknowledged and sometimes living up to this role was exhausting because of the expectations this included.

I used to love sports and the competitive thrill. I cared very much about the outcome and would strive for first place desperately. I thought I would be less liked, less important even in second place and obviously it would state I had not trained hard enough.

School was quite stressful also because of the grading system and how I graded myself as an individual based on that system. The grading system did not appear to allow us room for human error but underlined the word 'perfection,' a word very popular in my vocabulary at the time.

I was always worrying about my family, especially my little sister. I thought I should be largely responsible for her well-being and happiness and if something caused her any harm, I would blame myself for not coming to the rescue quickly enough. I also remember as a child checking all the windows, doors, the stove and toaster when my family was in bed at night to ensure that everything was secured and turned off. My fears and paranoia were obviously already manifesting at an early age. I wasn't inhibited or ashamed of myself at that juncture, but then things started to slowly change.

I became quite reclusive. Rarely would I get out with friends or family unless coerced and felt there was no alternative. I dropped out of all sports quickly and made many excuses as to why. I had no motivation because I was afraid of failure, afraid that people would judge and criticize me and I felt it necessary to have universal acceptance regardless of circumstances, differing opinions, etc.

I always wanted to be a good, compassionate and kind individual but somehow I believed I had been severely overlooked. Every time I attempted to do something that apparently was kind and thoughtful, I thought for sure I must have another motive and it definitely wasn't enough always. If someone else did a similar thing, it was genuine of course and beyond reproach. I used to lie awake in bed many nights, imagining all the horrible things that would befall those I loved if I once again allowed myself to venture out and be part of the world.

I started to exercise obsessively and eat less well, narrowing down the types of food I allowed myself. All the foods I loved were no longer on my menu. I started hiding food, pretending I ate it and would only eat with my family when given no alternative. I was ashamed that they would wonder why I thought I deserved to eat and especially in the presence of others. I denied myself pleasure in this aspect as well as many others because I believed myself unworthy of partaking in anything remotely enjoyable, especially since I had not given enough of myself to others and was not capable of mending the horrors of the world. The happiness of others was far more important than my own at any time.

The pressures inside my head were driving me crazy and I didn't know how to cope with them. I quite often contemplated suicide and after a few failed attempts, my imperfections were once again confirmed. I thought I was an absolute failure, as I couldn't even get that right. I had already accepted the fact that I had failed at life.

It is difficult going back to the place I have described above, only because today, I feel so far removed from how I felt then. The contrast between then and now is astounding. It's almost as if it were another lifetime. I feel like I have described someone else's previous life.

I have learned to work through things as they arise. I no longer worry unnecessarily or 'buy trouble' as some would say. I realize now that all things are not my responsibility, I can only do so much because I am imperfect. I have limitations and I do not have all the answers nor do I want them all. I have ceased caring about being the best at anything because it's irrelevant and only a matter of opinion.

I am still a sensitive human being but I can now put life in perspective. I am able to objectify situations quite well – well enough for me anyhow. I have a lot to offer the world but I can now balance that with my personal needs as well. Recognizing my potential has enabled me to love life again and I know without a doubt that there is no negative condition left. I am not coping or managing my life; I am truly living and intend to continue on in this vein.

*　　*　　*

I have now been well for seven years. It's hard to think back to when I was ill for I don't even remember who that person was. What I do know is how I feel now. I have greater understanding and acceptance of my uniqueness as a human being. I enjoy the small details of that that I never allowed myself to enjoy before.

*　　*　　*

I cannot express the difference of waking up in the morning and being glad that I am here, as opposed to waking and wishing that I was dead. It is as simple as that and there is nothing more astonishing than comparing my state of mentality today to what it was 3 years ago. Today I can honestly say that if it hadn't been for a miracle, I would be 6 feet under and not have the slightest element of regret because at that point I saw no need to continue with a pointless, meaningless existence that caused everyone pain and suffering. I had no reason to live and not an ounce of hope left in my body, let alone strength to keep it there. Starving my body at the time made me feel [like] a better person although in reality the strength that I was desperate for was being reduced to non-existence and so I was inflicting more pain on myself both mentally and physically.

I saw no need to try to defeat the negativity that was growing day by day; or hour by hour because whatever I was doing was never enough for me to concentrate on and time went past so painstakingly slowly that I lost interest in life. Nothing I did was good enough and although I craved praise and congratulation for everything, nothing ever reached the point of satisfaction. A feeling of emptiness became the only way of making sure that I had been 'good' that day and in the end it became a feeling of comfort and reassurance that I had not rewarded myself undeservingly. I wished every day for some kind of triumph that would either take it all away and let me live without permanent punishment or kill me so that I wouldn't have to begin to deal with ridding myself of the negativity and never-ending hopelessness that filled the void that someone still called 'life.'

Today I finally have a 'life' and I can honestly say that every element of every arduous day of recovery has been worth the feelings I have now. The tantrums over eating another mouthful of chickpeas and the black depression that I hopelessly sank into having caught sight of my reflection in a mirror seem inconsequential compared to the happiness and joy that I can experience now.

I don't have to sit for hours calculating exactly how many calories I have eaten or when I next need to go to the gym in order to force my body to undergo more exercise and grueling calorie-burning activity. I no longer walk around supermarkets wishing that I could eat all the things on the shelves and putting things in my mouth to get the taste and spitting the whole lot out because I was not only going to look like more of a hideous balloon than I already did, but someone might see and think that I was obviously treating myself unnecessarily and without reason.

Not only does the difference within myself seem incomparable but the reaction of people around me, especially my family and close friends who instead of distancing themselves now ask me out to dinner and no longer feel worried about giving me a hug. Physically there are still good days and bad days but having the strength to deal with them is more than enough to pull through and realize that there are far better things to worry about.

For years the fashion industry has been accused of brainwashing women with its images of super-slim perfection, and being confronted with skinny models pasted on bus stops every day no longer affects me. Thanks to Peggy and Montreux I now accept the fact that if people can't like me for who I am rather than what I am or look like then they are valueless, hopeless people themselves.

The difference of being able to sit around the table and not have to worry about pushing food around my plate, make sure that I am interesting and ensure that everyone else looks happy is fantastic. And the biggest difference of all is being able to just sit down and relax because I am who I am, and in my mind I have acquired the strength that means I can learn to deal with almost anything at all!

*   *   *

It seems that the person that I was when I was sick did not resemble me as I knew myself to be. It has been ten years since I felt so pathetic, hopeless, and detached from the world as I knew it back then. I vividly remember cursing when I awoke each morning that I had to manage another day – not understanding what was wrong with me. I knew that others did not appear to feel the way that I did and I secretly wished to share my thoughts to know for sure. I remember watching others and wondering what made them so different from me.

Through the understanding that Peggy gave me, I

learned that I saw myself in my life and the lives of those around me through clouded eyes and a shattered soul of mixed up feelings and distorted ideas. With her perspective, I was able to see that I was the person I always wanted to be but was unable to see it in myself.

Since then, I no longer feel I have been singled out to be punished but allow myself to be human, make mistakes, and learn along the way. I take life for what it is and play with it rather than always trying to 'fix it.' Most importantly, I accept myself for who I am and enjoy learning more about myself and the world I am part of with every year that has gone by since I have been well.

*　　*　　*

Four years ago I led a bleak existence; trapped in the living hell of a bulimic's life. My days were preoccupied with a series of private rituals and activities consisting of bingeing and purging, obsessive exercise, and laxative abuse. Obsessive concerns about my body, looks, and weight were just the tip of the iceberg; there was no aspect of my personality that didn't disgust me. I felt that who I was, was worthless and without this bulimic identity, I was nothing. Often, frustration and self-loathing would lead me to acts of self-abuse and violence against others, and the guilt I felt would reinforce my beliefs that I was a horrible person.

I used to wonder what I had done to deserve such torture, but the ugly voice in my head would tell me I was getting what was coming to me and that this is what my future held for me. Deep down in my heart, I knew that wasn't who I was and who I wanted to be. I wanted to see what my life would be like without that horrible negative voice screaming at me every day.

Then I met someone who made me realize that I wasn't worthless, that it wasn't my fault, and I certainly didn't deserve these things for the rest of my life.

Today I live a life free from anxieties about food and body image and I love myself unconditionally. I can now look in the mirror without wanting to smash my head against it in disgust for what I see there. I no longer live my life to please other people, I know who I am and I realize that I can be anything or do anything I want to do; I have no limitations or fears now. I am in control of my destiny and look forward to wherever my life may lead me and I am happy to know myself.

I feel a great sadness in my heart when I hear people say that eating disorders can't be fully cured, because I know that I am living proof that they can. I was no different from anyone else, no exception to the rule, and I know that there is hope for a life free from this terrible thing and hope for a future.

*   *   *

I wrote a final exam last night, and when I went for a drink of water, a whole wave of memories swept over me. Ten years ago, I'd been at the same fountain, having written my final. I recall having an incredible thirst, and the panic and terror I experienced when I accidentally actually swallowed some of the water I was so desperately swishing in a futile attempt to moisten my mouth. Terrified, I took off for the tallest building at the university where I spent the next hour or so running up and down the stairwell in an attempt to burn off the effects that water would have on me. (I had traveled up and down so often between classes that the details of the floor and walls along that staircase are indelibly etched into my mind. To this day, though, I'm still not sure what lies beyond the top-floor doorway . . .)

The fear and depression and sadness of those last years of university are only memories now. As I attend lectures and write exams there once again, visions and events of those hellish years often flash through my mind. But that is all they are. That uncontrollable urge to exercise; that intense fear of food; the unceasing desperation and fear; they're all gone now. And Peggy saved me from that living hell. All the 'specialists,' psychologists, drugs, programs, and medical models used by these 'professionals' only made the condition worse over time. Without Peggy's patience, understanding, and love, I know I would not be here today to experience the life I lead.

And what a wonderful life it is! My job is terrific. It's challenging, interesting, and I'm valued for the contribution I make. My employers and coworkers are the best of friends. Days are filled with laughter and fun. School is also going well; only three courses remain until I graduate. Exams are hard but I enter into them confident of my capabilities; the psychologist that ruined my confidence (the little that remained after anorexia stripped most of it away, that is) by repeatedly stating that the brain damage caused by malnutrition meant I would never again amount to anything (because I would be unable to pass such grueling exams) has been proven wrong. (Indeed, I received 98% on my last exam!)

Weekends and after-work time are spent reading, on the computer, and biking – a hobby I continue to love and enjoy. It's such a relief to do it for fun again! (Those 12-hour-long sessions of non-stoppable pedaling are just a bad memory now.) Better yet, I often go home at night and do nothing but watch a movie or listen to music. Best of all, when I look at life, I can think of nothing I would choose to change. There's a feeling of laughter inside my chest that regularly erupts into laughter and joy again. It's great! I can honestly say that I couldn't possibly be happier. I have proven all the doctors wrong. I am happy and I love life!

*　　*　　*

I have suffered from anorexia nervosa for almost fourteen years. In those years I have tried to commit suicide many times and have spent many years in different hospitals. I hated my life and my only goal in life was to die. I lost my social life and contact with all my friends. I tried to look after other people but did not care about myself. I went through years of depression.

My Life After Anorexia Nervosa

I have been recovered now for two years. I am enjoying my life, have a social life back and spend a lot of time with my friends. For over a year, I have taken care of my friend's baby, as my friend went through a bad time of her own. I like helping people and do what I can for them, and I care a lot more about myself. I [want] to work with people with eating disorders or to be able to work with children as I have always adored children. At present, I am doing a lot of voluntary work which I really enjoy doing.

I can't get back the years that I missed out on due to

my illness and I don't regret that as I am making up for those lost years now.

*   *   *

I was eleven years old when anorexia entered my life. Anorexia was a monster. He would never leave me alone. Anorexia constantly told me I was fat and if I was skinny, people would like me. Instead the only friend I had in my mind was the scale. Each day I weighed myself about twenty times, hoping the scale would be less, thought if I did weigh less, anorexia was still not satisfied. I isolated myself from my family, consuming my head with calories, wanting to exercise constantly, and only seeing a massive image in the mirror. Doctors considered me a statistic; just waiting until I weighed sixty-five pounds so they could admit me to the hospital.

Suddenly my life instantly had a sense of hope when I met a lady named Peggy Claude-Pierre, who understood anorexia completely. I trusted her the first time I sat in her office because she looked into my eyes and told me, 'I know why you are rubbing your hands up and down your legs: for exercise.' That was a secret only anorexia and I knew. From that day on, I believed in Peggy. She took the responsibility of anorexia away from me, allowing myself to heal, so I could get strong and beat up anorexia until he vanished. Peggy also helped my parents understand anorexia, which brought me closer to them. Peggy became an angel because she saved my life.

I am now nineteen years old and going to the university. I have been able to go around schools and talk about anorexia so people have a better understanding of the monster that once lived in my head. I have been able to enjoy sports such as winning the county championships for rowing. Anorexia is no longer a part of me. I am never afraid of food and I am very happy. My family has become the most important part of me. I consider my mom and dad my best friends.

*   *   *

Before I came to Montreux, I was completely consumed by anorexia – it was my entire identity. The hooks of anorexia were embedded so deep in my mind and my body that I thought they would never loosen. I had no self-esteem, self-confidence, or sense of self-worth. The negative mindset and obsessive-compulsive behaviors of anorexia completely controlled every aspect of my life, as I lived according to a very strict and rigid set of rules created by anorexia to control every minute of the day, from my thoughts to exercising to my every action.

Suffering from frequent mood swings and depression, I was withdrawn and isolated from my family and society; I couldn't trust people, and was terrified of life and people. I felt completely unworthy of love and friendship because I was a failure as a person and could never be good enough to live up to the unrealistically high expectations I placed on myself and that I perceived were placed on me by others. I felt I had to be perfect at everything in my life, but constantly failed, and that I had to please everyone.

I was apathetic, not caring about life or living – I lived through and for other people, according to other people's expectations, because I wasn't worthy of living for myself and had to take responsibility for everyone else's life and problems, trying to solve everyone's problems and take away their pain.

Filled with self-loathing, I was on a path to self-destruction leading to death, constantly inflicting physical pain upon myself by bruising, burning myself with hot water, making myself bleed, and making my skin raw and sore. The anorexia filled me with an intense phobia of food, eating and weight gain (I weighed myself several times every day); constant nightmares and insomnia; defiant, secretive and manipulative behavior; frequent dizziness, fainting, and blackouts; constant never-ending inner and physical pain; constant, relentless daily exercising to the point of exhaustion and collapse, always working myself harder; atrophy of my muscles to the point of no longer being able to walk by the time I came to Montreux; and starvation to the point of severe emaciation and near death, looking like a skeleton.

I was in and out of hospitals for 2½ years, becoming even more severely anorexic each time. By the time I came to Montreux, the doctors and hospitals had given up on me – I had no blood pressure, an almost undetectable pulse, no hope.

Coming to Montreux saved my life, without a doubt; I could not have survived if I hadn't come here. I was horrified when I came here and thought it would be the same as the hospitals. I was convinced that the people here would give up on me and send me home, but they never gave up on me in their battle to defeat anorexia, no matter what the 'condition' did.

The whole atmosphere and treatment here is different from hospitals. At Montreux, I was under 24-hour care by people who understand the condition and are patient, loving, and caring. I was enveloped by *unconditional love*, positive reinforcement and objectivity in a home-like environment where I was totally made to feel safe and learn to trust people again. All my trust was put into the careworkers and the counselors.

I was on complete bed rest at first, and was not allowed to exercise or do any other self-destructive or self-harming behaviors. Responsibility for everything, including eating, was taken away from me and given to the careworkers to alleviate my guilt and shame. I was hand-fed by the careworkers for many months – liquid nutritional drinks at first, then slowly and gradually introduced to food. It was a long, hard battle but the careworkers were always there helping in the struggle and providing constant love, support, and encouragement. I was made to feel that I deserved and was worthy of love and friendship and happiness.

As time progressed, I went from being on 24-hour care to being in partial care to being off care and in counseling. Even though I was off care, my careworkers were still available for me to talk to. I had counseling sessions several times per week, at which we talked about many different topics, issues, and problems that I had to deal with, and how to conquer my many fears. I was given many projects to do, and taught many things – including how to live life again, and to discover myself. I've made many friends here.

At this point, I am living in my own place not far from the clinic; I am volunteering at a local charity and looking for a part-time job; I am going for weekend visits home to my family; and having sessions once a week, working on clearing the final hurdles.

I can't believe how far I've come and never thought it would ever be possible before I came to Montreux.

Everyone here is so special, and the best thing to come out of my becoming anorexic was coming here and meeting all the neat people, making great friends, and being given a chance to live.

* * *

I started loathing myself when I was 11. It started by waking up every morning and picking apart every flaw I thought I had. This escalated to my cringing every time I heard my own voice. I thought I talked too much or not enough, I was evil or I was a doormat. It didn't seem to matter what I said or did, nothing was good enough.

If I ate, no matter what it was, it was too much and I had to get it out of my body. My knuckles were raw from stuffing them down my throat; my teeth scraped off skin. There was about five minutes after I purged where I felt a numbness. The pain inside subsided. Only to return stronger shortly thereafter.

Being sick was like being drunk for seven or eight years, although I was that too. I don't like to use the overused words 'out of control.' . . . I think 'loss of being' is a better description. No sense of myself existed. I was what each different individual in my life wanted me to be. 'I' had disappeared. All I wanted to do was die and even in that I saw myself as a failure.

When I entered into the program, I didn't even know who or what to believe. The more these people described this condition to me, the more at ease I felt. For the first time in my life I felt understood. I wasn't better overnight and it wasn't as though I woke up one morning and yelled, 'Yay! I'M WELL!' It took a lot of time and effort by both myself and those who helped me at the clinic. And slowly but surely I started to find out who I really was, and to my amazement, I began to accept myself.

Today, which is now 3½ years after I finished the program, I work 40+ hours per week, am living with someone, and am no longer a half of a whole. I feel complete inside and out. When I look back at what my life was like when I was sick, it only makes me look forward to all that I now have the chance to enjoy.

*   *   *

BEFORE
BEFORE I came here and during the times when I felt most TRAPPED, whilst I was here I was so SUICIDAL.

I was a BURDEN to the world, USELESS and an IMPOSITION on everyone. I felt GUILTY for living, for using ELECTRICITY. I WASN'T ALLOWED ANYTHING. NO LIGHT, NO HEAT, NO BED. NO SHELTER from a building, a BUSH was too GREEDY. NO MUSIC, NO TELEVISION. I was not allowed WARM baths or showers. NO WARM CLOTHES or COVERS. I felt GUILTY for the MONEY it cost to refrigerate my FOOD, when I was too FAT and too OBESE to ever need to eat another CALORIE in my life.

I was so INTRINSICALLY BLACK, so deeply, deeply EVIL I COULD NOT EVEN BE HUMAN. No human being could be so BLACK INSIDE, so INCREDIBLY EVIL.

I would CUT myself with RAZORS or KNIVES, 100s of times. Each time, the BLACK liquid within me, so much thicker than any tar, could NOT be RED. It could not be. There was ONLY BLACK inside me. WHY was it still RED? *WHY?*

IF I was even a little human, I wanted so badly to DONATE MY ORGANS, so that good people could live and do good things in the world. I NEVER could, despite wanting to HELP PEOPLE MORE THAN ANYTHING in the world.

I was a SELFISH, SELF-CENTERED, FAT BITCH. I didn't and COULDN'T even WANT TO WANT TO GET BETTER.

I was NEVER allowed to enjoy anything and must CONSTANTLY HURT MYSELF. I couldn't open letters as I enjoyed it but it might also confirm that SOMEONE OUT THERE MIGHT CARE. No I couldn't allow that. I must BURN, CUT, SCAR, STARVE, BINGE, PURGE, EXERCISE, ABUSE LAXATIVES, PAINKILLERS, ANTI-DEPRESSANTS, ANTI-PSYCHOTICS, SEDATIVES, CALMING PILLS, anything to NUMB the PAIN. I would SHUT my EYES as I walked along, pretending LIFE WASN'T HAPPENING. I'd go to bed hoping and praying I'd be DEAD by morning. The SCALES were never low enough. The CUTS and BURNS, never NUMEROUS ENOUGH or DEEP ENOUGH. The clothes SIZE never SMALL ENOUGH, the GRADE never HIGH ENOUGH, the CALORIES were always TOO HIGH, my DANCE never GOOD ENOUGH. I wanted everything to be PERFECT, but it NEVER could be.

I was USELESS, HOPELESS, WORTHLESS. I was IMPRISONED in my MIND. All I wanted was to HELP PEOPLE. But I was a USELESS, SELFISH BITCH.

I deserved NO ONE. I deserved NOTHING. And SELFISHLY to end the PAIN, I saw DEATH as a door to PEACE.

The WORLD would be BETTER WITHOUT ME. Family, friends, the world would be better with me DEAD.

AFTER

AFTER 23 months, I am now understanding, truly, for I think the first time in my life, what 'HAPPINESS' means.

I'm FREE. I'm SAFE. I'm INDEPENDENT. When I go for a walk, I DON'T wish I was under a car. When the SUN is out, I love the way the world looks. I LOVE my FRIENDS, I TRUST people and I have people who are so KIND to me.

I am so GRATEFUL I have people who UNDERSTAND me and KNOW the REAL ME.

I LOVE DANCING. I love going out for BREAKFAST or a LATTE. It's so fun to go for a *WALK* just because it's so beautiful outside. It's FUN to be SPONTANEOUS and to enjoy being SOCIABLE. To be honest, I do still feel like a burden and I worry that people feel obligated to take me out, but it DOESN'T rule my life, and is something I have to work on still.

EMOTIONS are so much STRONGER. I am NO LONGER numb or fighting to sub-exist. I'm NOT on drugs, and I'll NEVER have E.C.T. [electroconvulsive therapy] again, or have people threaten to lock me up.

When I SMILE, it's GENUINE.

When I LAUGH, I MEAN it.

I have ENERGY. I'm NOT in physical or emotional pain. I ENJOY MUSIC, I ALLOW MYSELF so much more. I DARE TO RISK. I LOOK FORWARD to making plans, I want to travel. I want to spend QUALITY TIME with my FAMILY, especially my FATHER and GOD-CHILD.

I'm so much more OBJECTIVE and can put things into PERSPECTIVE, quicker and easier or ask for help to.

I'm finding out who I am.

I'm discovering what I LIKE, and when I think of things I WANT TO DO, NOT everything and everyone I would never see again.

Now I go to bed because I have to sleep, NOT to escape, and I LOOK FORWARD to getting up in the morning and to TOMORROW. I don't know what TOMORROW will bring, but I DON'T fear it or worry. It's EXCITING and DIFFERENT, yet SECURE.

I know I will see or talk to people I CARE ABOUT. Not every day is a breeze, but I TRUST those I know and can now ASK FOR HELP.

I'm BEGINNING to find PEACE, and I'm very HAPPY.

It's a long road and it's not an easy one, but I like where it's taking me and it's incredibly WORTH-WHILE.

I'm very HAPPY, LUCKY, AND GRATEFUL I'm still ALIVE. Now I have the chance to START to *LIVE* my life.

*   *   *

Ever since I can remember, I was a very caring person. I used to take every little thing that someone said about me personally. I was worried about my parents and felt badly about spending their money, taking their time. Four years ago, food started to become an issue; I stopped eating and felt good being hungry all the time. I used to care a lot about what other people ate, and I was always in the kitchen making food for others, but never for myself. I wanted to eat but I just couldn't. Something in my head was stronger than I was, and controlled the way I acted and what I ate or thought.

287

Now that I am better, I see life in a different way. I don't worry about little things, and I accept myself and my body the way I am. I am happy now and I have many interests and ideas. Food is not an issue anymore, and I can eat anything I ever wanted and was not allowed to have. This feeling is great.

*   *   *

Food was a dear friend from an early age. It was a steady chum to turn to; it was accessible, reliable and sweet, and after an hour in its company, I felt calm and sedated. Food was something controllable, and in a world that was spinning too fast to figure out, it was the eye of the hurricane.

But when, as a teenager, a burgeoning body led to a more mature world than I was prepared for, food became the enemy, and I was to continue a love/hate bulimic relationship with it for another twelve years.

There is a graphicness about anorexia and bulimia that only a guy like Oliver Stone could do justice to. Perhaps you have to experience it or witness it at close range to realize that it truly is a war. My friends and family had a lot of difficulty understanding why I'd enlisted. Trying to explain it to someone was always the most difficult part of intimacy.

Obsessed by my world of alcohol, cocaine, ipecac, and Dulcolax, I became equally compulsive about learning what I could about eating disorders, hoping I would discover the magic formula that would end the madness. I needed tools to apply my energy positively, rather than to my demise. My motivation to recover from bulimia was never lacking; however, my bleak financial picture from years of practicing my illness did little to encourage professionals to want to work with me.

My great fortune was in meeting people who understood my strange interior life without judgment and who, at a time when I didn't feel there was anything to live for, were there to lend me their vision and pull me through the grueling journey of recovery. I'd never been afraid of hard work and perhaps it's that 'work ethic' that finally worked for me rather than against me. Recovery is arduous – coming back from being that far 'out there' is a deep emotional and spiritual challenge.

I almost consider my struggle with bulimia an alchemical gift – I'm thankful for the opportunity it afforded me to take a cool, discerning stare into the contexts that were running my life and identity, contexts I didn't invent, but I went along with unconsciously. Driving the right car, wearing the right clothes, dating the right men, or impressing the right authority all seemed to matter when I was ill and trying to prove to the world that I had worth. The paradox was that when I stopped trying to prove myself externally, I realized I already had.

Now I look back on my illness without the veil of denial that is so characteristic of anorexia and bulimia, and I stagger when I think of what I did to my body, mind, and spirit for so many years. I now live a life where the important things are my husband, family, and friends and the comforting love we all share, not calories, exercise, secrecy, and shame. I gave up a life of chaos and drama, filled with constant thoughts of striving and achieving, for a gentle inner peace – traded the BMW mentality for a cardigan.

I hope someday to look back on this time in our

history and only read about the curious phenomenon of anorexia and bulimia to be touched by it, not have to witness its destruction and ruin on the bodies and faces I pass on the street. Thank God one woman witnessed her daughters' pain, soothed it, and now tells others how she did it. I hope they'll listen. . . .

*　　*　　*

Everything in life is a process; or at least it is in mine. I didn't become anorexic overnight. Nor is there a definite time when I can say I realized I was sick. It all happened gradually for me.

As long as I can remember I hadn't liked who I was in any facet or sense. To me, I was a terrible, despicable, and ugly human being who had been created simply due to negligence. I was a mistake from the beginning. I convinced myself that I didn't deserve anything, least of all love. I didn't allow myself to believe that I was loved, no matter what I was shown or told. I thought they must be lying, that I was unlovable. Over time, this negativity increased. I got to the point where I thought I didn't deserve to live. I thought I was such a terrible person that I deserved and was destined to die.

Food is one thing you definitely need to be alive. I didn't think I deserved anything that would facilitate life. I began to slowly starve myself. I slowly began to cut out things, but that wasn't enough. I deserved less and less every day. I eventually got to the point where I thought I shouldn't allow myself any food, that I had to get rid of it. This led to bulimia. Throughout this time, my opinion of myself plummeted even further. I thought I was a nobody and I hated myself for everything.

When I started getting better, I started believing that I deserved to be alive and happy. I no longer thought I was a terrible person who wasn't worthy of anything. I realized it was okay to make mistakes, and that I didn't need to blame myself for everything. I stopped focusing on imperfections and started to focus on the good parts of myself. In letting go of all my guilt for events in the past, I was able to start to like who I really was. I allowed myself to be happy and have fun and soon it became a natural thing.

I now look forward to getting up in the morning just because I enjoy being alive. I now like who I am as a person, and that means everything to me. I know that I can deal with anything that may come my way. I know what is out there in the world and what I can do, and what great fun it can all be.

*　　*　　*

No one should ever have to worry. I am a person who has spent years worrying. I've been worried for everything from my little sister's cold to the starving people in Africa and in my distress for every person, animal, and situation, I missed everything in life that is fun.

I am now sixteen and I finally feel like being a teenager can be a happy experience; it's too bad it's taken me so long to accept myself, to be content. So many unfair things happen in this world. I had wanted to fix everything, take away all pain, all hate. Save everyone!

Now I know I can use this will to be strong so I can go out in the world and just be happy. Instead of handling problems as I always did before – hopelessly taking out the world's problems on myself – I'm able to contribute a caring, but healthy and energetic personality to the people around me. At least I can actually get up in the morning looking forward to the day ahead of me, knowing that though things won't be perfect, nor will everything go exactly right, but I can do the best I can, and my positivity will rub off on others.

I use my powerful determination to actually get things done, instead of destroying my body in despair. With good health, my outlook has become so different; I get so enthusiastic about things. I've also noticed this attracts others, from school friends to the neighbors next door – people just seem drawn to happiness. It's awesome!

I was sick with anorexia since the fifth grade. Even before that, I remember carrying everyone else's burdens along with my own load and slowly being crushed harder and harder into a person filled with self-hatred and depression. I thought that everything was my fault; I didn't deserve to live. After all the suffering, the eating disorder manifested, and I went through all the traumas that go along with anorexia in our society. I saw the end many times, in fact, I'm amazed that I'm here today after all I've been through. Now I can be glad I've made it!

Somehow a little flame flickered inside, even through the very toughest moments. A little part of me still had hope and wanted somehow, to live. Then, with the help of understanding and unconditional love, things started to be put back in perspective. Time and patience are the biggest and most difficult parts in fixing such a negative mindset, but life does get better, as I can attest to now. It's a relief when you realize it's true – no one should ever have to worry.

*　　*　　*

When bulimia started, I was about thirteen years old. I had always had a low self-image. As the condition took over, I started to lose everything; the ability to look at myself objectively, a sense of self, a positive perspective on life, and most importantly, the will to live. At sixteen, the condition had really taken over and at seventeen, I was out of school and all I did all day was write in my diary about how I wanted nothing but death. My soul had almost completely deteriorated and I was overtaken by the demons inside of me. All I could think about was how I was going to end my life.

Luckily, my friends and family exposed my condition, and I got help. I started seeing Peggy Claude-Pierre and found someone who really understood me and my condition. I went through a difficult process of gaining strength, confidence, and a sense of self. I am now twenty-one and I have regained my soul, my confidence, and my will to live. I love life and appreciate every pleasure it brings me. I love living without that negative feeling lingering around me constantly. When people used to look into my eyes, they would tell me how sad and distant they seemed. When people look into my eyes today, they say that they glow, as I glow. Life is definitely worth living, and now I know how much I have to offer this world, to the people around me, as well as to myself.

*　　*　　*

Anorexia is the most indescribable pain anyone can ever experience, as well as the toughest hurdle to overcome. I know this to be true because I had lived with the condition for five years, until I overcame it.

Looking back, I can honestly say I had no life whatsoever. All I thought about every minute of the day was how unattractive I thought I was, at what time I would exercise, how I could get out of eating, what lies I would tell my parents and friends, how awful a person I was, etc., etc. These thoughts played like a broken record over and over in my head, to the point where all I wanted to do was to go to sleep and not wake up. I can remember getting so frustrated asking myself why I was going through such mental torture, that I would start screaming, pulling my hair, banging my head, anything to try to give myself a moment of peace.

The constant dictating or nagging to do what anorexia wanted me to do caused great loneliness and isolation. I withdrew from my family and friends and any social setting. I did not want to accept any help from anyone because I felt that I did not deserve it. I believed I was a horrible person for making my parents watch me slowly dying, thus, receiving help from them would be total selfishness.

Being able to see things realistically now, I can see that I did not purposely choose to be sick. Being overly sensitive from day one, feeling as though I had to take care of my family, feeling inferior to my friends, and having low self-esteem all contributed to my negative mindset. Thus, the act of starving myself not only from food, but of things that made me happy were the outlets or paths of my negativity. When I think about it today, how I treated my body and my mind, I am in complete shock and awe of how I survived. How I ate nothing for days on end, as well as not even drinking water, brings chills to my body when I think about it. However, feeling pain, hunger, fatigue, and weakness did not even cross my mind for many years, for it became my way of living.

I can now realize my true identity, separate from the condition, and what is normal for a 16-year-old girl. I promised myself I would overcome this hurdle, and I did. I feel like such a weight has been lifted off of me. No more do I base my worth on if I managed to exercise all day, eat nothing, my appearance, etc. I look at each day as a new one, and enjoy things again.

*　　*　　*

I was sick for most of the years of my adolescent life, with anorexia. Through my ninth year of school, I spent most of my days in hospitals and programs. I was a straight-A student, a dancer, involved in activities and in general, a pretty good kid; but inside I had a drowning feeling of worthlessness. I didn't know how to express my feelings and I strove to hurt myself instead of letting my emotions out. As I grew sicker, I began to have more hate for myself. I reached my goal; I was thin, but nearly dead, and I came to the realization that the thinner I became, the more unhappy I was.

One night, in the hospital, I had a dream where I was told by a heavenly power that I had a purpose to serve in life. The next day, I left the hospital and was on Peggy's doorstep. I made the choice – the choice to help myself. I learned to talk about my difficulties and work through them. Life is beautiful. Food isn't the issue, life is. When I stopped focusing my energy on food, I had so much more time for myself, for love and enjoyment of others. With the condition, I wasn't functioning to my full capacity. I now eat to be healthy and strong. The stronger I become, the more attractive I feel.

This year, my graduating class is the Class of the Phoenix. The Phoenix is a mythological bird that burns into ashes and transforms into a beautiful creature. I feel that the bird relates to us all; our struggles will help us grow, develop, and become stronger. I took the power within myself to help me transform.

*   *   *

Trying to recall the agony I went through when I was anorexic is at times easy because of the extreme state of torment it created. On the other hand, remembering becomes more difficult because I have not been in that negative frame of mind and body for over ten years. Over ten years without a hint of the anorexic condition left other than the understanding of what anorexia and bulimia means. This complex theory enables me to help any other victim of this horrible condition. . . . horrible though very reversible.

I am proof that you do not have to spend your life wondering if your heart will withstand one more evening or feel the desperation to torture yourself both physically and emotionally because you have made the wrong comment or perhaps have hurt someone's feelings. When I was ill with anorexia, I truly didn't think it was possible to be saved, I felt doomed 24 hours a day. I guess there must have been one percent of a seed of myself left to work with though it was not evident to me at the time. Now I know the road one must take to recovery, total recovery.

Coming through the painful tunnel to wellness has made me a complete person. Once I conquered the negative mindset I was much more objective, gently confident and fully aware of my surroundings. By surroundings I mean society and its motives. The type of knowledge I now have makes me feel rich and fulfilled instead of diminished, hopeless, and frustrated. I once saw life through a different set of eyes.

I trust people and not an imaginary voice being repeatedly negative. I trust myself. Though I am inherently sensitive, interacting in any circumstance or situation is completely comfortable for me. I exude optimism without having high expectations of anyone or anything, including myself. I adore my position in life and the many, many people immediately surrounding my life. Because I respect my purpose for existence, I ultimately respect myself.

*　　*　　*

There was a time when I was young, eleven years old to be exact, that I came up with an idea of how to stay skinny. I decided that if I ate and then threw it up, I could eat whatever I wanted but never gain weight. At first it was just a little diet, then it became an everyday activity, then that diet became a web of terror, filled with anxiety, self-hate, and self-worthlessness, which I no longer controlled. I hated life, never believed I deserved to live, to be loved or to eat; in my eyes I was a fat, worthless, horrible person who deserved nothing, not even love. When my eating disorder was at its worst, I could no longer take the self-hate and pain, but I didn't know what to do because I believed anorexia was something I had to live with. I believed life would hold nothing amazing for me, nothing except misery.

I was wrong. Life was worth living and anorexia is nobody, it just feeds in the minds of those who are too nice to say no to its nastiness. I'm glad I listened to Peggy and my family and my special friends because [otherwise] I wouldn't have become a success – because I beat it and am living my life the way I always should have. It is strange how life is so pleasant and full of love once you are freed from the iron grips of anorexia. I can actually love myself for all of myself, no longer spitting at the image in the mirror. I cannot imagine if I had died because life began when I found my own self, a self who loves to be loved, a self who is the strongest she's ever been.

I am now fulfilling all of my dreams, dreams anorexia made me believe that I was too worthless to have. Anorexia was wrong; we are all worthy. I am living proof.

*　　*　　*

During my struggle with anorexia, I felt an overwhelming concern with my self-image. I felt I had to be perfect in all areas of my life, yet I didn't even know who I was. I tried in vain to be what I felt others expected me to be, but always fell short in my eyes.

I absorbed the pain and suffering of [all] I came in contact with, soaking up all the negativity around me, finally sinking into despair and depression.

Meanwhile, consuming food resulted in nausea and bloating, convincing me that I was allergic to most foods. Further, I still became ill after what little I did find safe to eat, causing me to question the value of eating at all. I often found myself lying on the kitchen floor, physically weak and emotionally pained.

Everything in life required great effort and I found myself losing hope and security in society, people and my ability to succeed in anything. I wanted to isolate myself, to disappear or cease to exist in an attempt to escape the despair, fear, self-hatred, and imperfections that I felt were so active and evident in my life.

Today my view of life has become one filled with hope, courage and joy. I find myself respecting and loving myself and accepting imperfections as a part of being human.

I enjoy a balanced lifestyle of enjoyment and responsibility. I am now married to a wonderful wife and we anxiously await the arrival of our first child.

*　　*　　*

All of my life I lived for other people – not out of choice, but because I didn't know any other way. It wasn't until years later that I found out that I didn't actually have a self. I became what other people liked, thought, said and did; without respect for myself, going day by day trying to please other people so that I could be good enough. The breaking point was when I displayed the manifestation of anorexia, because all of the self-hatred and worthlessness became too much, and I began a slow, subconscious suicide. My life became a living hell; isolating myself from anyone who cared while I destroyed myself; thinking that I was crazy and yet holding on for dear life; clinging to it because I felt that I had no other choice.

When I came to Montreux, all control was taken away from anorexia, and I felt sad, terrified, depressed and very panicked. I didn't know how I could live without my only so-called friend – my condition. Because I had no self, and the only idea I had of myself was the anorexia, I felt like there was nobody there; I had no personality, and this was really scary. In the environment of unconditional love and acceptance, my personality, locked deep inside for so long, began to emerge, growing stronger by the day, until it grew stronger than anorexia. I could fight what it told me, by myself. Now, anorexia has no control of me. I know who I am and I like myself – something I never thought possible. I enjoy my days, and other people don't scare me – I love being sociable and making friends. Going through this experience has given me so much knowledge and wisdom about the world; I don't regret having been sick because otherwise I wouldn't know what I know now. My only regret is for all of the wasted years when I was so miserable. I'm making up for it now, by being doubly happy. My life has just begun and I'm finally ready to live it.

*　　*　　*

For most of my life, I changed or interpreted situations until they caused me worry, anguish, and grief. It is extremely difficult to explain because a lot of what went on was in the subconscious mind. I didn't realize what I was doing until it became so obsessive and uncontrollable that I became severely anorexic. Let me start by giving you a brief synopsis of my childhood. I was a very intelligent, cheerful girl with supportive parents, tons of friends, vacations every year, a dog and a pool in the backyard. Everything I ever needed was provided for me, including much understanding, encouragement, and love. Looking back, I realize that even then, at a different degree, worry was always inside and sensitivity was a major factor. As the years went on, my self-acceptance and worth gradually deteriorated, causing negative thinking patterns and anorexia to enter my mind. Nothing was logical, yet everything was incomprehensible; for it felt like even though I had eyes, I couldn't actually 'see,' I had ears but I couldn't 'hear,' I could talk but not 'listen,' and I could think but not 'understand.' It felt as though I was incapable of doing anything because of how unreachable my true identity really was. If my life was in the form of a ladder, I was desperately grasping the last rung. Inside, my mind was a series of webs, entrapped and intertwined with negative thoughts, causing me to become greatly confused and upset. My anger and frustration would then get turned against me and I would harm myself even more. My mind, body, and soul were never at peace; even sleep was disturbed with evil nightmares and pains. Nothing in the world was of any importance to me, except suffering.

Now, years later, my life is incomparable to how it was then. I can actually live, go to school, make friends, interact with family and most importantly, I can truly laugh and be happy. I am able to be logical and look forward to making my future dreams into a reality. I often ask myself 'why.' The only answer I can come up with is this: Everything happens for a reason and with courage, determination, faith, love, and understanding from others, the top of the ladder can be reached.

* * *

Dear Peggy,

In the year that I have been here at the clinic I have learned more about myself and about others, and have finally begun to accept the joy of life, the goodness of so many, and the very miraculous gift you have given me. I want so much to be able to glean from you all the knowledge and guidance you have demonstrated and bestowed upon those who work with you. I have been graced with the chance to experience new thoughts [that are] no longer debilitating me with fear and [are] unable to plague me with hatred. I cannot express to you my sincere thanks for it would truly take the very wonderful lifetime you have helped me discover. I only wish to use all the wisdom and the progress to come in the future to aid another to realize the magnificence and contentment I know now. You gave me a miracle far greater than I could have ever imagined.

*　　*　　*

When I was young
My father told me
Smile
So they think you're happy
And my smile became a mask
That I hid behind, ashamed to come out.
I didn't realize until too late
That the mask had become
Stuck to my soul
I couldn't take it off
I didn't know how
Until I started learning
To smile with my heart
And the mask began to crack
And I could slow, slowly step outside.
I left the mask discarded
Cracked and broken on the pavement
So I could turn my face to the sun.

*　　*　　*

If someone had asked me four years ago where I would be today, I honestly would not have been able to answer. I suppose at that time I would have hoped that I would no longer be alive, because I could not have imagined living another year trying to battle bulimia. Every day I woke up hating myself more and more, convinced that I was a weak person unable to control a disease that was ruling every minute of my day. I was purging at least five times a day, my face was swollen, my hair was falling out, and I was too ashamed to see my family and friends. I became withdrawn and secretly hoped that I would be diagnosed with some terminal disease so that I could finally end this torment. I had begun to think about suicide, but felt I could never disappoint my family with such a selfish action. I honestly thought that bulimia/anorexia was a part of my personality that I could never release and would have to learn to live with for the rest of my life. And then I met Peggy.

I remember walking out of my first meeting with Peggy and for the first time I had felt a small glimmer of hope. I had been to different physicians and counselors but had never experienced such a sense of compassion and understanding of eating disorders, nor had I ever been told that I would one day be free from living like a prisoner in my own body. Well, I am free, and I am stronger than I could have ever imagined. I have learned to love myself and, along with this, have learned to be loved.

I know that whatever I am faced with in the future, I will succeed, and I will be happy, because I am a wonderful, intelligent, beautiful individual who deserves the best that life can offer. The road to recovery is never easy but I am so happy that I have had all my experiences because they make me who I am and I'm pretty happy to be me.

There was a time in my life when I thought that I would never be freed from the 'shackles' of anorexia. So powerful were they, that I had inadvertently become a slave to an existence void of freedom by the obsessive darkness that controlled my every thought and action. So heavy were they that I was pulled further and further down into a state of despair. My acute sensitivity and ultimately my great lack of self-esteem had created a monster. Initially, this monster was my friend, my comfort, and the one thing in my life that I could control. It made me feel happy, strong, and safe from the disturbing injustices of society that surrounded me. Before long, 'it' had taken over. 'It' was no longer my friend; I no longer felt any joy, safety, or strength. All that I can remember feeling is terribly guilty, shameful, and powerless for having made my loving parents cry and suffer so.

I have been well for five years now, and rarely think of my illness, as I know it was an isolated incident of the past. In retrospect, it was probably the most influential experience that I could have gone through. The process of my recovery enabled me to let go of my false sense of and need for control. I learned how to love myself and how to live again. I feel empowered in a way that I never thought was possible. I've taken responsibility for my own happiness and future, as I have let go of all of the elements that are beyond my control. I wake up smiling and always look forward to the wondrous adventures that lie ahead. I feel strongly for those who are going through what I did, yet I am convinced that however dark their reality may seem (forgive the cliché), there is a light so brilliant at the end of the tunnel, that the darkness (with the right help) will soon fade away.

*　　*　　*

I leap into the world
Embracing the sunlight
Fearlessly chasing the shadows
Which before I would run from
I laugh at myself
At the pure joy
The smiling faces
Children caught in a spider's web
Of wonder and delight
At a world still fresh and new
It's only a normal day
But only if I want it to be.

A Final Message of Hope

A LETTER TO SOCIETY

Jesus Christ said, 'Verily I say unto you, Inasmuch as ye have done it unto one of the least of these my brethren, ye have done it unto me.'

Throughout history, societies stand by, time and time again, helpless, naive, or self-righteous, as human life becomes expendable; throughout history, death or murder are condoned or justified by mass inaction; boundaries of ethics are extended under the guise of morality to accept the unthinkable; societal desensitization evolves as a means of personal survival, and reason never did have a hand.

Throughout history, people have sought ways of identifying themselves by excluding others. Competition celebrates the individual or the few beyond the well-being of the whole. Race, religion, performance, or socioeconomic status decide who is valid in society and who is not. The natural imperfection of human nature is forever measured and made conditional.

Moreover, we humans cling to the traditional for the sake of stability, security, and continuity. We preserve kings beyond their time and create deities where none exist to validate our mores. Whichever way the trend, our perceived safety depends on our general adherence to the social norm. We bow to authority for its own sake sometimes, out of fear, confusion, or apathy. Doubt in our own abilities or acceptance of the status quo permits us to blind ourselves to questionable or inadequate leadership. We evade personal responsibility.

We naturally assume that society's members in some manner reflect it as a whole. Given the differences among people, it should be no surprise that many interpretations will develop from a seemingly equal premise. These many interpretations are not themselves the problem; it is our failure to understand and appreciate them that compromises the individual's sense of security and peaceful coexistence with his neighbor. If we do not understand another's motivation, at least let us not be unkind.

Fear that involvement in others' suffering might complicate our own forward movement can paralyze our inherent spontaneity to help those in need. Recall the case of Kitty Genovese, the woman beaten to death in New York City in 1964 as neighbors watched and heard her screams but did not come to her aid. (The term 'bystander apathy' was coined at that time.) Cannot the same be said of people with eating disorders? We witness their ordeal and ignore their need for help. Not only do we not help, but we blame them for their plight.

My daughter Kirsten's poem, written while she had anorexia, speaks to that experience:

. . . We are some, allowed error in minimum
Depending on who we are
Others would seem,
Have free rein
And with many disguises they strike and assume,
Always looking to lay blame

A title, a letter or two
Borrowed from those who lie behind the mind
Tools to flaunt
Improvise and misuse.

My correspondent Edna also writes about society's misinterpretation of the anorexic's plight:

. . . If I were to choose
the finest words
available to man,
and sculpt
these baffling strifes
so fellow minds
might understand;

Assuredly,
those words would drown
in the tides
of interpretation;
the Truth
a victim of witlessness,
and confused evaluation.

We have allowed an unkind, sometimes inhuman interpretation of eating disorders to prevail, and that interpretation has permitted the deaths of countless innocents.

Life and the living of it are an unpredictable struggle for balance. That the human race survives as well as it does is perhaps commendable. The lamentable thing is that kindness and compassion have become rare, exceptional, even remarkable. Therefore, however well society feels it moves from each decade to the next, the concept of progress is always only that of interpretation.

Our successful interaction with others depends on the social contract of respect even when we do not always understand one another. Surely, survival of the human race depends on the inclusion of all. Why has not everyone's child become our own? Why do differences not bring enlightenment and curiosity but fear and disavowal? How can we turn our backs on a segment of society – those with eating disorders – unfairly announce that they have brought this calamity on themselves, and allow them to die?

Recently in a Western European country, a young girl with anorexia was granted permission to kill herself because she and her care team believed her condition was hopeless. That the sufferer of an eating disorder can be so mistaken and forsaken as to resort to the incredible loneliness of euthanasia makes me think we live in a psychological ice age. That a person who has lived a mere twenty-four years, albeit part of it in intense psychological misery, has been validated in her despair and hopelessness is a nasty comment on how society values such people. That we have come to condone despair, even promote it, leaves one to wonder at the purpose of 'progress.' If we do not embrace humanism, then what is the point?

I am deeply saddened by our indifference to the plight of those suffering from CNC. When do we become responsible for those who see no other avenue but euthanasia or suicide? How is this not condoning murder, especially when we see that eating disorders can be cured? When does bystander apathy or ego with regard to eating disorders become a crime against humanity as great as the others profiled in history books?

What has happened to tolerance, understanding, and

compassion? Why is it so remarkable that any child is our responsibility? Modern society somehow adheres to a 'survival of the fittest,' a 'kick him while he's down' attitude. Would we be so uncaring if it were an animal that was frightened and hurting rather than a child? Why? Perhaps because we have no expectations of animals, because they are less complicated, because there are not so many societal variables in interactions with them.

Could bystander apathy be a conditioned response? Could watching violent movies and television programming have furthered our inability to realize that we are not helpless when dire circumstances are real and not the product of someone's overheated imagination? Have we become so paralyzed that most of our actions are internal and therefore in need of sedation? Could society have 'progressed' to such a state of internalized turmoil and anxiety that it needs to be sedated in order to survive?

What part does the widespread use of prescription drugs play in our value systems? Granted, the value of these drugs is irrefutable. But has their usage become an unnecessary norm and a precursor to social acceptance of illicit use? Does the sedation of society create isolation and shame for those unable to survive without it? When we prescribe a pill for every emotion, do we seek to eliminate emotion and responsibility for others? Does this not suggest that emotions are expedient, that people and humanness are expendable for the sake of the greater cause of efficiency and productivity? A pill may address all of the symptoms, maybe, of an emotional problem, but the message conveyed is that the human condition, with all of its frailties and foibles, is not to be supported.

Do modern societies find it inexpedient to take time for nurturing? Do we expect too much of our children too soon? Do our children have the tools and support to construct their lives? Do our external values really represent our selfish desires? If so, how then can the true humanists, those predisposed to a CNC mindset, survive except by exclusion from such a society?

To comprehend the phenomenon of eating disorders, we must understand their origin – the platform of modernity. Eating disorders are a complex negative interpretation of one's role in life. CNC is the culmination of negative assumptions about oneself in the caring of and responsibility for the world. Because of the hallmarks of this mindset – sensitivity, above-average intelligence, caring, compassion, and commitment – these children are sitting ducks for learning society too well for their own good.

How, then, can we castigate a segment of our population, who, being more caring and aware by virtue of their genetic endowments, have learned all they have been taught? They are guilty of the suggestibility and gullibility of the young trying to adapt to their environment. They are guilty of adapting without the maturity necessary for a proper perspective. Their sensitivity, caringness, and anxiety for their fellow man has created in them a subservience that precludes realistic existence. That these children are better equipped for learning society's lessons, are so vulnerable to sensationalism and marketing, has apparently worked as their worst enemy.

The victims of eating disorders are a devastating by-product of modern society. The responsibility for this contemporary social issue is the responsibility of all of us, not of the victim! The attitude of 'What are you going to do about your problem?' 'When are you going to comply?' places the onus of blame and responsibility primarily on the victim. And ultimately that is incompatible with their healing. If we direct ourselves to nurturing the humanness within ourselves, we can drive out the scourge of eating disorders.

A LETTER TO PARENTS

Dearest Parents,

I write this letter to you in answer to the thousands of missives I have received from you and have been unable to respond to personally. You have much company. Your helplessness and desperation haunt my every moment. Your courage and dignity, even so, charge me with determination beyond what is sometimes humanly possible. Please pardon my limitations and realize that could I take into care every person I hear about, I would gladly.

But, I thank you for the gift you have given me – that of knowing what I have always hoped was true. The world is full of wonderful people, even in their moment of direst need and misery.

Know that you are not at fault for your child's condition. Know that she may at times attempt to alienate you. In her darkest hour she cannot bear the pain of the burden of her love for you and her sense that she has somehow failed you and society. Be strong. Live the lesson she must learn for survival – that of objectivity.

To understand the world, one must observe it from apart – with compassion for the motivation, personality, and conditioning of each person, regardless of how he or she behaves.

Love your child unconditionally. Talk to her with calm

logic to offset the negative tape running constantly in her brain. Do not allow unkindness to her from any source. Try to teach rather than to condemn those who do not understand. The end of knowledge is wisdom; the end of wisdom, humility.

I have stood where you stand with my children; I stand there yet, with yours.

A LETTER TO SUFFERERS

My Dearest Ones:

Every day I receive letters from you or your loved ones on your behalf. Every day, my heart aches more for your pain. Daily, I read testimonials of despair:

'My darling child has had anorexia for ten years. Her organs are shutting down – she has been everywhere, she has tried so hard – if she dies, my heart will be buried with her. You are our last hope.'

'Even the central venous catheter which always saved my life when I was dangerously emaciated can no longer be used – my veins are ruined. I am twenty-one and have had this for twelve years. I cannot bear to live any longer like this. You are my only and last hope.'

'Our child is only eleven. How can he have become so sick in two years? We don't know him anymore. How can he want to die so young? He hasn't even lived yet. Please, please help us. We are desperate. He is the hardest case they have ever seen.'

'We were told to prepare for her death. They say that after five years in hospitals, she is treatment-resistant. She is only sixteen.'

I hear cries from the shrinking self:

'No one can see me or
Watch me watching myself walking
Into walls.'

I hear the despair:

'Scuffed faces stained with defeat observe
The still existence of themselves and others,
Everyone appears to be a watcher.
Watching life after life
Shuffle in their descent.'

If I have one purpose on earth, it is to make your plight understood by the masses. With this book, I have attempted to clarify the nature of CNC to those who may wish to know. Of those, there are many – professionals, educators, parents – who would wish to study and to mitigate this societal calamity. The world is full of good people who care about you.

You are not failures at life, merely at understanding your own value. Soon professionals across the globe will discontinue treating the symptoms of eating disorders as the cause.

You are altruistic angels who care more for the well-being of the world than you do for yourselves. If there are those who cannot lend themselves to positive caring, give them compassion and understanding. Though ignorance will always exist, don't be afraid of it. Don't allow it to defeat you.

There are two parts to the living of life. Yes, the first you are masters of: to be kind, always. The second and the more difficult, however, is not to condone ignorance. We all have the opportunity to be teachers. In another discourse, it could be said, perhaps, that your purpose here is to teach the world what it is beginning to forget – patience, tolerance, kindness, and compassion.

A girl with anorexia wrote to me: 'Know that my embrace of you is much larger than my arms are wide.'

I couldn't say it better. You are always in my heart. My every thought begins with you. Much love from your forever kind of friend.

Peggy Claude-Pierre

Resources

UK

RESTORE
51 Market Jew Street
Penzance
Cornwall TR18 2DZ

Helpline: 01736–360524
(Mon, Wed, Fri between
10am–2pm)
Admin: 01736–331726
(Mon, Wed, Fri between
10am–4pm)

NIWE
1 Pink Lane
Newcastle-Upon-Tyne
NE1 5DW

Tel: 0191–221 0233

**EATING DISORDERS
ASSOCIATION**
First Floor
Wensum House
103 Prince of Wales Road
Norwich
Norfolk NR1 1DW

Admin: 01603–619090
Fax: 01603–664915
Youth Helpline only:
01603–765050
(18 years and under,
Mon–Fri, 4pm–6pm)

**ANOREXIA
ANONYMOUS**
24 Westmorland Road
Barnes
London SW13 9RY

Tel: 0181–878 9199

IRELAND

**EATING DISTRESS
COUNSELLING**
6 Marino Mart
Dublin 3

Tel/fax: (353) 1–833 3126

**IRISH EATING DISORDERS
ASSOCIATION**
47 Harrington Street
Dublin 8

Office tel: (353) 1–475 3599
Donna: (353) 1–496 8887
Mary
Whelan: (353) 1–842 3975

BODYWHYS
PO Box 105
Blackrock
Co. Dublin

Helpline: (353) 1–283 5126
Fax: (353) 1–283 4963

SHINE
University College Cork
Students' Union
Cork City
Ireland

Tel: (353) 21–902 181

**OVEREATERS
ANONYMOUS**
Dublin

Tel: (353) 1–451 5138

For Further Reading

The following is a list of some of the books on philosophy and psychology that have been powerful influences on my own thinking. I found these and others extremely helpful in shaping my own perspectives on eating disorders. I invite my patients to explore them for themselves.

Adler, Alfred, *Superiority and Social Interest*. Norton, New York, 1979.

Ansbacher, H. L., and R. R. Ansbacher, eds., *The Individual Psychology of Alfred Adler*. Harper & Row, New York, 1964.

Bruch, Hilda, *The Golden Cage – The Enigma of Anorexia Nervosa*. Vintage, New York, 1979.

——, *Eating Disorders – Obesity, Anorexia Nervosa, and the Person Within*. Basic Books, New York, 1973.

de Chardin, Teilhard, *The Future of Man*. Harper & Row, New York, 1964.

Foucault, Michel, *Mental Illness and Psychology*, Alan Sheridan, trans. Harper & Row, New York, 1987.

Fromm, Erich, *The Anatomy of Human Destructiveness*. Holt, New York, 1992.

Fromm, Erich, *The Art of Being*. Continuum, New York, 1994.

——, *Man for Himself – An Inquiry Into the Psychology of Ethics*. Holt, New York, 1992.

Hegel, G. W. F., *The Phenomenology of Mind*, J. B. Baillie, trans. Allen & Unwin, London, 1966.

Horkheimer, M., *Eclipse of Reason*. Seabury Press, New York, 1974.

Koestler, Arthur, *The Sleepwalkers – A History of Man's Changing Vision of the Universe*. Penguin, Middlesex, 1982.

Lucács, Georg, *History and Class Consciousness*, Rodney Livingstone, trans. Merlin Press, London, 1983.

Marcuse, Herbert, *One-Dimensional Man*. Beacon Press, Boston, 1964.

Piaget, Jean, *The Construction of Reality in the Child*. Basic Books, New York, 1954.

Index

330

Notes

Notes